Proceedings of the INHALATION TOXICOLOGY AND TECHNOLOGY Symposium

Sponsored by
The Upjohn Company

Kalamazoo, Michigan
October 23–24, 1980

Proceedings of the INHALATION TOXICOLOGY AND TECHNOLOGY Symposium

Sponsored by
The Upjohn Company

Kalamazoo, Michigan
October 23–24, 1980

Edited by
Basil K. J. Leong
Senior Research
Industrial Toxicologist
The Upjohn Company

ANN ARBOR SCIENCE
PUBLISHERS INC / THE BUTTERWORTH GROUP

230 Collingwood, P.O. Box 1425, Ann Arbor, Michigan 48106

Library of Congress Catalog Card Number 81–67510
ISBN 0–250–40414–1

Manufactured in the United States of America

Butterworths, Ltd., Borough Green, Sevenoaks, Kent TN15 8PH, England

CONTENTS

AEROSOL TECHNOLOGY

INHALATION TOXICOLOGY

Welcoming Address

R. H. DENLINGER
Manager, Pathology and Toxicology Research
The Upjohn Company
Kalamazoo, Michigan 49001

It is a pleasure to welcome you to The Upjohn Company and to have you participate in The Symposium on Inhalation Toxicology and Technology. This Symposium was planned in concert with the opening of a brand new inhalation toxicology facility which we are very proud to show to you. The history of Inhalation Toxicology at The Upjohn Company goes back a number of years, although this new facility represents the first major advance in the area.

The need for inhalation toxicology was recognized in the development of agricultural, chemical, and pharmaceutical products and in evaluation of potential hazards of the workplace environment. In 1967 Dr. Richard Johnston organized a group of people to visit several laboratories to determine the state-of-the-art of the field of inhalation toxicology and bring such technology into the company.

In 1968 a small laboratory was developed for acute inhalation studies. A plan was adopted to expand the capability in acute inhalation toxicology; to develop capability of chronic inhalation studies; to generate data for safety evaluation by Occupational Health and Safety; and to familiarize others in the company of the merits of inhalation technology.

In 1976, a new 7-story, multimillion dollar research building was constructed here at The Upjohn Company. Only part of the total floor space was allocated to be completed at that time. Additional floor space was planned for completion over the next several years to coincide with the growth of research and development activities. As the number of governmental regulations began to proliferate, we saw the need to move ahead rapidly to develop a new, inhalation toxicology facility. In December, 1978, we were very fortunate to have Dr. Basil Leong join our staff. Many of you know him personally, since he has spent his entire professional career in the field of inhalation toxicology. He was given the responsibility to coordinate the efforts in designing the facility and developing a program in Inhalation Toxicology. The personnel from the Inhalation Toxicology Unit, the Facilities Planning and Environmental Regulatory Affairs Unit and the Engineering Division worked together closely in designing and constructing the facility that you will be seeing later today.

The new laboratory was opened last week, so the animal rooms and exposure chambers have not yet been occupied by animals on studies. However, the equipment is in place and is operational to demonstrate their functions for you on the tour. You will also see the operation of two new devices - a new dust generator and new inhalation exposure chambers. Patents have been filed for both so that discussion and demonstration of these instrument and equipment are possible.

We are happy to have so many people attend this Symposium and to help us celebrate the opening of what we consider a top notch facility. I was told that this is probably the first time that such a large group of Inhalation Toxicologists have convened. Most of the major laboratories doing work in this field are represented either in the audience or as speakers. Again, I say welcome. If there is anything that I can do to make your visit more pleasant, please feel free to let me, or anyone else from the Upjohn staff, know.

Opening Remarks

B. K. J. LEONG
Industrial Toxicology Laboratory
The Upjohn Company
Kalamazoo, Michigan 49001

In inhalation toxicological investigations, experimenters tend to develop exposure techniques and equipment to meet their needs for animal studies of airborne toxicants, which may be gas, vapor, mist or dust. Consequently, the "art" of inhalation toxicology is in a state of continuous evolution of inhalation technology. The purpose of this Symposium is to review the state-of-the-art of this dynamic discipline and to extend the dialogue between investigators on the recent achievements and the existing problems. Hopefully, through gentle persuasion or vigorous discussions, the usefulness of some new techniques and apparatus may be recognized and the frontier of knowledge may be pushed a little distance in the right direction.

It is a great pleasure to acknowledge those who made this meeting possible. First and foremost, the contributors who agreed to take an active part, not only in their presentations at the Symposium, but also in the preparation of the manuscripts; The Upjohn Company whose support makes this meeting a pleasant reality; and last but not least, those who assisted in the administrative preparation of the Symposium and the subsequent publication of the Proceedings of the Symposium.

EXPOSURE TECHNOLOGY

Hazard Containment in an Inhalation Toxicology Laboratory

W.B. REID
Facility Planning and Environmental Regulatory Affairs

J.R. KLOK
Client Engineering
Pharmaceutical Research and Development

B.K.J. LEONG
Industrial Toxicology Laboratory

The Upjohn Company
Kalamazoo, Michigan 49001

ABSTRACT

The design of an inhalation toxicology laboratory required consideration of hazard containment. Effective planning required complete communication between the inhalation toxicologist and the engineers on the philosophy, regulatory requirements and economic impact of conducting inhalation experiments. After this exchange of ideas, the toxicologist and the engineers discussed the technical details and visited other established inhalation laboratories.

The final design incorporated as much as possible the latest technology in floor plan design for proper isolation of functional areas, ventilation, and most important of all, the containment and elimination of chemical and animal wastes.

INTRODUCTION

Until recently the pharmaceutical industry was concerned primarily with protecting drugs intended for human consumption from contamination by employees during the manufacturing process. However, the industry is increasingly aware that workers should be protected from the possible harmful effects of overexposure to drugs. The Occupational Health and Safety Act of 1970 made a safe environment for the workers a legal obligation of the employer.

The Upjohn Company's standing policy and practice has been to comply with the law and to minimize the environmental impact of drug manufacturing on employees and the surrounding community. For the evaluation of hazards and toxic effects from exposure to drugs and chemicals in the workplace, the company built an industrial toxicology laboratory with the most up-to-date facilities for conducting inhalation toxicology studies.

PLANNING

Before the drawings for the inhalation toxicology laboratory were started, the effects of working with potentially hazardous materials had to be considered (Steere, 1971; Sansone, 1980). First, The Upjohn Company engineering staff, already quite experienced with the unique requirements of designing pharmaceutical laboratories, and the inhalation toxicology personnel had to establish communications. The inhalation toxicologist explained to the engineers the philosophy of inhalation toxicology and reviewed the techniques for testing gases, liquid aerosols and dust generation and procedures for performing inhalation experiments. The detailed explanation was in terms that people outside the field readily understood.

The design team visited several inhalation laboratories, discussed their function with the scientists using them, the problems encountered and the changes the scientists would make. The latest technology and planning were incorporated in the layout drawings. Following careful review and discussion between the inhalation toxicologist and the design team, the design approved for field work was developed.

HAZARD CONTAINMENT

Floor Plan

The inhalation toxicology laboratory suite was built in an isolated corner of a research building. The building's general traffic pattern is outside the suite which has only one entrance, and yet other facilities like the building ventilation system, utility service shafts, animal waste disposal and cage-washing are convenient. Furthermore, a floor-to-floor dimension of 14 1/2 feet in this section of the building permits all service conduits or cables to be installed overhead, keeping the floor traffic and work area free of obstacles.

Traffic flows from the clean to the contaminated parts of the suite (Figure 1). The clean areas include rooms for animal quarantine before experiments begin, office space,

AC = Acute Exposure Chamber

S = Subchronic Exposure Chamber

C = Chronic Exposure Chamber

H = Animal Holding Room

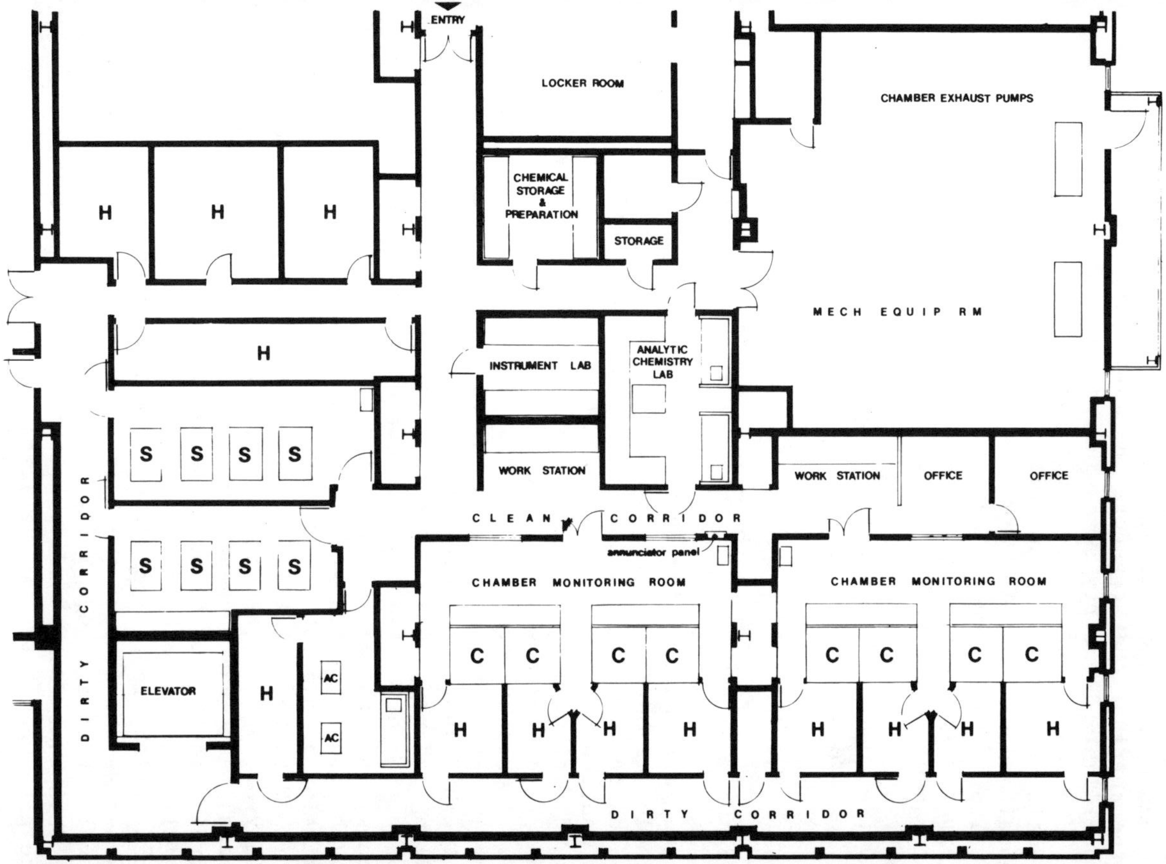

Figure 1. Floor plan of The Upjohn Company Inhalation Laboratory

the rooms housing analytical equipment for exposure chambers and the corridor that connects the suite with the rest of the building. The dirty areas include the exposure chambers, the postexposure animal-holding rooms and the corridor connecting the holding-rooms with the elevator to the waste disposal and cage-washing areas on the floor below.

The animal exposure facilities follow the one-room one-experiment and the double-corridor concepts (Leong, 1977; Sansone & Losikoff, 1979). Animals from each exposure chamber can be isolated in separate holding-rooms after each daily treatment. The temperature and humidity of each holding room are controlled by zone thermostats and humidistats.

LABORATORY VENTILATION

One air-conditioning unit serves the inhalation toxicology laboratory. Air drawn from the outside of the research building is filtered and regulated to 74° ± 2° dry bulb and rehumidified to 50% ± 5% relative humidity before being distributed to other sections of the laboratory. All animal holding-rooms are provided with 20 air changes per hour. A pressure gradient is created so that all air flows from clean to dirty areas in a one-pass system (Figure 2). Within the laboratory suite in the rooms designed for handling and preparing chemicals, conditioned air flows through the perforated ceiling toward the laboratory benches. All the air entering from the ceiling is exhausted through hoods equipped with two-stage filtration systems consisting of bag-out filter housings. The first-stage filter is 90 to 95% efficient according to the ASHRAE (American Society of Heating, Refrigerating, and Air Conditioning Engineers) test, and the second-stage filter is 95% efficient according to the DOP (dioctyl phthalate test).

All exhaust hoods also have airflow-sensitive alarm systems which are activated when the linear velocity of airflow across the face of the hood drops below a specified ft/sec value (Witheridge, 1967). Exhaust hoses which we fondly call "elephant trunks" are provided for local removal of waste gases generated by analytical instruments such as gas chromatographs and chemical storage cabinets.

The air exhausted from the laboratory suite is discharged into the central exhaust system. Then it passes through the heat exchanger for energy recovery before being released outside.

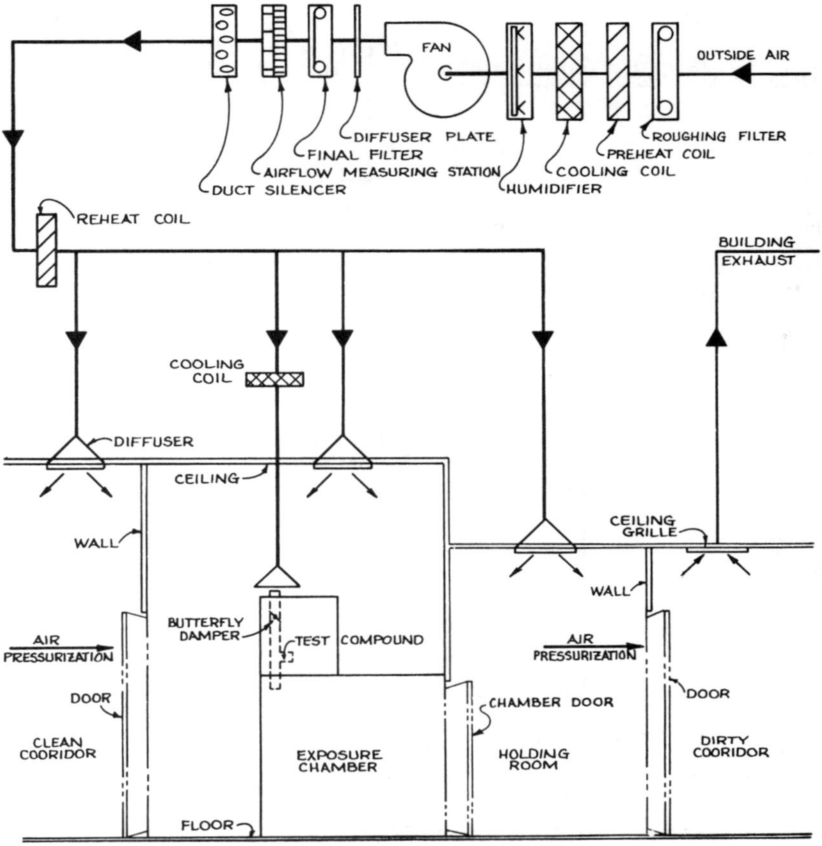

Figure 2. Schematic diagram showing the direction of airflow within the Inhalation Toxicology Laboratory.

EXPOSURE CHAMBER VENTILATION

Air from the laboratory air-conditioning system is drawn through branching ducts into individual chambers. At each branch, an additional heating and cooling system permits further adjustment of temperature and humidity to meet the needs of individual experiments (Figure 3). The design temperature points are 55°F dry bulb temperature for the supply air, 54°F wet bulb for the cooling coil and 75°F for the reheating coils. Temperature in the chamber is monitored by a high and low thermostat connected to an automatic pneumatic controller with manual override.

If the temperature varies from the range selected for a particular experiment, a signal is sent to the microprocessor which triggers an alarm in the work and office areas. The light flashing on a panel indicates the chamber which

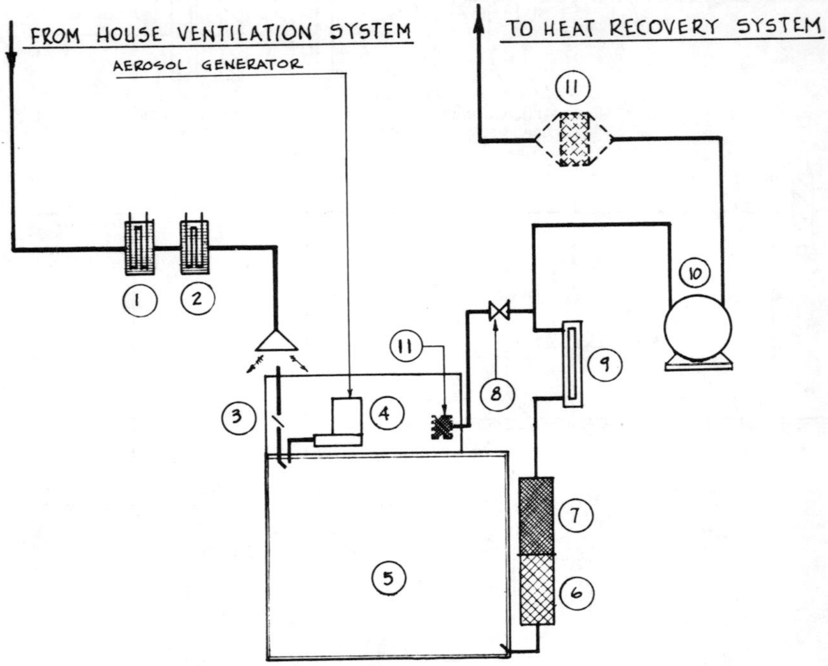

EXPOSURE CHAMBER AIR FLOW DIAGRAM

1. REHEAT COIL
2. COOLING COIL
3. BUTTERFLY DAMPER
4. AEROSOL GENERATING CHAMBER
5. EXPOSURE CHAMBER
6. ROUGHING FILTER
7. HEPA FILTER
8. BY-PASS VALVE
9. FLOW METER
10. VACUUM PUMP
11. FUTURE HEPA FILTER

Figure 3. Schematic diagram showing the air supply and exhaust for an exposure chamber.

caused the alarm. While the alarm can be silenced by pushing the silence button, the pilot light will continue to flash until the problem has been corrected. During the silence, failure of another chamber will sound the alarm as before.

CHAMBER PRESSURE CONTROL

All chambers operate under dynamic air flow at a negative pressure of 0.1 to 0.2 inches of water. This is accomplished by restricting the supply air entering the chamber by throttling the butterfly damper in the chamber air inlet. The total chamber airflow equals the sum of the volume of air ejected from an aerosol or dust generator and the volume of air drawn into the chamber to make a specified concentration of test compound. Airflow is read on the flow meter and adjusted to the proper rate (cubic feet per minute) by throttling the manual bypass valve. Two differential pressure switches (DPS) within the chamber monitor the pressure. The first DPS is wired to the microprocessor alarm system. If, for any reason, the chamber is not properly sealed and the negative pressure is not within the proper limits, the first DPS will sound a local alarm within 30 seconds, depending on the specified program (Figure 4). If a pump fails, a back-up pump can be switched on manually to restore airflow and the slightly negative pressure in the chamber.

CHAMBER EXHAUST PUMPS

Rotary sliding-vane pumps (Furtado, 1978) with the capacity to create various vacuums exhaust the animal exposure chamber atmosphere. This type of exhaust pump has a stable volumetric efficiency over a wide range of vacuum pressure and, therefore, reliably maintains a constant airflow in each chamber. The pump is also durable for continuous operation for a long period of time. One pump is used for each chamber so that the chamber airflow can be individually regulated.

EXPERIMENTAL ATMOSPHERE GENERATION

A compartment at the top of the chamber houses all vapor or aerosol-generating equipment. The compound to be tested is added to the air stream entering the air inlet at an upper corner of the specially designed chamber (Leong, 1981). This compartment also operates under a slightly negative pressure relative to the ambient pressure to ensure total containment of the test compound. A DPS connected to the exposure chamber controls the power supply to the generating equipment. All generating equipment operates only when the chamber atmosphere reaches a specified negative pressure. Thus, the hazard from accidental dispersion of airborne toxicants can be eliminated.

CONTAMINANT AND WASTE CONTROL

For ease of decontamination, the wall and ceiling finishes in the animal and chamber rooms are coated with epoxy paint. The floors are made of inlaid epoxy. All

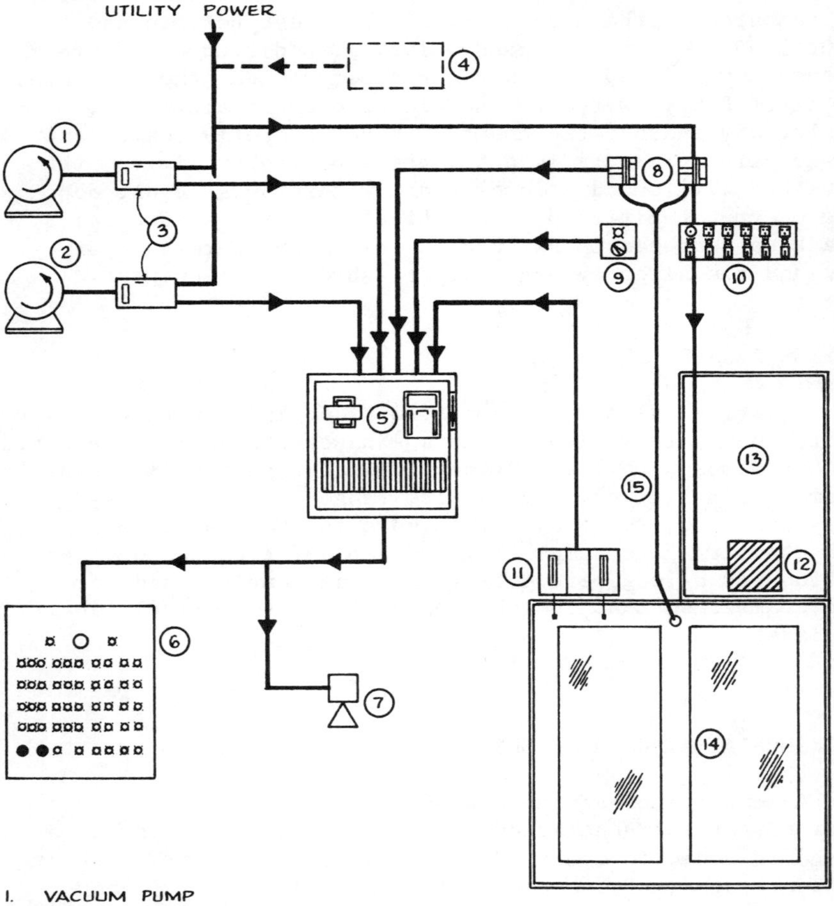

1. VACUUM PUMP
2. VACUUM PUMP (STAND-BY)
3. PUMP CONTROLLER
4. FUTURE EMERGENCY GENERATOR
5. MICRO PROCESSOR
6. ANNUNCIATOR PANEL
7. LOCAL ALARM
8. DIFFERENTIAL PRESSURE SWITCH
9. REMOTE START/STOP VACUUM PUMP SWITCH
10. EQUIPMENT OUTLETS FOR AEROSOL GENERATING CHAMBER
11. HIGH - LOW THERMOSTAT
12. AEROSOL GENERATOR
13. AEROSOL GENERATING CHAMBER
14. EXPOSURE CHAMBER
15. PRESSURE SENSOR PROBE

Figure 4. Schematic diagram of chamber temperature and pressure monitoring-alarm system.

doors, frames, case work and exhaust hoods are enameled steel. Thus, all the finishes used are based on durability, ease of maintenance and impermeability.

The airborne toxicant in the experimental atmosphere is exhausted through a filtering system which consists of successive filters of fiberglass, foam, high efficiency particles and activated charcoal. The filtered waste air is then discharged into the central exhaust system previously described. The entire filtering system can be disassembled easily, and the various filters can be pushed into a bag and disposed of by incineration without contaminating personnel.

The non-airborne wastes such as deposited particles, ex reta and fur of animals in the exposure chambers or the animal-holding rooms can be hosed into drains leading to the company sewage disposal system. If necessary, the drainage can be diverted to a holding tank in which a hazardous compound can be neutralized, inactivated or retained until being pumped into suitable containers for further treatment.

SAFETY

In general, the safe operation procedures follow the guidelines for chemical laboratories (Steere, 1971, Manufacturing Chemists Association, 1972; McKusick, 1981; and Sansome, 1980). Standard safety equipment such as fire extinguishers, eye washers and emergency showers are provided at strategic locations in the laboratory. In addition, all emergency showers are connected to pneumatic horns which sound when the shower is turned on. Furthermore, all the inhalation exposure rooms and the corridors are provided with breathing air supply lines and hood attachments to be used routinely during animal transfer and chamber cleaning or during emergencies.

SUMMARY

The Upjohn Company has built and is operating an inhalation toxicology laboratory which has incorporated the most up-to-date technology of floor plan, exposure chamber designs, animal and chemical wastes control for safe operation and personnel protection.

ACKNOWLEDGEMENT

The authors gratefully acknowledge the contribution of J.O. Haeger, S.N. Moerman and R.C. Patel, members of the

Engineering Design Team; J.R. Cushman, the Field Engineer; and the editorial assistance of S.K. Moyer of the Scientific Publications unit of The Upjohn Company.

REFERENCES

Furtado, V.C. (1978). Air movers and samplers, in Air Sampling Instruments for Evaluation of Atmospheric Contaminant 5th Edit. by the American Conference of Governmental Industrial Hygienists, p. K5.

Leong, B.K.J. (1977). The current state of chamber design and inhalation toxicology instrumentation, Proceedings of the 7th Annual Conference on Environmental Toxicology, pp. 141-149. AMRL-TR-76-125 National Technical Information Service, 5285 Port Royal Road, Springfield, Virginia.

Leong, B.K.J., Powell, D.J., Pochyla, G.L. and Lummis, M.G. (1981). An active dispersion inhalation exposure chamber. See page of this volume,

Manufacturing Chemists Association (1972). Guide for Safety in the Chemical Laboratory, New York: Van Nostrand Reinhold Company.

McKusick, B.C. (1981). Prudent practices for handling hazardous chemicals in laboratories. Science 211:777-780.

Sansone, E.B. and Losikoff, A.M. (1979). Potential contamination from feeding test chemicals in carcinogen bioassay research: Evaluation of single- and double-corridor animal housing facilities. Toxicol. Appl. Pharmaco. 50:115-121.

Sansone, E.B. (1980). Particulate and vapor contamination in experiments with carcinogens. In Generation of Aerosols and Facilities for Exposure Experiments. Edited by Willeke, K. pp. 541-551. Ann Arbor Science Publisher, Inc., Ann Arbor, Michigan 48106.

Steere, N.V. Ed. (1971) CRC Handbook of Laboratory Safety, (Cleveland, OH: Chemical Rubber Company).

Witheridge, W.N. (1967). Ventilation in Industrial Hygiene and Toxicology, Vol. 1. Edited by Patty, F.A. pp. 307-310. Interscience Publishers, New York.

A Problem and a Non-Problem in Chamber Inhalation Studies

H.N. MacFARLAND
Gulf Science & Technology Company
Pittsburgh, Pennsylvania

ABSTRACT

When samples of the atmosphere in a dynamically-operated chamber are withdrawn for analysis, an artifactually low result may be obtained. This will arise when the total flow through the chamber is maintained constant by a pump on the exhaust side and agent is supplied positively at constant rate at the inlet. When the sampling pump is turned on, total flow at the inlet is increased and the agent, supplied at fixed rate, is now more highly diluted, i.e., its concentration is reduced. The problem is eliminated by a simple piping arrangement.

Many investigators appear to be unduly concerned about the uniformity of distribution of agents, especially aerosols, in dynamically-operated chambers. This arises because of a failure to appreciate the actual conditions in a chamber when it is essentially equilibrated. An interpretation of the conditions will be provided which will show that these concerns are largely unnecessary.

THE PROBLEM

Figure 1 shows schematically the arrangement most commonly employed in the conduct of dynamic inhalation studies in exposure chambers. The main pump on the exhaust side of the chamber demands a fixed total flow through the chamber. Agent is supplied from some generating device at a fixed, and relatively low, rate. The make-up air, entering the main inlet pipe, automatically assumes a flow rate such that it, plus the agent flow, equals the flow demanded by the main pump. In the example shown, values have been selected to yield a concentration of 100 ppm at equilibrium.

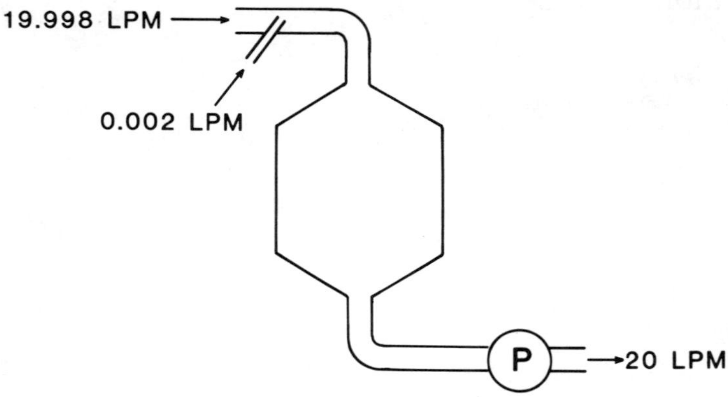

$$\text{AT EQUILIBRIUM, } C = \frac{0.002}{19.998 + 0.002} \times 10^6$$

$$= 100 \text{ PPM}$$

Figure 1. Common Arrangement for Dynamic Inhalation Chamber Studies.

If it is further given that the volume of the chamber is 100 liters, the equilibration characteristics of the system are given by the equation:

$$C_{t_1} = \frac{f_o}{F_o}\left(1 - \varepsilon^{-\frac{F_o}{V} t_1}\right) \tag{1}$$

where C_{t_1} = concentration at time t_1,

f_o = flow rate of agent,

F_o = total flow through chamber,

V = volume of chamber.

Silver furnished this equation, utilizing weight, rather than volume, units (1). In Figure 2, the plot of the equation is shown up to t_{99}, which is 23.03 minutes when the values shown in Figure 1 are utilized in a 100-liter chamber. The concentration at this time is 99 ppm and,

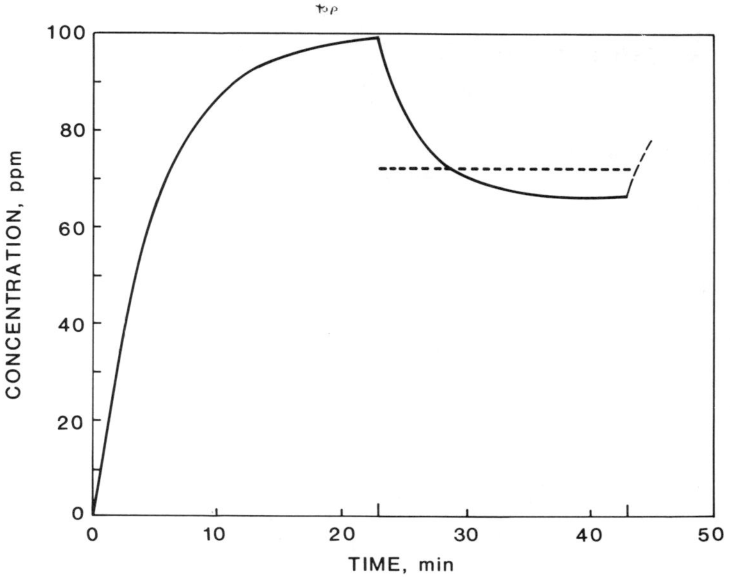

Figure 2. Equilibration Curves in a Dynamically-Operated Inhalation Chamber.

although the equilibrium concentration of 100 ppm is theoretically never reached, we note that no matter how long the chamber is operated after t_{99}, the concentration of agent will increase by less than 1%, i.e., it is essentially constant.

In critical inhalation studies, it is essential that samples of the chamber atmosphere be taken for analytical determination of agent concentration. In Figure 3, a typical arrangement is shown, with a sampling probe leading from the chamber, through an absorber or analytical instrument. The sample is drawn from the chamber by means of a small pump, the discharge from which is usually vented into the room. If the sampling pump operates at a flow of 10 lpm, the total demand at the inlet is increased to 30 lpm. Thus, the fixed flow of agent is now being dispersed in a larger flow of air, so its concentration in the chamber begins to equilibrate towards a new and lower concentration, which is readily shown to be 66.67 ppm.

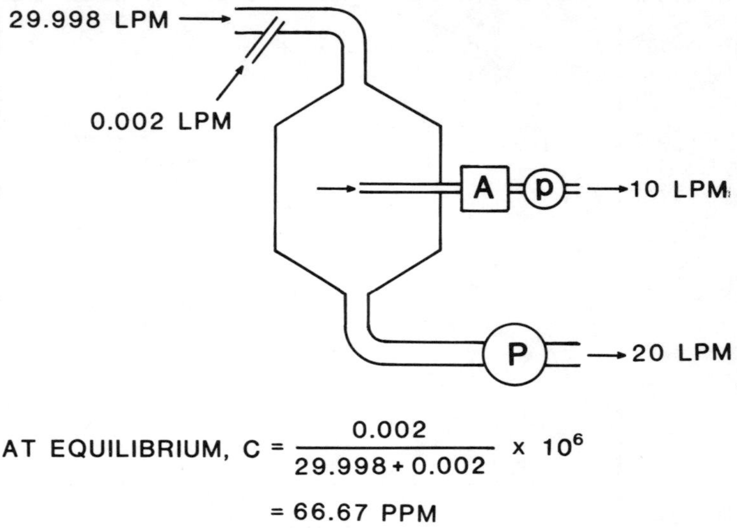

Figure 3. Common Arrangement for Sampling is a Dynamic Inhalation Chamber.

In Figure 2, the curve of declining concentration is shown, starting at 23.03 minutes. Investigators may not start sampling just when the original equilibration of the chamber is 99% complete but, as already noted, the concentration at any time after t_{99} will not be essentially different from its value at t_{99}. The equation of the declining concentration is:

$$C_{t_2} = \left(C_{t_1} - \frac{f_o}{F_1}\right) \varepsilon^{-\frac{F_1}{V}(t_2 - t_1)} + \frac{f_o}{F_1} \quad (2)$$

where C_{t_2} = concentration after $(t_2 - t_1)$ minutes of sampling,

C_{t_1} = concentration after t_1 minutes of original equilibration,

f_o = rate of flow agent,

F_1 = sum of flows of main pump and sampling pump,

V = volume of chamber.

If sampling is continued for 20 minutes, i.e., 43.03 minutes after the start of the study, the concentration of agent will be 66.75 ppm. The average concentration for the duration of the sampling period, $\overline{C}$, may be calculated from Equation 2, rearranged into the more convenient form:

$$\overline{C} = \left(1 - \frac{1}{\tau}\right)\frac{f_o}{F_1} + \frac{1}{\tau}\, C_{t_1} + \frac{1}{\tau}\left(C_{t_1} - \frac{f_o}{F_1}\right)\varepsilon^{-\tau} \qquad (3)$$

$$\text{where } \tau = \frac{F_1}{V}(t_2 - t_1)$$

In the example chosen, the average concentration is 72.07 ppm, and this is the result obtained on analyzing the sample. This may surprise the investigator who expected 99 ppm, based on nominal calculations that omitted the effect of the sampling pump.

Two solutions may be offered to this problem. Equation 3 can be rearranged to the form:

$$C_{t_1} = \frac{\tau}{1 + \varepsilon^{\tau}}\left[\overline{C} + \frac{1}{\tau}\,\frac{f_o}{F_1}\,\varepsilon^{-\tau} - \left(1 - \frac{1}{\tau}\right)\frac{f_o}{F_1}\right] \qquad (4)$$

Knowing $\overline{C}$, the concentration at the time sampling was started, C_{t_1}, can be calculated. However, this decline in concentration is real and the experimental animals have been exposed to it. It would be better if the sample could have been obtained without lowering the concentration of agent in the chamber. This preferable solution to the problem is obtained by the simple modification of the equipment arrangement shown in Figure 4. The discharge from the sampling pump is fed back into the main exhaust line upstream from the main chamber pump. Flow conditions at the inlet of the chamber are now the same as they were in Figure 1, the agent concentration in the chamber is unaffected by operation of the sampling pump and the analysis reveals the expected concentration of 99 ppm.

The magnitude of the effect discussed above is increased when the sampling pump flow is a high proportion of the total flow, and when sampling is continued for a long period. The example discussed above was a more extreme, but not a completely unknown, case. However, if the equipment is arranged only as in Figure 3, even a sampling pump of low flow rate operated for a short time must cause some lowering of the concentration of agent in the chamber.

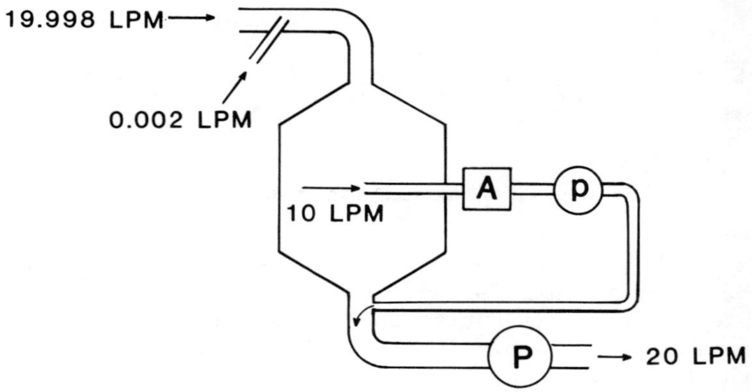

Figure 4. Arrangement to Circumvent the Sampling Artifact.

THE NON-PROBLEM

Almost every investigator who contemplates conducting a dynamic chamber inhalation study wonders whether or not inequalities in distribution of the agent in the chamber, reflected in different concentrations in different locations in the chamber, will be a problem under his planned operating conditions. His concern is at a maximum when the airborne agent is an aerosol, solid or liquid, and less so when a gas or vapor. One of the first investigators to consider this matter was Silver (1), who studied the distribution of a gaseous agent in a cubic chamber, operated under normal and appropriate conditions. He observed no significant differences in concentrations among samples taken from the eight corners of the cube and the body center. Thus, there were no inequalities of distribution in the chamber, i.e., it was a non-problem.

Unfortunately, many investigators, contemplating this hypothetical problem, have behaved in a most unscientific manner and have proceeded to make changes in design or operating conditions without ascertaining in advance whether or not they were, in fact, faced with a demonstrable problem.

Silver examined the case of a gaseous agent, but it may be thought that results would have been different if the agent had been an aerosol. To show that this will not alter the conclusion, the argument will be restricted to what are called "respirable" particles, i.e., particles having an MMAD of 5 micrometers or less. It is such particles which are of interest in the majority of aerosol inhalation studies. To a first approximation, such particles can be regarded as behaving almost like gas molecules. They are close to being permanently suspended particles. The settling rates of 5 micrometer particles are shown in Table 1, based on Stokes' Law with the Cunningham correction factor.

Table 1. SETTLING RATE OF 5 MICRON MMAD PARTICLE

Sp. gr. = 1	0.08 - 0.09 cm./sec.
Sp. gr. = 2	0.2 cm./sec.

Stokes' Law with the Cunningham Correction Factor.

These are settling rates in absolutely still air. But the atmosphere in a dynamically operated chamber is in a state of continuous turbulence, hence the particles may be regarded as essentially permanently suspended under these conditions.

If samples are collected from various points in a chamber, small differences in concentration from location to location are usually found. But, the important point is that these differences do not remain constant, but are continuously fluctuating over a limited range. A concentration gradient detected at one time does not remain constant, but shifts around as time elapses. In fact, it is difficult to see how one could maintain a constant concentration gradient in an exposure chamber of normal configuration operated at an appropriate flow rate.

The following facts should be kept constantly in mind. First, it is impossible for a local concentration in a chamber to exceed the equilibration concentration, regardless of the physical form of the agent (gas, vapor, solid or liquid aerosol). Fluctuations, if present, will always be below the equilibration concentration. Secondly, after t_{99}, the concentration in the chamber will increase by less than 1% no matter how long the chamber is operated. The corollary of this is that the concentration of the agent in the atmosphere entering the chamber at the inlet differs by less than 1% from the agent concentration already in the chamber. This is why there is no mixing problem in the chamber after t_{99}.

Most dynamic chamber studies are performed by closing the animals in the chamber, turning on the main pump and then introducing the agent, allowing the chamber to equilibrate in accordance with Equation 1 and as shown in Figure 2. The exposure period should be quite long in comparison with t_{99}. This matter has been discussed by the author (2). If there are stagnant spots in the chamber that have a slightly longer t_{99}, this will be of no significance if the total duration of exposure is sufficiently long. If t_{99} constitutes a large fraction of the total duration of exposure, then the investigator should use a different form of dynamic chamber for the study, one utilizing some type of air lock or other mechanism (2).

In conclusion, if a hypothetical problem of uneven distribution of agent in a chamber is envisioned, the investigator should determine whether or not it is a problem and not make changes to deal with what may well be a non-problem.

ACKNOWLEDGEMENT

The author wishes to thank Prof. W. C. Rheinboldt for developing Equations 2, 3 and 4.

REFERENCES

(1) Silver, S. D. (1946). Constant Flow Gassing Chambers: Principles Influencing Design and Operation., J. Lab. Clin. Med. 31, 1153-1161.

(2) MacFarland, H. N. (1976). Respiratory Toxicology in Essays in Toxicology, Vol. 7.

Comparison of Three Methods of Evaluating Inhalation Toxicology Chamber Performance

OWEN R. MOSS
Biology Department
Battelle
Pacific Northwest Laboratories
Richland, Washington 99352

ABSTRACT

Three approaches are used to demonstrate the degree of air-mixing throughout an exposure chamber designed at Battelle-Northwest. The innovative feature of the chamber design tested is that the location of the excreta pans directs the air flow in such a manner that an aerosol is uniformly distributed throughout the chamber without mixing devices. The three tests used in this evaluation are: modeling, full-scale/point tests and full-scale/dynamic tests. A model of the chamber can be dynamically scaled for use with water, instead of air, as the fluid medium. Dye is injected for flow visualization and infused for point tests of buildup and decay. Point tests are made either by sequentially moving a single sampling probe throughout the chamber, or by simultaneous sampling with multiple probes. Uniformity of concentration buildup, decay and distribution are measured. Dynamic tests are performed by simultaneously sampling inlet and exhaust flow to obtain concentration-time curves for a bolus of tracer compound injected into the chamber inlet line. These curves are compared to output predicted for an ideal, perfectly mixing box of the same size as the chamber. The results of these tests in our chamber showed that uniform air mixing was maintained in the chamber when the excreta pans were in position. The relative usefulness of each of these approaches for rapidly testing chamber design criteria is discussed.

INTRODUCTION

Exposure chamber performance is usually described by showing test concentration buildup or clearance curves. This information is used to predict how much time it will take to reach 90 or 95% of the equilibrium concentration

(Drew, 1973; Silver, 1946). The general assumption is that the chamber behaves as a reactor vessel or a perfectly mixing box (Silver, 1946). It is assumed that, as material (uniformly distributed in the inlet line) is first injected into the exposure chamber, it is instantaneously and uniformly mixed throughout the chamber. Under such constraints, in a dynamic system, the concentration (C) of the material in the box at any time (t) is an exponential function of the mass (W) of the material injected per minute, the flow rate (F) through the chamber, and the volume of the chamber (V):

$$C = \frac{W}{F} (1 - e^{-Ft/V}) .$$

The presence of dead zones (zones of little or no air movement) changes the shape of these buildup curves and, therefore, the performance of the chamber as an efficient air mixing box (Himmenblau and Bischoff, 1968).

The three tests we have used to demonstrate the degree of mixing throughout an exposure chamber are called, for the purpose of this discussion, "dynamically similar model tests," "full-scale/point tests" and "full-scale/dynamic tests." The dynamically similar model tests used in our particular chamber were first discussed in a presentation, "Can We Design Chambers for Uniform Exposure to Particulates on Several Tiers With Catch Pans?" This was given at the first Inhalation Toxicology Symposium, at Brookhaven National Laboratory, Upton, Long Island, NY in October 1978. The proceedings of that conference are now in the final stages of preparation as a Brookhaven National Laboratory document (Bob Drew, Editor). The full-scale/point test consists of samples taken at different locations and times to measure concentration buildup, uniformity and clearance. Presented here is a review of independent work as published by R. L. Beethe, et al. (1979), and of our work, "Aerosol Mixing in An Animal Exposure Chamber Having Three Levels of Caging with Excreta Pans," presented at the 1980 Industrial Hygiene Conference, Houston, TX. (This material is currently being prepared for publication in the American Industrial Hygiene Association Journal.) The full-scale/dynamic test consists of injecting a bolus of test material into the total chamber air flow and sampling continuously at the inlet and exhaust lines. The work was first presented by D. R. Hemenway, "Inhalation Toxicology Chamber Performance: A Quantitative Model," at the 1980 Industrial Hygiene Conference, and is also in preparation for publication in the Journal.

Background

A model of the chamber can be dynamically scaled for use with water instead of air as the fluid medium. The fluid flow in the model duplicates the flow in the full-scale chamber, provided that the Reynold's number, N_{Re}, of fluid flow is equal in both systems (Whitaker, 1968). The Reynold's number is a function of a system's characteristic velocity and dimension (for example, the mean fluid velocity, V, and diameter, L, of the chamber inlet tube) and the kinematic viscosity, ν, equal to the viscosity, η, divided by the density, ρ, of the fluid medium. If a one-sixth-scale model is used, with water instead of air as the fluid medium, then the characteristic velocity in the model must be 0.4 times the characteristic velocity in the full-scale chamber in order for the Reynold's numbers to coincide. A water flow of 3 ℓ/min through the model inlet line has the same Reynold's number as 283 ℓ/min of air flow through the 7.62-cm diameter inlet line of the full-scale chamber (given η_{water} = 0.01002 g/cm·sec, η_{air} = 0.000183 g/cm·sec, ρ_{water} = 0.99823 g/cm³ and ρ_{air} = 0.001189 g/cm³ at 20°C; (West, 1976). Besides being less expensive to build and modify, the main advantage of using a model rather than a full-scale chamber is that fluid flows can be clearly visualized by dye injection, and can be recorded on film or video tape.

Point tests of concentration buildup, decay and distribution are made either with a single sampling probe moving sequentially throughout the chamber, or by simultaneous sampling with multiple probes. Such tests are easier to do in the full-scale chamber but can also be done in the model, provided that the sampling volume is proportionally reduced. In multiple-point sampling, the main difficulty is in demonstrating that all the probes operate correctly at the same time. Multipoint sampling can also be used to determine whether upstream mixing of the test material and the chamber inlet air is complete. The build-up and decay curves can be compared against the expected exponential curve for a perfectly mixing box of the same volume as the chamber.

Dynamic tests on a full-scale chamber are performed by simultaneously sampling inlet and exhaust flow to obtain concentration versus time curves for a bolus of tracer compound injected into the chamber inlet line. These curves can be compared to the output predicted for an ideal reaction vessel or perfectly mixing box of the same size by calculating the mean time, $\bar{t}$, and variance, s^2, of the concentration versus time profile as it passes the inlet and exhaust sampling points ($_1$ and $_2$, respectively, in the following equations). This comparison can be expressed:

$$\bar{t} = \frac{\sum_{i=1}^{n} C_i t_i}{\sum_{i=1}^{n} C_i}$$

$$S^2 = \frac{\sum_{i=1}^{n} (t_i - \bar{t})^2 C_i}{\sum_{i=1}^{n} C_i}.$$

If the theoretical residence time, $T = \frac{V}{F}$, for flow in the chamber and the distance, L, between sampling points are known, the percent dead space, %DS, and dispersion coefficient, D_L, can be calculated:

$$\%DS = \left(\frac{T - T_m}{T}\right) 100$$

and

$$D_L = \frac{L^2 \, (s_2^2 - s_1^2)}{2 \, T_m^3}$$

where $T_m = \bar{t}_2 - \bar{t}_1$ is the measured residence time.

The percent dead space is a measure of the amount of streaming of material through the chamber. The larger the percent of dead space, the greater the proportion of material that streams through the chamber without mixing.

The dispersion coefficient gives only a partial indication of chamber performance. In a laminar (horizontal) flow chamber having a perfect plug flow, it would be zero. In a perfectly mixing box, the dispersion coefficient should be very much greater than zero (Himmelblau and Biskoff, 1968). A chamber having well-mixed airflows and exhibiting minimal waste of test material would have a low percent dead space and a dispersion coefficient greater than zero.

All three types of tests were used in testing a chamber developed at Battelle. Each test showed that the chamber performed very much like a perfectly mixing box, and that air-mixing was uniform when the excreta pans were in position. The full-scale/dynamic tests were the easiest and least expensive to perform and gave a general basis upon which to base decisions on improving chamber performance.

MATERIALS AND METHODS

The modified chamber (Moss, 1980; Figure 1) was first fabricated according to our specifications by Hazelton systems (Aberdeen, MD). It is 1.35 m wide (outside dimensions) and 2.08 m high to the top of the male quick-

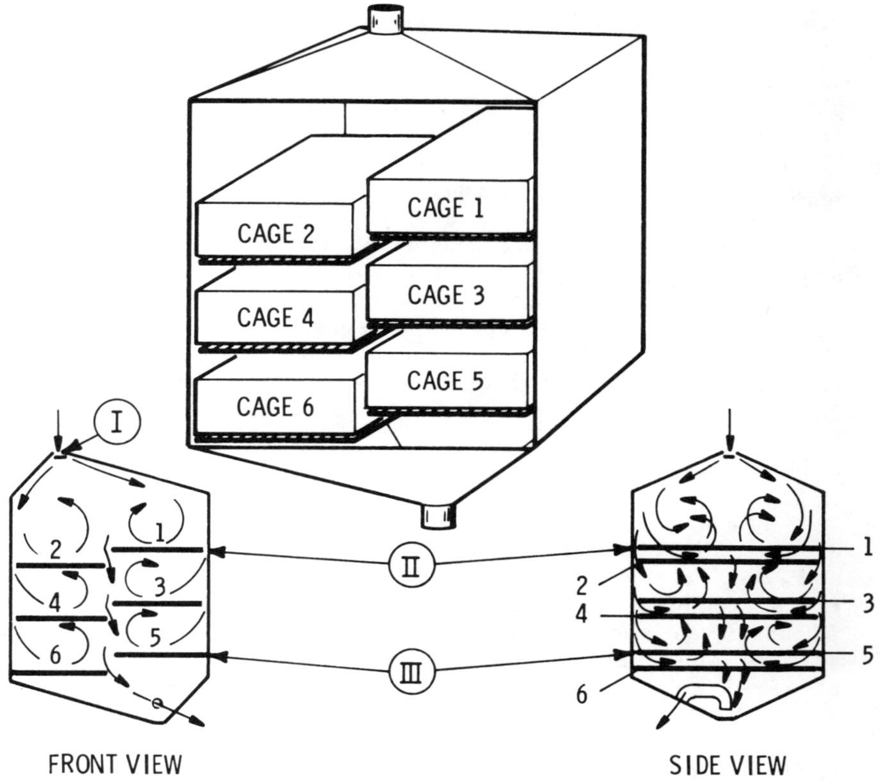

FIGURE 1. Sketch of Battelle-designed exposure chamber, showing air flow lines and placement and numbering of caging units and excreta pans. I. deflection disk; II. spacing of excreta pans with respect to walls; and III. filled space for lowermost pans.

disconnect on the inlet line. Excreta pans are 53 cm wide by 122 cm long, and are 35.6 cm apart, vertically. Outer edges of the pans are 3.2 cm from the chamber walls. This space (III in Figure 1) is filled with a metal strip for the two lowermost catch pans. The right column of three catch pans is offset 2.54 cm horizontally and 10.2 cm vertically from the left column of three catch pans. A 7.6-cm-diameter flat disk is suspended 2.54 cm below the air inlet line. The volume of the cubical portion of the chamber is 1.7 m^3; the volume of each transition piece is 0.33 m^3. In all tests, flow through the chamber was 283 ℓ/min with a vacuum of 1.27 cm of water between chamber and room.

Dynamically Similar Model Tests

The 1/6-scale model of the chamber was constructed of plexiglass. The top and bottom transition pieces were formed by taping plastic pieces together and pouring plastic mold compound over the structure to form a solid block. Side pieces were then screwed to the blocks containing the negative impressions of the transition piece. Flow was visualized by injecting a concentrated solution of potassium permanganate dye into the water flow. The passage of dye through the chamber was recorded either continuously on black and white videotape, or sequentially on 35-mm film through a green filter (to enhance the contrast). Buildup and decay of sodium fluorescein dye continuously injected into the model was measured with a spectrofluorometer.

Full-Scale/Point Test

Ammonium fluorescein (approximate mass median aerodynamic diameter and geometric standard deviation, 0.8 μm and 2.2, respectively) was used as an aerosol in these tests. Concentration buildup and uniformity were measured in the area above each of the six catch pans, where the animals would be suspended, with an aerosol mass monitor attached to a coaxial aerosol sampling probe (Cannon et al., 1979). Six simultaneous filter samples were also taken with a 2.4-cm, open-faced filter holder (sampling rate, 0.5 ℓ/min) placed above the middle of each shelf.

Full-Scale/Dynamic Tests

Sampling probes were placed in the inlet and exhaust ports, just outside the main chamber cavity. The distance, L, between probes was 188 cm. The tests consisted of injecting 1.5 ml of acetone into the inlet air line and measuring the concentration as a function of time at the two sampling points with a photoionization detector (PID). (Because the detector had only one sampling port, repeat acetone injections were run with the PID alternately monitoring the two sample lines.)

RESULTS

Three techniques were used in evaluating the operating characteristics of our inhalation exposure chamber. These were dynamically similar model tests, full-scale/point tests and full-scale/dynamic tests.

Dynamically Similar Model Tests

The photographs in Figure 2 show that the dye, 20 seconds after injection into the water stream, outlined

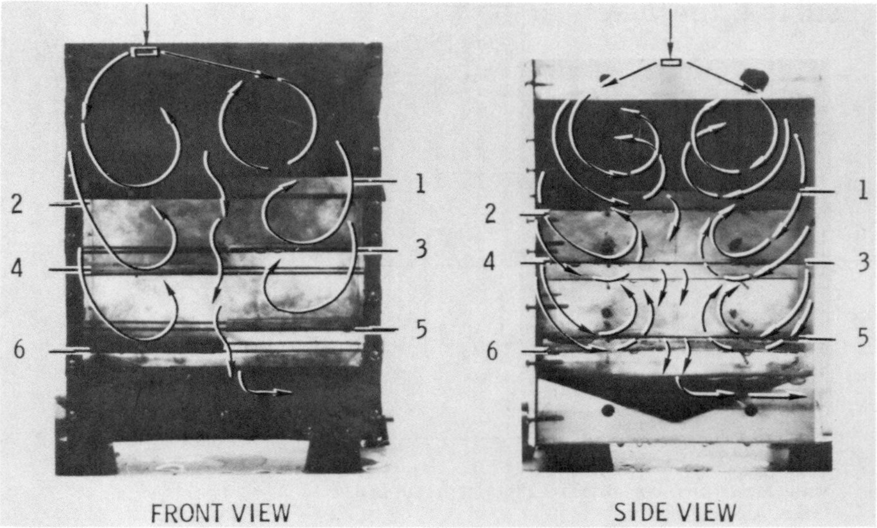

FIGURE 2. Visualization of eddies in a dynamically similar, 1/6-scale model of the inhalation exposure chamber. (Photos taken 20 sec after injection of dye bolus into model; total water flow = 3 ℓ/min)

eddies at each level. The clearance half-time, $t_{\frac{1}{2}}$, of dye at each level was: 88, 88, and 100 sec for levels 1 and 2, 3 and 4, 5 and 6, respectively. Onset was delayed 7, 30 and 60 seconds, respectively, after infusion of dye was stopped. (Events in the full-scale chamber would probably take 2.5 times longer.)

Full-Scale/Point Tests

Buildup and decay curves for level 4 are shown in Figure 3; points where the generator was adjusted are also shown. The sketch above the curve shows the location of the sampling probe above the excreta pans. The buildup and clearance portions of the curve were used to calculate the clearance half-time above each excreta pan. For levels 1 through 6, the clearance half-times were, respectively, 4.5 ± 0.2, 4.6 ± 0.1, 3.4 ± 0.5, 5.0 ± 0.9, 4.2 ± 0.1 and 4.2 ± 0.7 min; delay times were 0, 0, 1.3, 0.5, 1.5, 2.0 min. The indicated deviation in each measured half-time represents the calculated extremes in half-times between buildup and decay curves. In replicate experiments, values for six simultaneously taken samples, one from above the center of each were, respectively, 2.03 ± 0.07, 2.17 ± 0.13 and 2.04 ± 0.08 μg/ℓ. Similar results were observed by Beethe et al., 1979) in a more complete experiment.

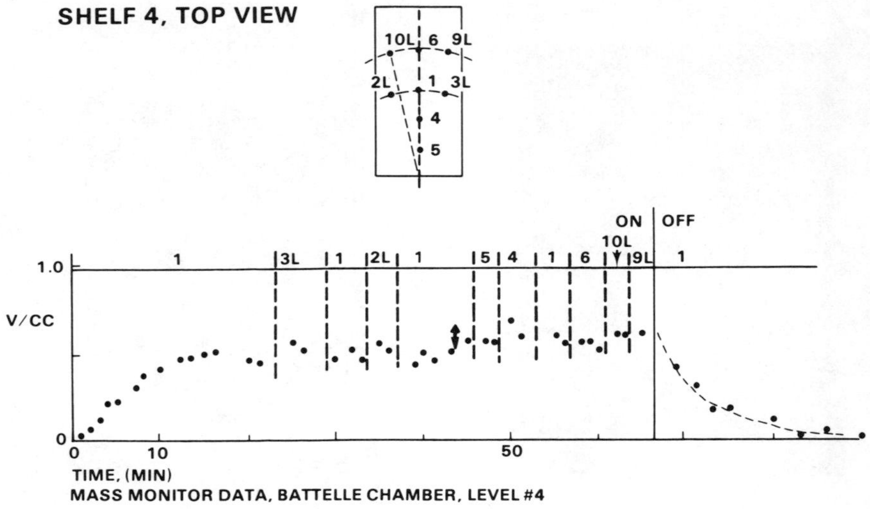

FIGURE 3. Buildup and distribution of aerosol above shelf #4 in the inhalation exposure chamber. Δ indicates where aerosol generator was adjusted. (Sampling locations indicated in drawing above graph.)

Full-Scale Dynamic Tests

The concentration time profile for a bolus of acetone and air passing the inlet and exhaust probes is given in Figure 4. The mean residence for time, T, for the total chamber volume was 7.8 and 8.9 min, measured on repeat runs. The average axial dispersion coefficient, D_L, was 0.12 m^2/min. The percent dead space was between 0 and 6, based on a theoretical mean residence time of 8.3 min.

DISCUSSION

By using the three tests described, many ideas can be tested in a short period of time. Each test provides useful information; each requires different amounts of effort. The dynamic model tests took approximately 4 manweeks, since (1) the design of the model was simplified so that we could rapidly construct it in our lab, and (2) a video camera was used to view and review dye injection test runs. This approach is particularly useful in testing ideas when designing new chambers.

The full-scale/point tests, normally used to measure chamber performance, requires considerable effort to insure that all sampling units are operating properly. (See, for example, the detailed work by Beethe et al. [1979] to

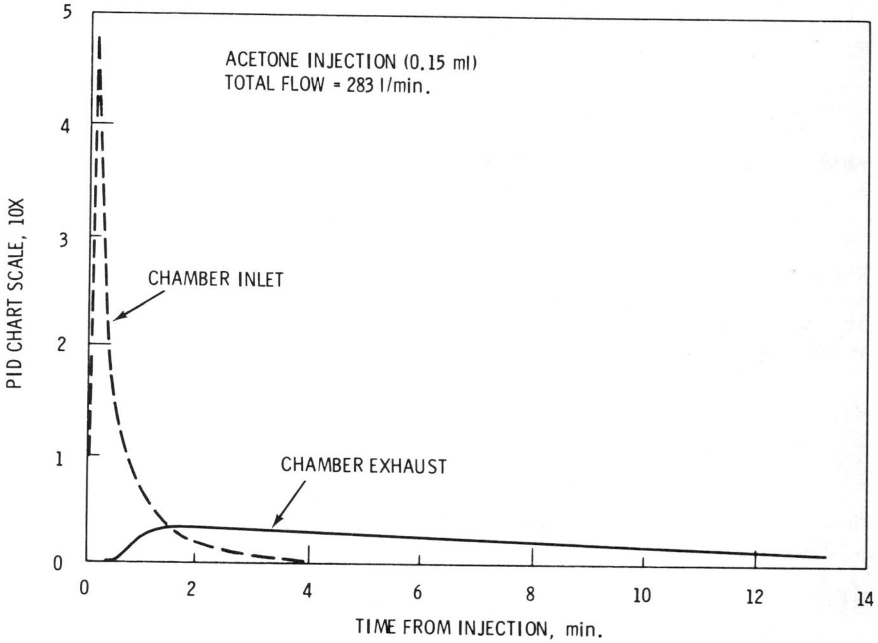

FIGURE 4. Concentration time profile of a bolus of acetone and air passing chamber inlet and exhaust probes.

evaluate a chamber similar to ours for use in their laboratory.) The information obtained from this test is especially useful in pinpointing failure of the chamber or atmosphere generating system to function as devices for uniform mixing of aerosols.

The full-scale chamber/dynamic test gives the most information for the least effort: the calculations (the difference between the measured residence time, T_m, and the theoretical residence time, T) give the percent dead space, a direct measure of (1) how well air is mixing in the chamber, and (2) the fraction of test material that streams through the chamber and is therefore wasted. In our opinion, dynamic tests should be the tests of choice to quickly evaluate the usefulness of modifications in existing chambers.

REFERENCES

Beethe, R. L., Wolff, R. K., Griffis, L. C., Hobbs, C. H., and McClellan, R. O. (1979). Evaluation of a Recently

Designed Multi-Tiered Exposure Chamber. Lovelace Foundation (Inhalation Toxicology Research Institute), LF-67, NTIS, Springfield, VA.

Cannon, W. C., Moss, O. R., Garrity, B. R., Laidler, J. R., and Ostler, O. (1979). A dilution probe for an aerosol mass monitor, In PNL Annual Report for 1978 to DOE, Part 1, Biomedical Sciences, February 1979, pp. 3.5-3.7. Pacific Northwest Laboratory, PNL-2850, NTIS, Springfield, VA.

Drew, R. T. and Lasken, S. (1973). Environmental inhalation chambers, In Methods of Animal Experimentation, Vol. IV, Environmental and Special Senses (W. I. Gray, ed.), pp. 1-42. Academic Press, New York.

Himmelblau, D. M. and Bischoff, K. B. (1968). Process Analysis and Simulation: Deterministic Systems, pp. 1-88. J. Wiley and Sons, New York.

Moss, O. R. (1980) Exposure Chamber. United States Patent 4,216,741.

Silver, S. D. (1946) Constant gassing chambers: Principles influencing design and operation. J. Lab. Clin. Med. 31, 1153-1161.

West, R. C. (ed.) (1976) Handbook of Chemistry and Physics. CRC Press, Cleveland, OH.

Whitaker, S. (1968) Introduction to Fluid Mechanics. Prentice-Hall, Englewood Cliffs, NJ.

Design, Operation and Characterization of Large Volume Exposure Chambers

R.M. SCHRECK, T.L. CHAN, and S.C. SODERHOLM
Biomedical Science Department
General Motors Research Laboratories
Warren, Michigan 48090

ABSTRACT

The Biomedical Science Department of the General Motors Research Laboratories operates a chronic inhalation exposure facility which includes an air treatment system and four 12.6 m^3 exposure chambers. The facility and its operation are described, emphasizing the capability for chronically exposing animals to aerosols and/or gases for 20 hrs/day. The facility's principal features are equipment for rapid animal care, unattended particulate and gas sampling, and automatic control and surveillance of key chamber parameters. In addition to routine measurements, the chamber atmosphere has been characterized by measuring noise levels, the size distribution of the background aerosol, and the spatial distribution of a submicron diesel exhaust aerosol generated for a recent study.

INTRODUCTION

Large numbers of exposed animals are required to provide statistically significant results in many health effects studies [Phalen, 1976]. Large populations of animals are exposed more efficiently in large chambers with one chamber per dose level than in multiple small chambers. This is based on the time per animal required to provide proper animal care and to clean the facility, and the time to generate, deliver, control and characterize the test compound in each chamber. Consequently, a chamber having a volume of over 10 cubic meters was designed in which over 250 rats could readily be housed. For other species, the number of animals housed per chamber depends on the size of the animal.

In order to minimize operating costs, the exposure chambers are designed to be easily serviced. This includes automatic watering of cage units, high pressure washing systems and animal cages designed in compliance with the accepted standards for each test species. The chambers are also designed to operate at a negative pressure to prevent leakage of test material to neighboring chambers and surrounding laboratory areas.

The entire chamber exposure system has been designed for continuous unattended operation, using a control strategy which emphasizes simple control elements and some redundancy. Basic control of the chamber utilities is achieved by relatively simple pneumatic controllers and actuators to regulate environmental parameters such as temperature, flow rate and relative humidity. Control of a separate environmental and chamber air monitoring system is programmed into a small computer which can oversee the chamber operational parameters. The computer performs the following general tasks:

a) calibrate and operate instruments in the Chamber Air Monitoring System,

b) monitor chamber air temperatures, flow rates, relative humidities and concentrations of several gases in each chamber,

c) tabulate, summarize and report data daily, and

d) set off alarms if critical control parameters deviate from preset ranges.

In case of system malfunction or failure, a separate electronic alarm system will alert operating personnel to exercise corrective actions.

FACILITIES

Exposure Chambers

The exposure facility is built around four large chambers designed and built for chronic inhalation exposure testing. A Rochester-type design [Laskin et al, 1970] was used to promote efficient aerosol mixing and distribution throughout the chamber. Gaseous mixtures are also distributed well in this type of chamber due to their higher diffusivities.

The chambers (Figure 1) are constructed primarily of stainless steel and glass to minimize interaction between interior surfaces and reactive compounds in the atmospheric mixtures under study. The major wall panels are of 304 stainless steel sheet with load-bearing elements constructed of stainless structural sections. Wire reinforced glass is used in the door panels to provide good lighting and visibility during an experiment. In addition, the chambers are equipped with internal lighting from two fluorescent fixtures installed in the top cone (Figure 2).

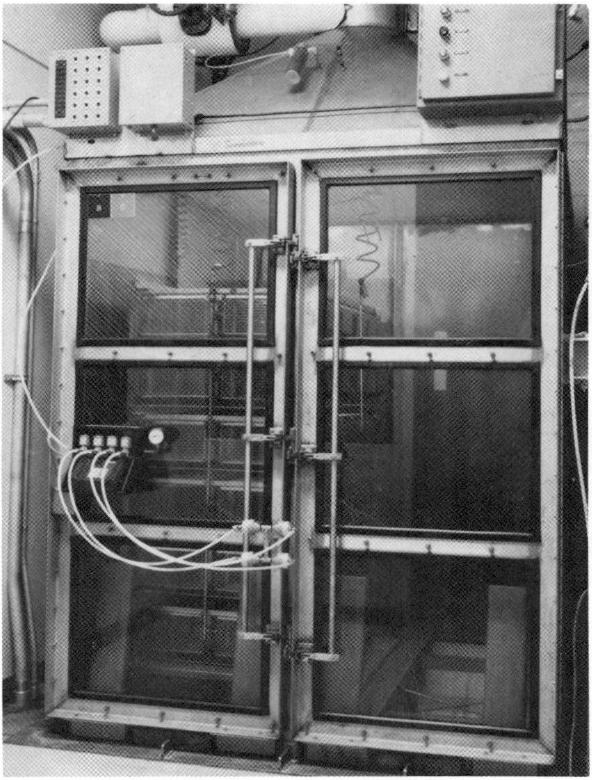

FIGURE 1 Frontal view of one 12.6 m^3 chronic inhalation chamber showing the air inlet section at the top, animal cages and cage racks with feeders, and internal automatic water supply. The entry track ramps are visible at the bottom of the chambers.

Visible at the top of the chamber in Figure 1 are the watering system lines (black tubing) which pass into the chamber via the top cone and connect to the cage racks as shown to provide continuous watering *ad libitum* to each cage unit. Fittings attached to the door front are for measuring pressures and aerosol mass concentrations within the chambers.

The lower cone assembly includes a suspended track structure within each chamber which supports the mobile animal racks. Each track has a hinged portion at the front of the chamber which is dropped when the doors are opened to form a ramp for moving the animal racks into and out of the chambers.

As part of their easy serviceability requirement, these chambers were suspended between floors. This feature allows

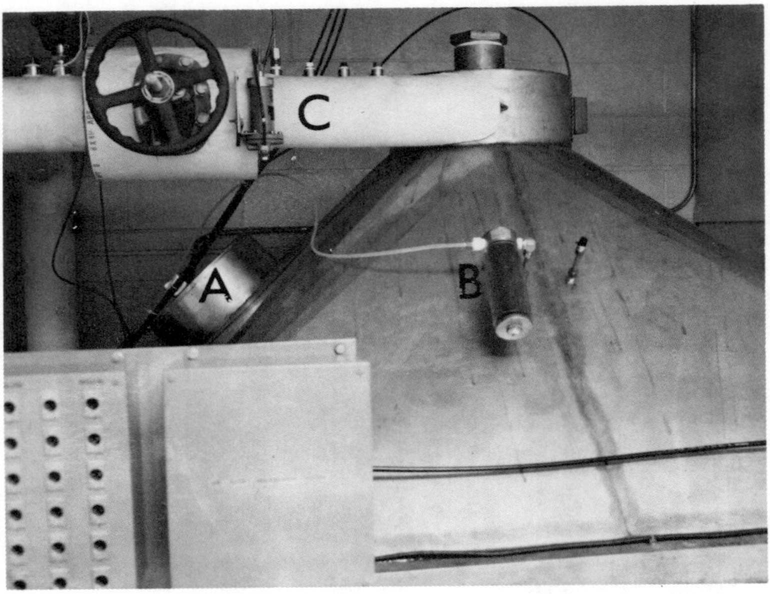

FIGURE 2 Top cone of chamber showing one lighting fixture (A), absolute filter on gas sampling line (B), and insulated inlet ducting and throttle valve (C).

easier access to the chambers than a raised floor and offers advantages in maneuvering heavy racks of animal cages up to as well as in and out of the chambers. Proper sanitation and housekeeping in the area under the chambers can be performed easily and effectively since the service area below the chambers is almost 6 meters high. Service access to chamber utilities is also facilitated since the chamber's air cleanup system and other wiring and plumbing are installed in this area. These facilities are visible for inspection and openly accessible for maintenance.

Caging and Cage Racks

Special stainless steel caging (Figure 3) was designed for aerosol exposure studies. The cages are constructed of welded wire mesh with latching mesh doors on top, water spigot inlets at the back, and covered pellet feed hoppers in the front. The caging units are provided with removable partitions allowing them to be used for individually housing six rats or three guinea pigs or other large animals per caging unit. Each unit has tracks on either side, permitting it to be suspended in large mobile stainless steel cage racks as shown in Figure 4. Attached to each cage rack is a water distribution manifold supplying drinking water *ad libitum* to

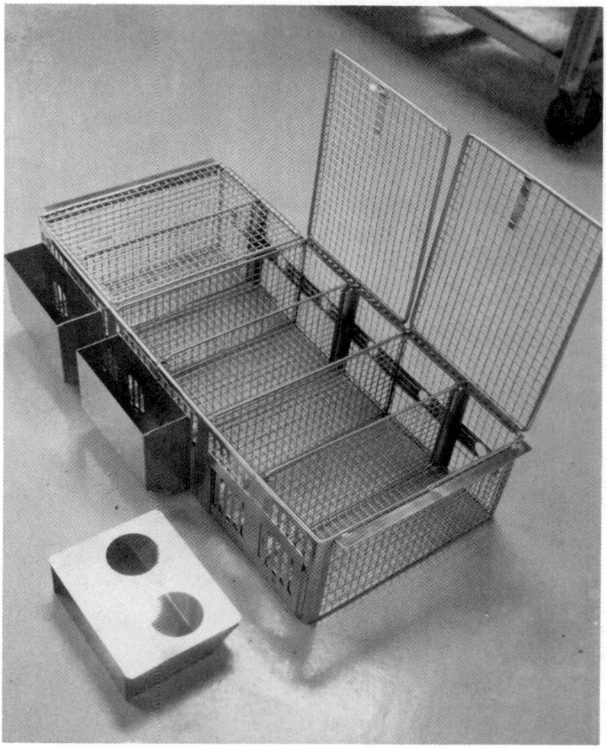

FIGURE 3 Individual stainless steel animal inhalation caging unit used in the chambers has feeders in the front and water spigot inlets at the back. Each module individually houses six rats or three guinea pigs (with dividers removed) and hangs suspended from tracks in a mobile cage rack.

144 demand spigots which enter each caging unit in the rack. Below each caging unit are stainless steel catch pans which fit into the racks to protect the animals below. The mobile rack of cages is designed to be rolled into or out of the chambers via the tracks shown in Figure 5 to minimize the effort required to load and empty the chambers each day. This feature, plus the automatic watering system, save a considerable amount of time each day and have been major contributors to the short daily cleanup period required for normal operation. Depending on the animal load, this usually requires one man-hour per chamber.

Air Delivery System

All air drawn through the chambers is clean building air

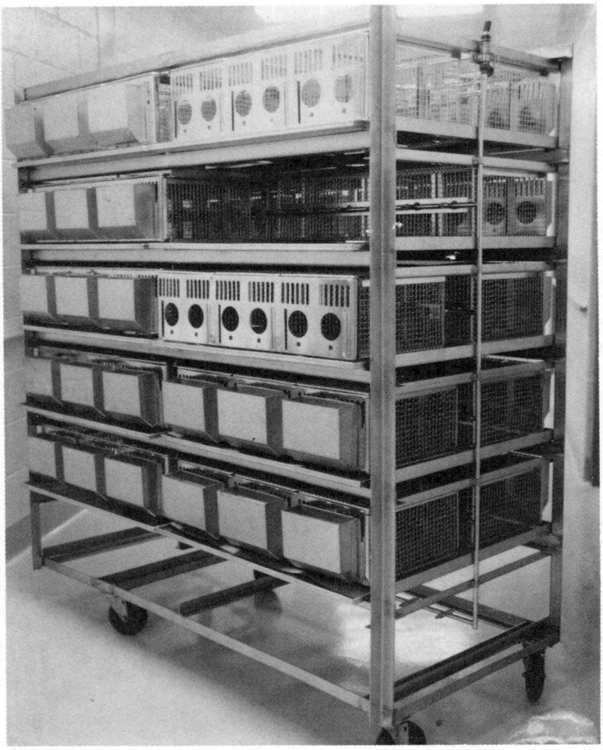

FIGURE 4 Stainless steel mobile cage rack showing cages in various states of assembly installed in the rack. The automatic watering system manifold and catch trays are also visible.

which is first cooled in a 10-ton chilled-water heat exchanger to a temperature of 6°C. The air is then prefiltered and contaminant gases such as ammonia reduced by passage over a 54 kg bed of potassium permanganate and a 22.5 kg activated carbon filter in a Purafil Model PC-22C air purification unit. Finally, the air is humidified and reheated as necessary to maintain a healthy chamber environment and filtered again with a HEPA filter before it enters the chamber (Figure 6). All air handling equipment after the heat exchanger is insulated to permit better temperature control of the delivered air.

The test material is injected into the clean air at the top of the chamber, Figure 6. The resultant diluted mixture is drawn through the chambers and connecting manifold before being exhausted from the laboratory by a single Buffalo Forge 1.5 kW (2 hp) blower located on the roof. In the event of a fan failure, the exhaust system is automatically switched over to a backup fan and an alarm sounds to alert the operators of the changeover.

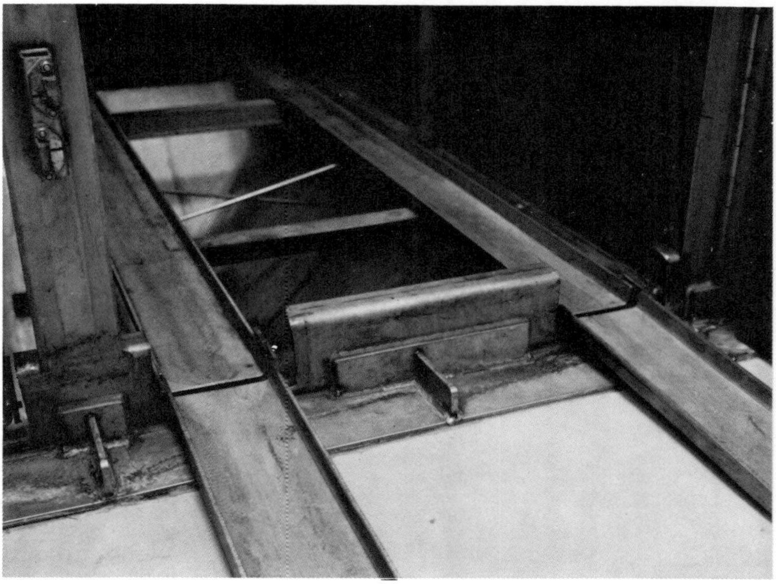

FIGURE 5 Fold-out tracks in lower cone of exposure chamber to support roll-in cage racks.

Air Flow Control

The total flowrate in each of the chambers is usually set at 2.8 m^3/min, corresponding to 13 air changes/hr. This chamber flowrate is monitored by calibrated venturi flowmeters mounted at the clean air inlet section of the chambers (Figure 6). Adjustment of airflow can be made manually by a pneumatically actuated exhaust throttle valve. A pressure switch in parallel will sound an alarm if the flow falls below 70% of the normal value. In the future, the computer will use a pressure transducer to monitor the airflow and provide a backup alarm for flow failure.

Pressure Control

Chamber internal presure is set to the desired negative value by throttling a stainless steel gate valve in the inlet air section (Fig. 6). The settings of this valve can be balanced with the exit throttle valve to obtain the required internal pressure at the desired total flow rate. Normally, the chambers are operated at a negative pressure of approximately 2 cm of water.

Temperature Control

As depicted in Figure 6, the chamber inlet air is reheated by individual heat exchangers after it is dehumidified and cleaned in order to maintain a desired temperature in the animal cages. The amount of heat supplied is regulated by pneumatic valves which are controlled by signals from pneumatic temperature sensors in the inlet of each chamber. Typical operating temperature in the chambers is 22°C. A thermocouple also monitors the temperature inside each chamber and provides a continuous readout of chamber temperature. When the temperature goes beyond ±3.5°C of the desired set point, an alarm is triggered to alert the operating staff.

Relative Humidity Control

Relative humidity is measured in each chamber by a pneumatic sensor which controls the introduction of distilled water steam into the inlet air as diagramed in Figure 6. The

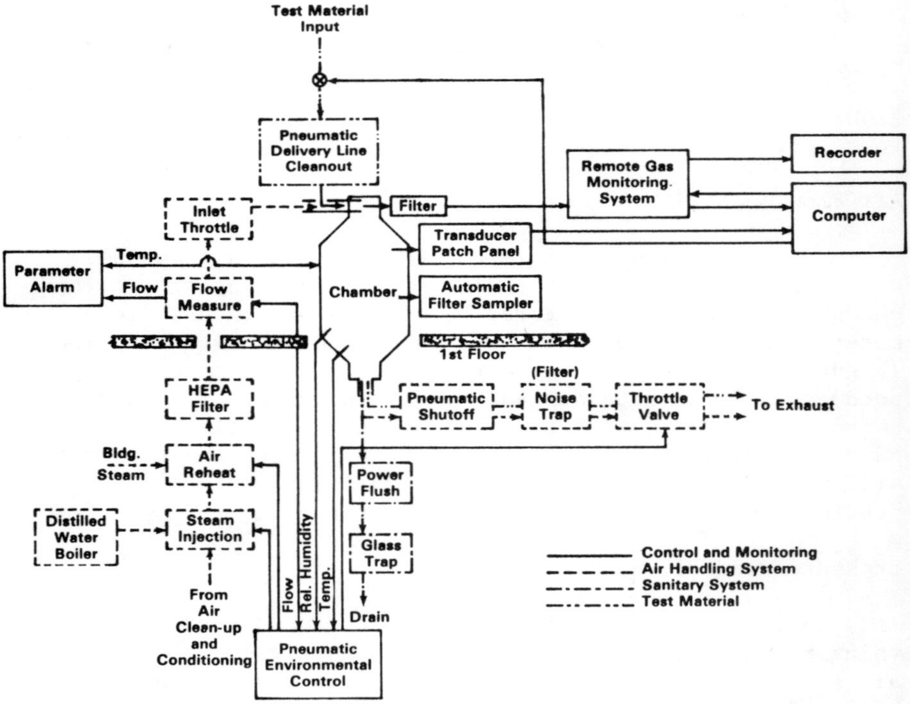

FIGURE 6 A single chamber showing the major associated fixtures. The inhalation unit consists of four such chambers operated in parallel.

relative humidity is displayed at each chamber by a calibrated pneumatic readout, and is measured independently by a dew point hygrometer in the Chamber Air Monitoring System. Relative humidity information is entered into the computer for recording and tabulation.

Chamber Air Monitoring System

Certain gases in the four inhalation atmospheres are measured by a Chamber Air Monitoring System (Figure 7). It consists of a console of instruments to determine CO, NO_x, S, hydrocarbons, and ozone concentrations, as well as the dew point of the air in each chamber. The system also includes a General Automation GA 16/440 computer for process control functions, data logging, and data analysis. The gas analyzers are all maintained in accordance with the manufacturer's recommendations except where experience dictates more frequent service. Calibration mixtures of gases are checked against standards traceable to the National Bureau of Standards. Zero and span checks are made daily on all analyzers.

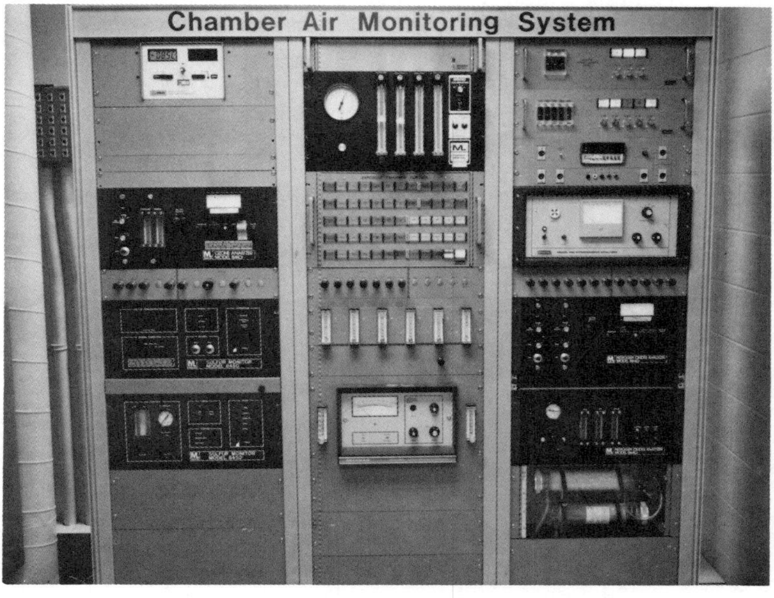

FIGURE 7 The chamber air monitoring system console containing instruments to monitor CO, NO_x, NO, NO_2, S, hydrocarbons, ozone, and dew point. Span, zero, and sample gases may be routed by manual or computer control.

Samples of gas are sequentially drawn from each chamber through an absolute filter (Figure 6), and into a 4L glass plenum from which the analyzers draw their samples. The gas is pumped through Teflon lines from each chamber to the central plenum to ensure no dilution of the concentrations being measured. After switching to a new chamber, the gas analysis instruments reach a steady state reading of the plenum concentration within one to four minutes. The value is recorded for that chamber by the computer, and the monitoring system switches to a new chamber. To assure rapid filling of the plenum with a fresh gas sample, the lines from each chamber pump a sample to the gas console for several minutes before it is switched to the plenum for measurement. All sample line switching is via solenoid valves controlled by the monitoring computer. As a backup to the computer, the gas analyzer outputs can also be monitored on a multiplexed paper chart recorder depicted in Figure 6.

Aerosol Concentration Measurement

During exposure to aerosols, samples are routinely drawn to determine the chamber mass concentration directly (Figure 6). The present system is convenient for unattended operation. Four filters are loaded into a holder assembly and mounted on the chamber door. A programmable timer (Figure 8) opens a solenoid valve behind each filter for a specified period. The flow rate is set by a critical orifice connected to the house vacuum. In the control chamber, a single filter is drawn during the entire exposure period. Aerosol mass concentrations determined from these filters are entered into an open-ended computation of the means and standard deviations of the concentration in each chamber. This computation can be used to determine the average exposure concentration in any chamber between any two days of the experiment, permitting convenient documentation of the exposure of any group of animals regardless of when they entered or left the chamber.

In addition to the gravimetric measurements, a TSI 3030 Electrical Aerosol Analyzer provides a fast indication of aerosol concentration. The channel 1 value should be proportional to the mass concentration of the aerosol, assuming the size distribution is constant from day to day.

Alarms

For unattended operation, each chamber is equipped with flow and temperature transducers which are connected to alarms (Figures 6 and 9). During a test, variations of any of these parameters beyond control limits trigger an alarm in the work area, departmental administrative office and the

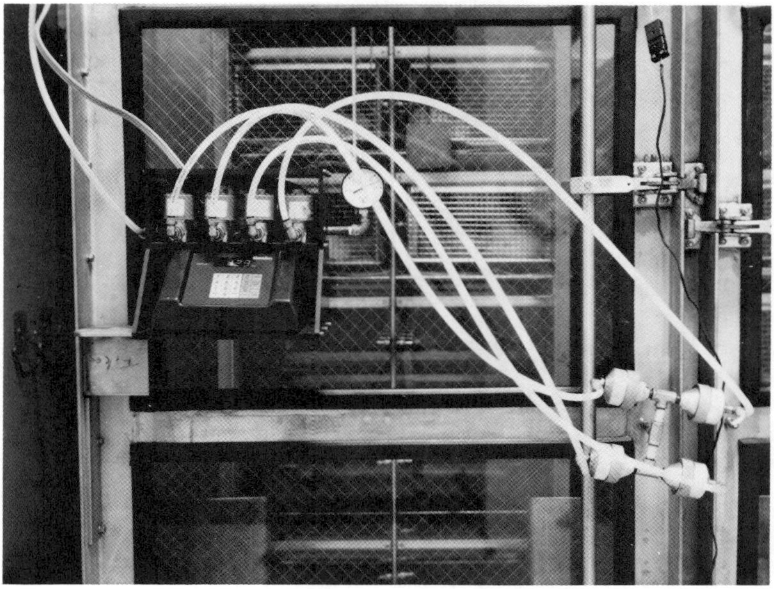

FIGURE 8 Programmable timer for filter collections during unattended operation of the chambers.

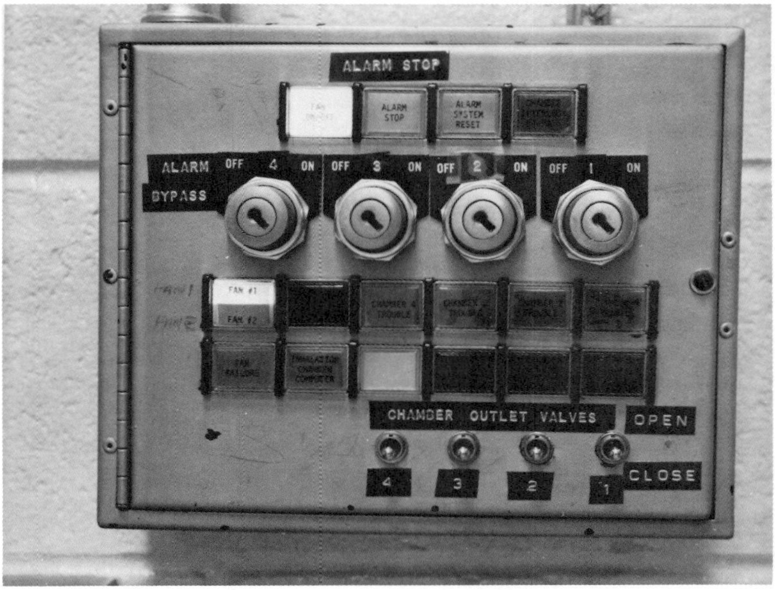

FIGURE 9 Parameter alarm which can electro-pneumatically monitor temperature and flow in each chamber, locked on during the entire test day, and turned off for clean-up. The alarm also controls and monitors the dual exhaust blowers.

Plant Security office, resulting in an emergency call to an experienced system operator who assesses the problem and directs corrective action. The alarm control box has a key switch on each chamber's circuits which permits the alarms to be disabled during cleanup and locked during unattended operation. In its final form, the computer will monitor an even broader range of control variables and send independent alarms when necessary as a backup for the electro-pneumatic alarm system.

Additional Data Channels

To allow for future experiments which may require a variety of measurements to be taken at the chamber, a transducer patch panel, visible in Figure 1 and depicted schematically in Figure 6, was installed on each chamber and is connected to the central computer. Both digital and analogue data can be transmitted via this route, enabling the experimenter to monitor temperatures, test material concentrations or even physiological parameters during the course of an exposure experiment.

OPERATING EXPERIENCE

The facilities described are in a continuous state of evolution and improvement; however, experience has been gained over twenty months of continuous operation and the overall performance of the system in this work will be discussed in this section. Operational experience thus far involves a chronic exposure study of diluted diesel exhaust. A GM 5.7L diesel engine produced the exhaust aerosol. Figure 10 is a schematic of the exhaust delivery system. To simulate passenger car emissions, the exhaust was drawn from a manifold located downstream from the muffler at a point where the end of a normal exhaust system would be. It passed through a valve assembly for adjusting the flow rate and into stainless steel delivery lines. These lines were heated to a temperature of 100±15°C to keep the exhaust at tailpipe temperature until it was rapidly diluted at the top of the chambers.

Spatial Uniformity of the Test Aerosol

Millipore® 25 mm filters were used to assess the spatial uniformity of the particulate mass concentration. Thirty-two sampling ports, visible in Figure 1, allow sampling at four levels in a chamber. The top and bottom rows of ports (Levels 1 and 4) allowed sampling above and below the cage racks. The middle rows of ports (Levels 2 and 3) allowed filter holders to be placed between two cage levels out of reach of the animals. Open-face filter holders connected to different lengths of 1/4" copper tubing provided a three-dimensional sampling array inside the chamber. All the filters were weighed to the nearest microgram on an electrobalance (Cahn Model 25) after electrically discharging them.

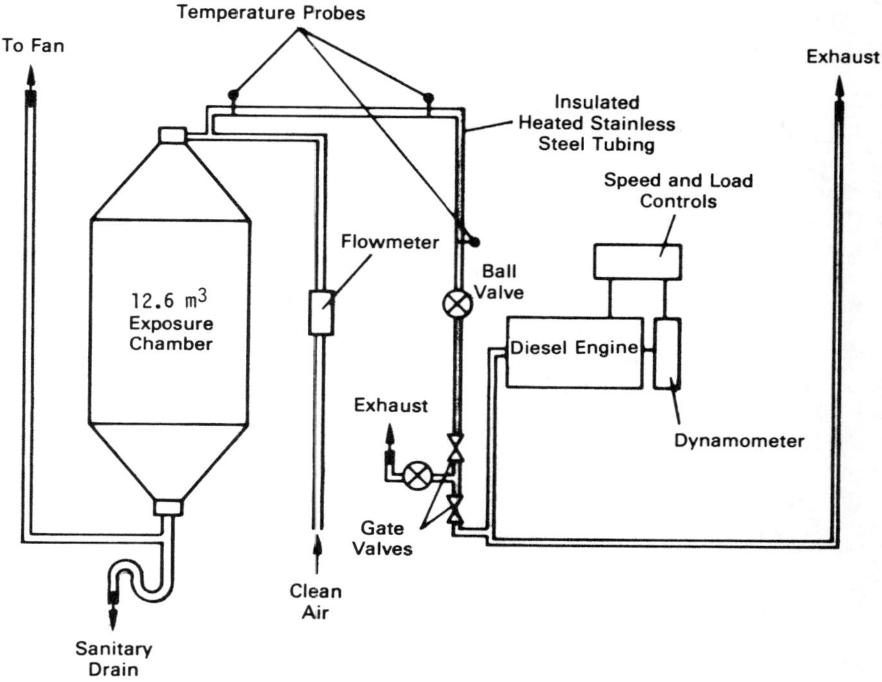

FIGURE 10 Schematic of the delivery system for a recent study of diesel exhaust showing the exhaust flow path through heated delivery lines from the engine to the chambers. For simplicity, only one chamber is shown.

Four sampling trains were assembled so that four filter samples could be drawn during the same sampling period. During each period, one of the four filters measured the "reference concentration" near the front center of the chamber above the racks (Level 1). Most of the measurements were made at a volume flow rate of 5 L/min with at least 250 L of air drawn through each filter. The concentration variation along a line was measured during each sampling period. The line orientations were 1) horizontal, parallel to the chamber doors, 2) vertical near the back of the chamber, 3) horizontal along the diagonal of the chamber, and 4) diagonal from top-back to bottom-front of one rack. The final set of filter samples was drawn at scattered locations, one on each level.

Due to particulate losses to surfaces, the particulate mass concentration near the bottom of the chamber (outlet) might be expected to be lower than near the top (inlet). In addition, the feeders on the sides of the cages and the catch pans below them might disturb the airflow in the chamber and cause a decrease in concentration inside the cage racks. To explore whether significant concentration non-uniformities existed, four different analyses of the data follow:

1) Figures 11a and 11b show some of the observations from the 5 L/min sample rate filter. The mean and standard deviation of the routine filter measurements for that day are also shown. One fact apparent from these graphs is that the reference concentrations (solid symbols) were not systematically higher than the others as would be expected if particulate concentration gradients existed. This observation holds true whether or not the catch trays and feeders are on the racks.

The apparent lack of concentration non-uniformities might have been due to excessive ventilation of the cages near the filter by the 5 L/min sample flow rate. Three sets of measurements of four filters each were made at a reduced sample flow rate of 1 L/min. Figure 11c shows some of the concentration data from the 1 L/min sample rate filters. The lack of concentration non-uniformities seen with the 5 L/min sample rate data was confirmed at the lower sampling rate.

FIGURE 11 Particle mass concentration data from filter samples. The solid symbol in each group is the "reference concentration" measurement. The point on the right is the mean and standard deviation of the routine filter samples for that exposure day.

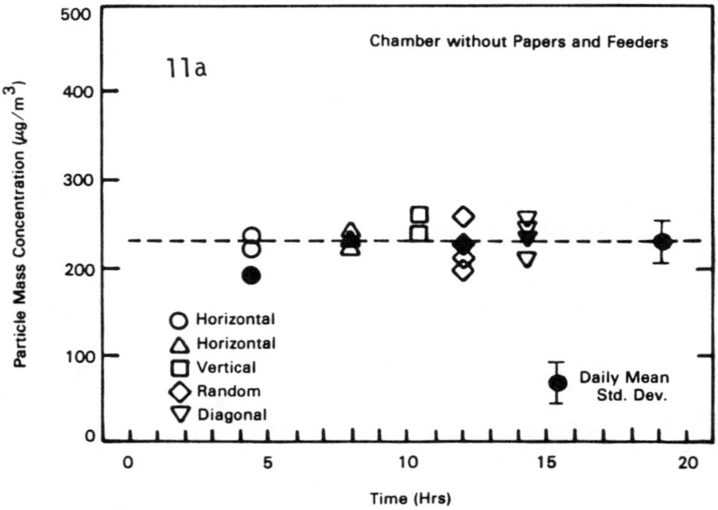

a) 5 L/min sample flow rate, without papers and feeders.

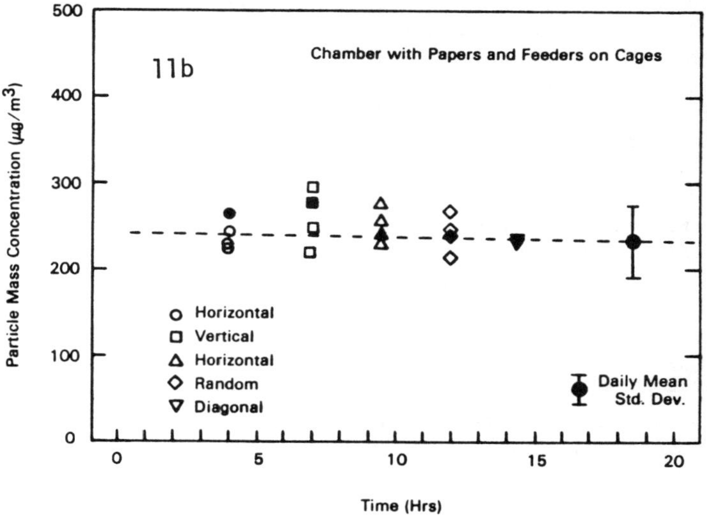

b) 5 L/min sample flow rate, with papers and feeders.

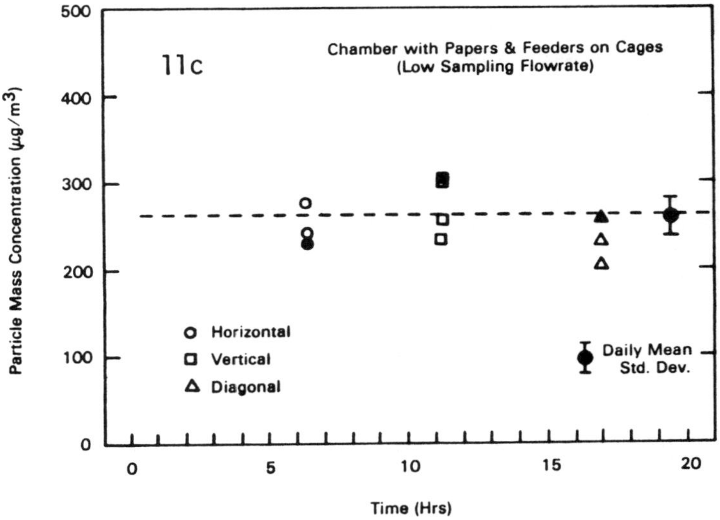

c) 1 L/min sample flow rate, with papers and feeders.

2) The overall variation of particulate mass concentration throughout the chamber was quantified by computing the mean and standard deviation for each set of filters drawn simultaneously. Sets were not included in this analysis if fewer than three of the four filter measurements were successfully completed. For the filters drawn at 5 L/min, the standard deviation of 3 or 4 simultaneous filter measurements drawn from different parts of the chamber was about 9% of the mean, whether or not papers and feeders were on the racks.

3) Table 1 presents another analysis of the filter data intended to show whether there is a top-to-bottom gradient of particle mass concentration. The means and standard deviations for filter samples obtained at each sampling level and chamber configuration are presented. Each filter measurement was divided by the "reference concentration" measurement taken above the racks (Level 1) to normalize the data sampled over one time interval for comparison with measurements taken at different times. There is no consistent pattern of a vertical concentration gradient throughout this data. The chamber appears quite well mixed, even with the racks in the chamber and the catch trays and feeders on the racks.

4) Another summary of the results is intended to detect differences between the concentrations inside and above the cage racks. All the filter data (5 L/min and 1 L/min) for Levels 2 and 3 (samples from inside the racks) were grouped and a mean normalized concentration calculated. With no catch trays or feeders on the cages, 14 measurements gave a mean normalized concentration of 0.91 with a standard deviation of 0.11. The measurements were not independent, so standard statistical tests to determine whether the mean values are significantly different from unity do not apply. However, there is an indication that the mean concentration in the cages was about 10% lower than the concentration above the racks when the papers and feeders were in place.

Summarizing the spatial uniformity data, no large concentration non-uniformities were detected, whether or not the catch trays and feeders were in place and whether the sampling flow rate was 5 L/min or 1 L/min. The observed non-uniformities on the order of 10% of the mean were considered acceptable for a chronic exposure study.

Size Distribution of Test Aerosols and Background Dust

The particle size distributions above and in a cage rack were measured simultaneously with seven-stage cascade impactors. Impactors were constructed following a previous design [Mercer et al, 1970], but the choice of jet diameters differed from the original. One pair of impactors had nominal flow rates of 4 L/min, making it possible to collect parti-

Table 1

SPATIAL DISTRIBUTION OF DIESEL AEROSOL IN THE CHAMBER

CONCENTRATION NORMALIZED BY CONCENTRATION IN UPPER (INLET) CONE

	5 L/min Sampling Flow Rate			1 L/min Sampling Flow Rate	
Empty Chamber	Catch Trays	Catch Trays	Catch Trays and Feeders	Catch Trays	Catch Trays and Feeders
1.00±.015 (5)	1.16±.14 (6)	1.01±.05 (4)	0.89±.03 (5)	0.90±.03 (2)	0.95± (1)
1.02±.06 (5)	1.04±.09 (3)	0.98±.11 (5)	1.03±.08 (5)	0.95±.18 (3)	0.82±0.10 (5)
1.05±.08 (5)	1.02±.13 (3)	0.82±.05 (3)	0.96±.15 (3)	0.82±.06 (2)	1.00±0.29 (2)

( ) Number of samples
± Standard Deviation

cles with aerodynamic diameters greater than 0.23 μm. Another pair of impactors operating at 1 L/min had similar collection characteristics. The collection surfaces were 22 mm diameter glass cover slips which could be weighed with high precision on the Cahn Electrobalance. To take a sample, one impactor was placed above the cage racks near where the "reference concentration" was measured. The second impactor was placed inside a cage near the center of the rack. No animal was in the cage with the impactor, but the surrounding cages were populated with rats. Samples were taken both in the "clean" chamber and in the chamber containing the test aerosol diesel exhaust.

One of the "reference" size distributions is shown in Figure 12. The mass median aerodynamic diameter, for which half of the mass is on larger particles and half on smaller, can be read from the intersection of the experimental curve with the 50% cumulative mass concentration line. The percent of mass on particles having aerodynamic diameters less than 1.0 μm can also be determined from this type of plot. Table 2 compares the size distributions above and inside the cages both with and without catch trays and feeders. There were no major differences in the size distributions in any of these cases. At the lower sampling flow rate of 1 L/min, impactor samples also showed no difference between the size distribution in a cage or above the racks, whether or not the catch trays and feeders were in place. This indicated that the usual sampling flow rate of 4 L/min was not excessively ventilating the sampled areas.

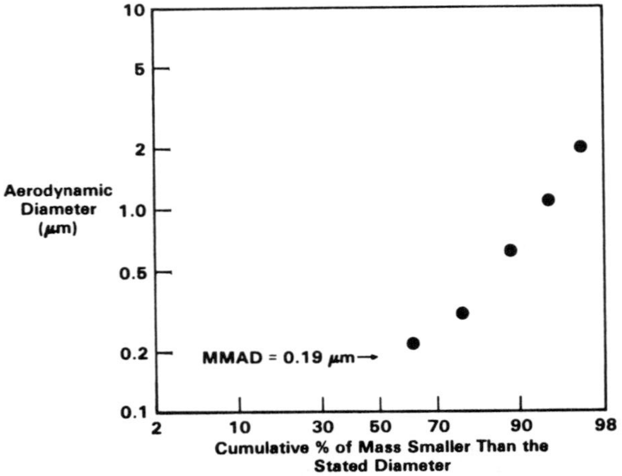

FIGURE 12 Typical set of cascade impactor data obtained in this study from the "reference" position. The mass median aerodynamic diameter (MMAD) and % of mass on particles smaller than 1 μm are obtained from this graph.

Table 2

CASCADE IMPACTOR* DATA

	Above Cages		Inside Cages	
Chamber Configuration	MMAD (μm)	% Mass Below 1 μm	MMAD (μm)	% Mass Below 1 μm
No catch trays or feeders	0.20	85	0.21	84
Catch trays and feeders in place	0.19	93	0.19	92

*7-stage multijet cascade impactor at a sampling flowrate of 4 L/min.

Size distribution measurements were also made in the control chamber. Since the air supplied to the chambers was filtered before entering the chamber, the aerosol in the "clean" chamber was attributed to the animals and any small leaks into the chamber from the room. One impactor was placed near the front of an empty cage. This position should have maximized the collection of food dust generated by the animals in adjoining cages. A second impactor was placed above the cage rack, as usual. Figure 13 shows the two cumulative concentration plots. The impactor inside the cage measured a mass concentration of 40 $\mu g/m^3$, but the impactor above the racks measured 20 $\mu g/m^3$. These results indicate the presence of some large size dust which was not uniformly dispersed in the exposure chamber. The mass concentration of these "background" particles smaller than 1 μm in the "clean" chamber was only about 10 $\mu g/m^3$.

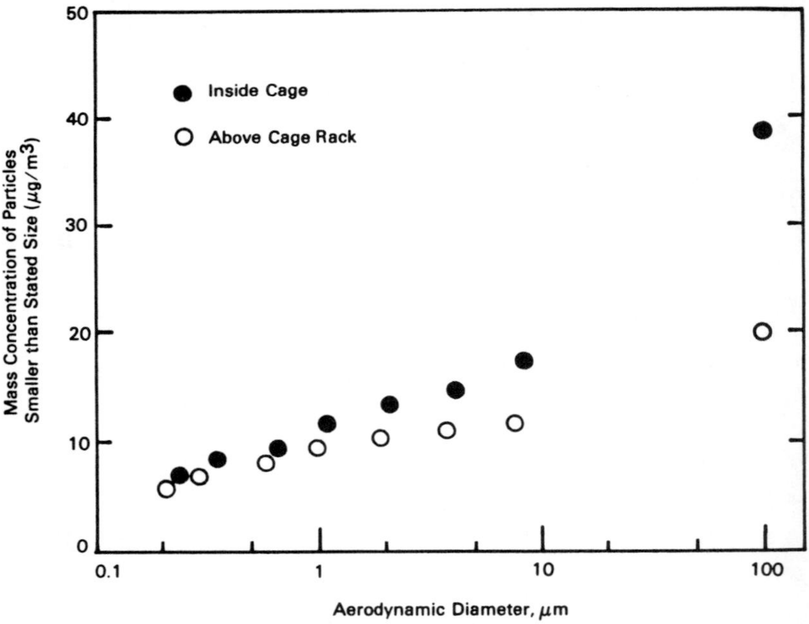

FIGURE 13 Cascade impactor data from samples inside and above the cage rack in the "clean chamber." In each case, at least half of the particles by mass have an aerodynamic diameter greater than 8 μm, and the mass concentrations of particles smaller than 1 μm were about 10 $\mu g/m^3$.

Chamber Noise

During the initial testing period, noise levels as high as 75 dBA were measured inside the chambers. Prolonged exposure of test animals to this noise stress is undesirable in a chronic exposure study [Holt, 1978]. The causes of the chamber noise were found to be the exhaust fan and aerodynamic sources in the chamber exhaust system. Noises from the engine test cell adjacent to the inhalation facilities contributed only 1 dBA to the chamber noise. Side-to-side resonance in an empty chamber added another 2 dBA with a distinct frequency at 160 hertz.

Acoustic panels will effectively reduce the noise but complicate air flow patterns and cleanup in the chambers. Instead effective noise control was achieved by adjusting the fan operation to avoid pulsations of the ventilating air at low fan speeds. Modifications in the chamber exhaust system were also made. These included the use of acoustic baffles inside a plenum (Figure 6) and the replacement of gate valves by damper valves to control chamber airflow. After the completion of the noise control program, a background sound level of 62-65 dBA was measured and judged to be acceptable for chronic inhalation studies. The improvement in the chamber noise level is illustrated in Figure 14.

Chamber Air Flow Rate

The volume flow rate of clean air into the chambers was reached and reset manually at least three times per exposure day. The values were stable and required little readjustment over the twenty months of testing.

Chamber Air Temperature

As pointed out by Bernstein et al, [1980], the temperature of the room containing the chamber has an important modulating effect on the chamber air temperature. As long as the room temperature is constant, the inlet air temperature is not critical for chambers with uninsulated walls such as these.

Over one 6-month period of exposure to diluted diesel exhaust, the average rack temperatures as measured by a glass thermometer hung on the end of one rack in each chamber were between 20.8°C and 21.7°C with standard deviations of less than 1°C.

Because the computer was not initially ready to monitor temperatures, a four-channel thermocouple recorder was used to continually record chamber temperature. It would set off the alarm if any chamber temperature was outside the range of 22±3.5°C. This system worked reasonably well.

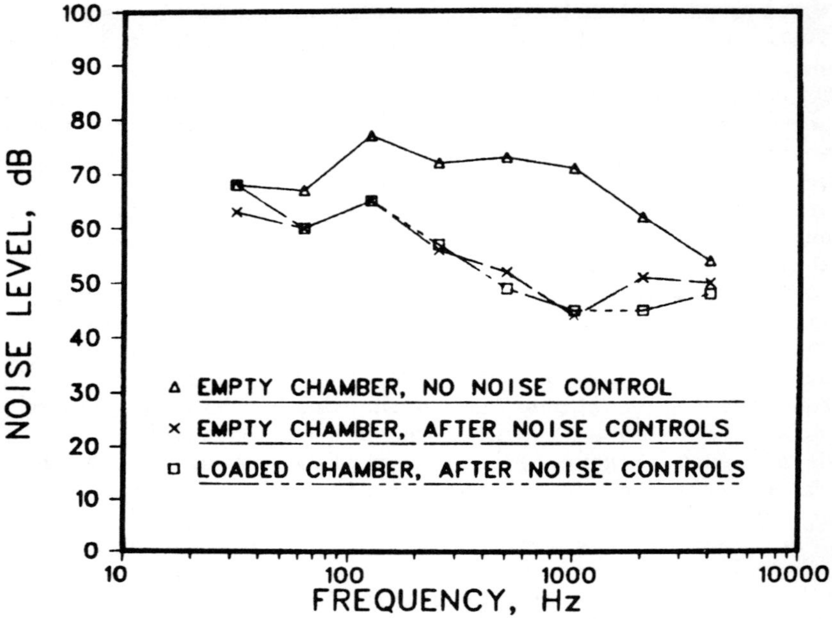

FIGURE 14 The noise level in the chambers was reduced considerably through operation of the blower in an optimal flow-pressure region of its performance curve, elimination of sources of aerodynamic noise in the lines and the installation of a noise trap between the blower and the chambers.

The same alarm could also be set off if the pneumatic temperature sensor in the outlet air line of any chamber exuded a preset value. This temperature measurement did not reflect the in-chamber temperature as well since the exiting air tended to equilibrate with the room temperature as it passed over the metal surfaces upstream of the sensor.

The pneumatic sensor controlling the amount of reheating each chamber's inlet air received was located in the duct upstream of the inlet cone. It did not accurately measure the in-chamber temperature either and was influenced by the exhaust which entered the duct just upstream from it. Despite these handicaps, the pneumatic temperature control system performed well in the large inhalation chambers as evidenced by the close control of temperature during the test.

Chamber Relative Humidity

The principle relative humidity measurement was by an

EG and G Model 911 dew point hygrometer sampling from the Chamber Air Monitoring System plenum. Over a six-month period the relative humidity in the control chamber was measured to be 56±6%. This instrument performed well with routine cleaning and maintenance for over one year but eventually the sensing element required replacement. This degradation may have been due to compounds in the test atmosphere despite the fact that the instrument was protected with an absolute filter.

The relative humidity control system was only used for short periods during the early months of testing since it showed a tendency to overshoot the control point. This was attributed to problems with the control characteristics of the steam injection valves and the pneumatic relative humidity sensors. New components will be installed in the system for further evaluation in the coming months.

Despite this problem, the relative humidity of the animal exposure environment was maintained within desired limits by condensing airborne water in the inlet chiller to balance the water vapor added to the air by the animals in the chamber.

CONCLUSIONS

An inhalation exposure facility has been constructed having the capacity to expose large animal populations to four exposure levels (including zero) of a test compound for 20 hours per day continuously for durations of one year or more. Automated equipment provides environmental control and monitoring throughout the day, permitting unattended operation of the chambers except for a short cleanup period. After over twenty months of round-the-clock operation, the facility has demonstrated its ease of maintenance, accurate environmental and test compound control, and a reliable alarm system.

REFERENCES

Bernstein, D.M., and Drew, R.T., 1980. The major parameters affecting temperature inside inhalation chambers. Am. Ind. Hyg. Assn. J., 41(6):420-426.

Holt, P.G., 1978. Auditory stress and the immune system. J. Sound and Vibration, 59:131-132.

Laskin, S., Kuschner, M., and Drew, R.T., 1970. Studies in pulmonary carcinogenesis. In: Inhalation Carcinogenesis, M. G. Hanna, Jr., P. Nettesheim and J. R. Gilbert, Eds., U.S. Atomic Energy Commission, Oak Ridge.

Mercer, T.T., Tillery, M.I., and Newton, G.J., 1970. A multistage low flow rate cascade impactor. J. Aerosol Sci., 1:9-15, 1970.

Phalen, R.F., 1976. Inhalation exposure to animals. Environmental Health Perspectives, 16:17-24.

An Exposure System for Toxicological Studies of Concentrated Oil Aerosols

R.W. HOLMBERG, J.H. MONEYHUN, and W.E. DALBEY
Oak Ridge National Laboratory
Oak Ridge, Tennessee 37830

ABSTRACT

An exposure system for the study of diesel oil aerosols is described. An evaporation-condensation generator capable of producing sub-micron sized aerosols of diesel oil in the concentration range of 0.5 to 20 g/m^3 has been designed and interfaced to Rochester style exposure chambers. It was found that the existing chamber design was not adequate to provide a uniformly distributed aerosol. Modifications to these chambers to develop a uniform distribution of the diesel aerosol are described. Photographic and instrumental verification of the uniformity are presented. Stripping of the spent aerosol from the chamber exhaust by coalescing filtration is described.

INTRODUCTION

The military has shown a renewed interest in the use of smokes and obscurants for screening purposes in warfare. This coupled with present day concerns for environmental and occupational exposure safety has prompted the Army to investigate the risks associated with passive and/or accidental exposures to these smokes. As part of this program, we have undertaken an investigation of the inhalation toxicology of one of these obscurants. This smoke is produced from diesel powered tanks from diesel oil in a system designated by the military acronym VEESS for Vehicle Engine Exhaust Smoke System. Briefly, the same oil that powers the tank is pumped into the hot manifold directly after the engine where it immediately vaporizes. The vapors are carried through the exhaust system and forcibly ejected, along with the normal exhaust gases, into the air where they condense to form a dense aerosol that is used for screening purposes. The size and cost of a military tank, as well as the amount of aerosol the VEESS system produces, precluded its use in our laboratory environment. This report then describes our efforts to develop a generator which adequately simulates this process, but on a much reduced scale and the modification of existing Rochestor-type exposure chambers to form a complete exposure system for bio-testing.

MATERIALS AND METHODS

The chambers used (figure 1) were of the Rochester type, rectangular with tapered end sections and having a total volume of 1.4 cubic meters. They have a capacity for 45 rat cages hung in five tiers. Conditioned air is fed to the chambers from the top, exhausts at the bottom and is filtered through absolute filters provided as a building facility before exiting into the atmosphere. Typically, the chambers operate with an air throughput of 420 l/min and at a slight (1 cm water) negative pressure. At the outset it was deemed important to be able to build into the laboratory generator a

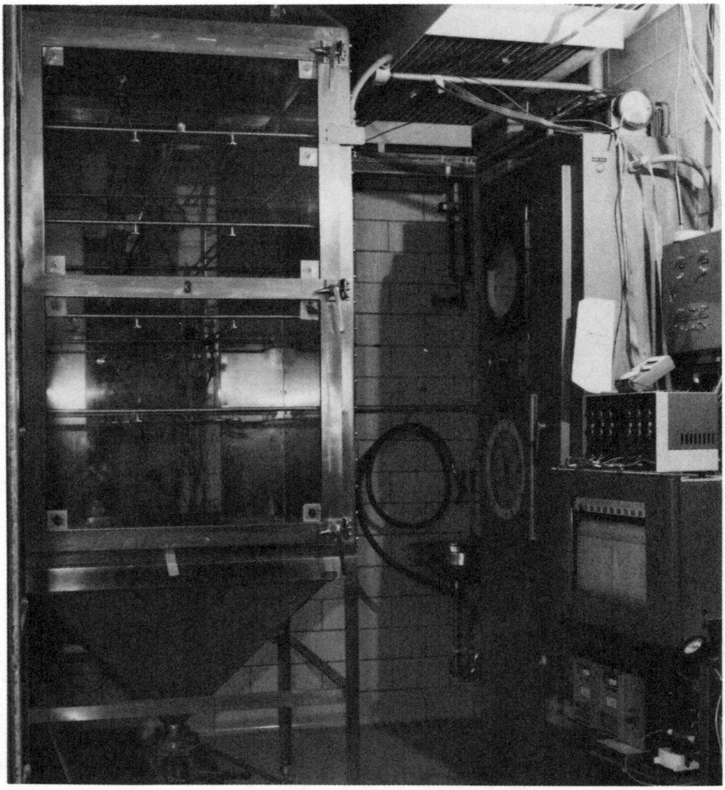

Figure 1. Exposure Chamber and Control Equipment.

chemical environment similar to that which exists in the exhaust system of the tank. It should be emphasized that the white obscurant smoke primarily consists of droplets of diesel oil in the micron and below size range. The black, sooty particles and the gaseous constituents of normal diesel exhaust are only a minor fraction of it. Nevertheless, the ability to study the chemical interactions of the oil with exhaust gases, for example partial oxidation of the oil, to form constituents of toxicological consequence were part of the design criteria of the generator. The generator (figure 2) consists of a one meter long section of stainless steel tubing of 2.5 cm I.D. A one kilowatt Vycor immersion heater is mounted inside the tubing to simulate the "manifold" heating. A carrier gas to simulate the exhaust gases passes along the heater where it is heated to 600°C. (Presently we are using nitrogen flowing at 10 l/min as the carrier gas. The chemical effects on the diesel aerosol of gases that better simulate the exhaust of the tank are underway, but will not be discussed here.) The temperature is controlled by means of a thermocouple controller. Diesel oil is pumped into the manifold impinging on the end of the heater where it is volatilized and then carried down the tube. Since the chamber system operates at constant air flow (420 l/min), the aerosol concentration is regulated by varying the injection rate of the diesel oil using low volume metering pumps. Oil flow rates from 0.5 to 10 ml/min produce aerosol concentrations 1 to 20 g/m^3. A thermostatically controlled heater surrounding the last two-thirds of the manifold is used to keep the exiting vapors at 350°C primarily to prevent premature condensation, but also to simulate approximately the exhaust temperature of the tank. The generator is interfaced to the chamber air supply through a glass pipe tee (figure 3). The hot gases and vapors enter countercurrently into the downflowing air supply where they mix turbently and rapidly cool to form a dense aerosol.

RESULTS AND DISCUSSION

It was found that the existing chamber design was not adequate to distribute the aerosol uniformly throughout the exposure volume. The aerosol stream did not at all follow and spread out in the tapered top section as might be naively expected. Rather it entered as a discrete plume (figure 4) flowing to the bottom of the chamber. It filled the chamber to a uniform concentration only very slowly and almost exponentially. It should be noted that this phenomenon, easily visualized in our experiments with a highly concentrated aerosol, is probably quite general with chambers of this design. The tapered entry section is of little value in dispersing the aerosol uniformly. This of course posed a serious threat of non-uniform exposure of animals. Not only is the build-up

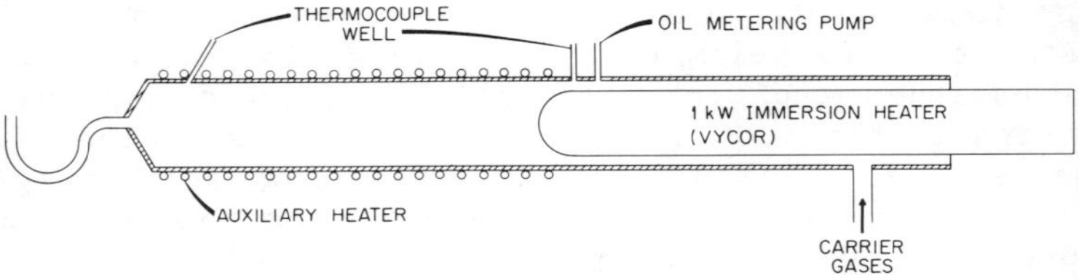

Figure 2. Schematic Diagram of Diesel Fuel Aerosol Generator.

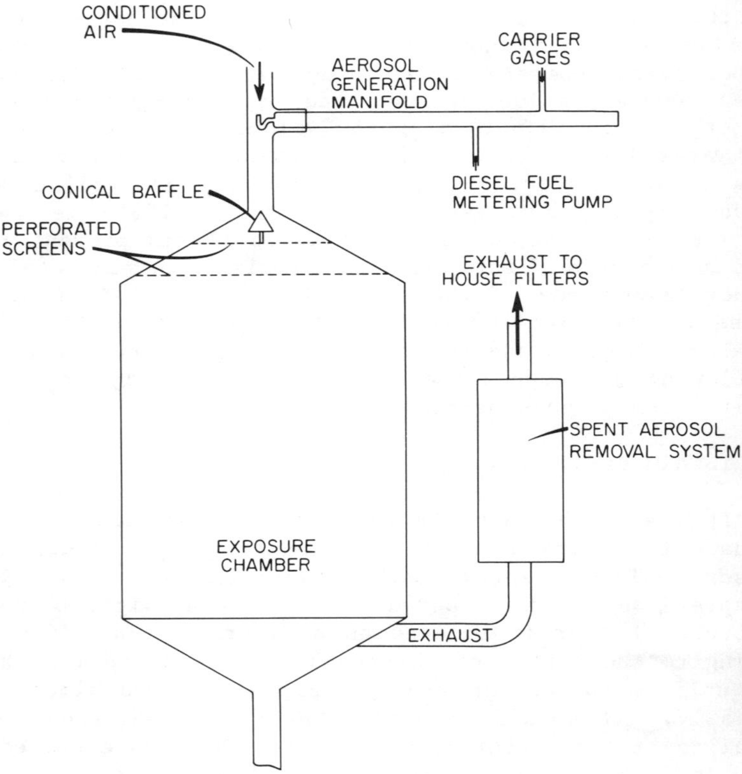

Figure 3. Schematic Diagram of Complete Exposure System.

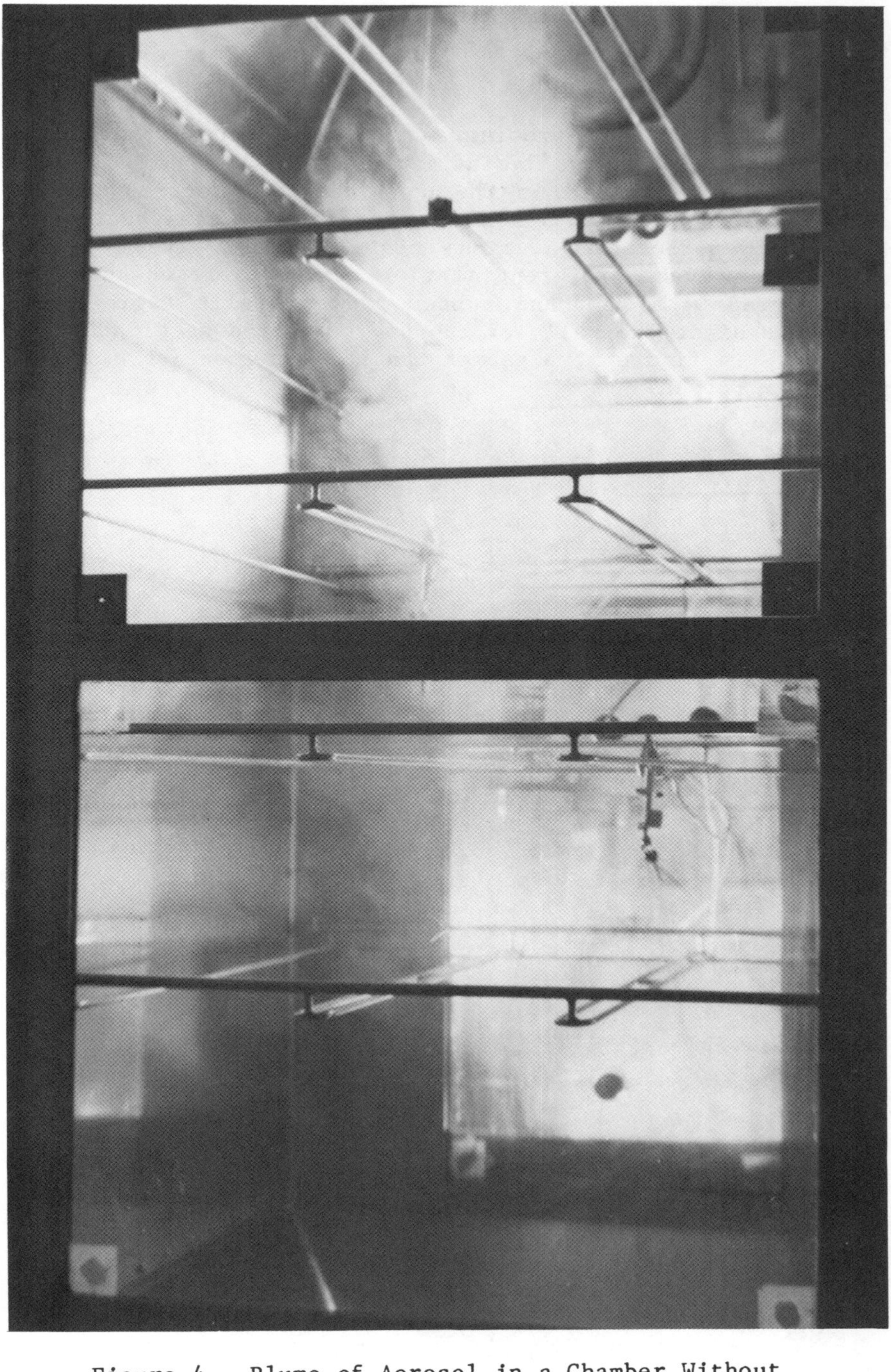

Figure 4. Plume of Aerosol in a Chamber Without Laminarizing Screens.

to a uniform concentration slow, but the somewhat warm aerosol plume impinges preferentially on the animals in the top center tier of cages.

To correct this problem, an assembly consisting of a dispersing cone and two laminarizing screens (figure 5) were designed and installed in the upper tapered section of the chamber (see figure 2). The screens were constructed of 0.080 inch perforated aluminum plate with 10% free opening area. To prevent preferential flow around their edges, they were fitted with neoprene rubber gaskets (slit tubing) and pressed against the walls of the upper tapered section of the chamber. In figure 5, a gasket had not yet been installed on the upper screen.

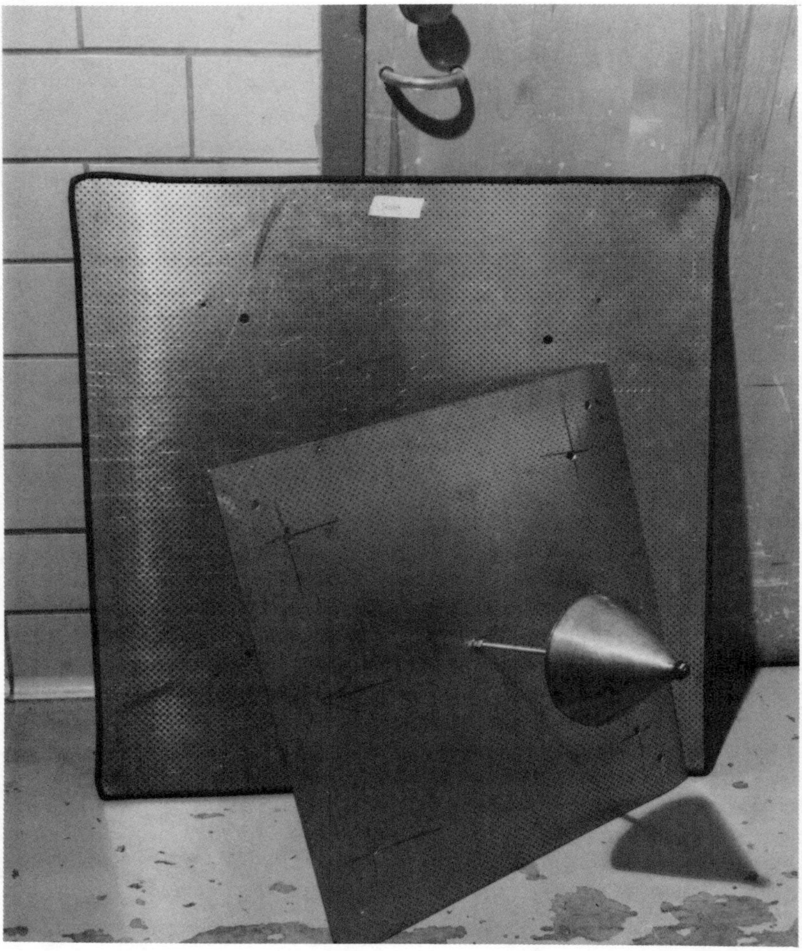

Figure 5. Cone and Screen Structure Before Installation.

With the screens in place the flow through the chamber was nearly laminar. This is illustrated (figures 6A and 6B) by photographs of the chamber taken shortly after the start of generation and as the chamber empties. In both cases the front of the advancing or retreating smoke cloud can be clearly seen. Because the aerosol laden air is somewhat more dense than the air that it displaces, there is more mixing, and the boundry is more diffuse, in the advancing front than in the retreating front. The filling/emptying chamber dynamics can also be illustrated more quantitatively (figure 7) with the use of Gayle/ORNL aerosol particle sensors (Gayle, 1979). Two matched sensors were mounted in the chamber, one just above the first tier of cages and one just below the bottom tier. The response of the sensors is essentially linear with aerosol concentration.

The homogeniety of the aerosol concentration throughout the chamber during exposures has also been investigated with the Gayle/ORNL particle sensors. For this experiment, 6 sensors were calibrated to respond equally to the aerosol concentration and then arrayed in a horizontal plane. Their output was fed to a multipoint recorder. In five separate runs, the response at each cage level was recorded. The recordings, at three levels, are shown as figure 8 and exhibit a spread from the average concentration of about 10%. We have observed that care must be exercised to preclude even small leaks into the chamber else a homogenious aerosol concentration is difficult to maintain. With the chamber operating at negative pressures, tiny leaks manifest themselves as jets of incoming air which extend for long distances into the chamber. These local disturbances in aerosol concentration, if unfortunately located, can result in nonuniform exposures at the site of some of the cages. Again, we feel that this observation is quite general for chambers operated in this mode, but is not easily detected unless detailed on-line monitoring is carried out.

The exposure facility must accommodate the lengthy exposures to highly concentrated diesel oil aerosols that may occur during these studies. The spent aerosol, that which passes through the chambers must be properly disposed of. Under some realistic exposure conditions over one liter of liquid diesel oil is consumed in a single chamber in a six hour exposure. We have found the diesel oil aerosol plugs the high efficiency particle filters of the existing facility in a fraction of that time. It would be unacceptable to directly vent these fumes into the crowded laboratory environment. We have found that coalescing filters are ideally suited for this application. The coalescing filters used in this work were supplied by the Balston Co., Lexington, MA. They consist of tubular arrays of thick fibrous filters. A

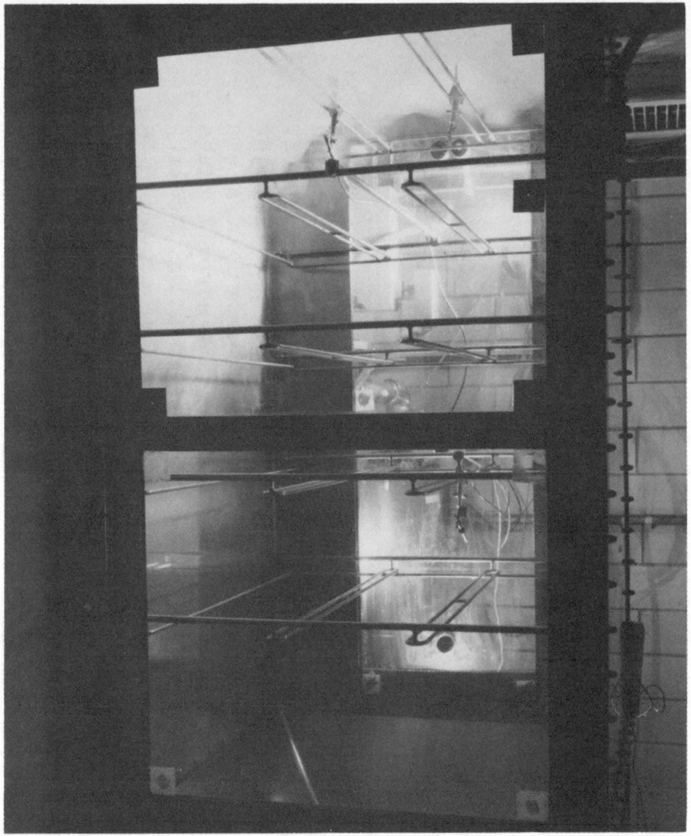

A

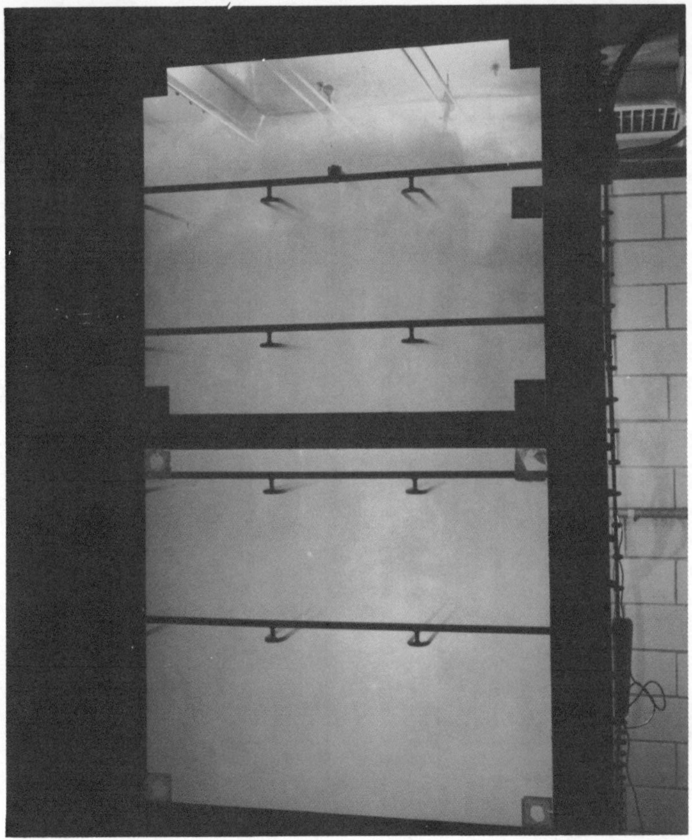

B

Figure 6. Aerosol-Air Boundries in Chamber With Screens.
A) Advancing front on startup of generator.
B) Retreating front as chamber empties.

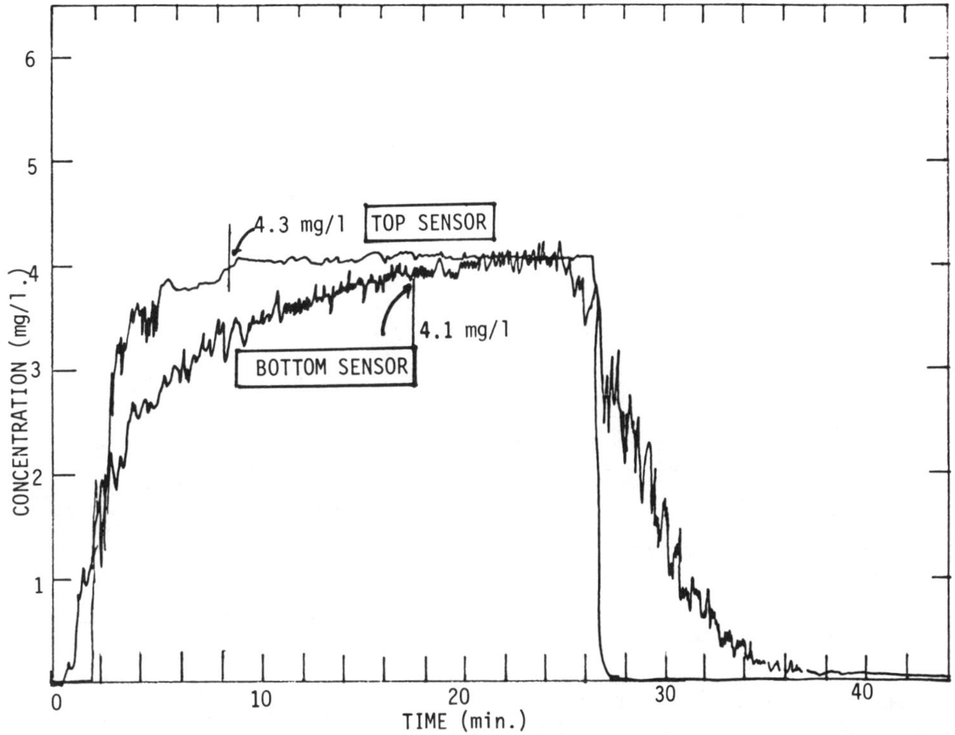

Figure 7. Two Channel Recording of Particle Concentration from Diesel Oil Aerosol in a Rochester Chamber.

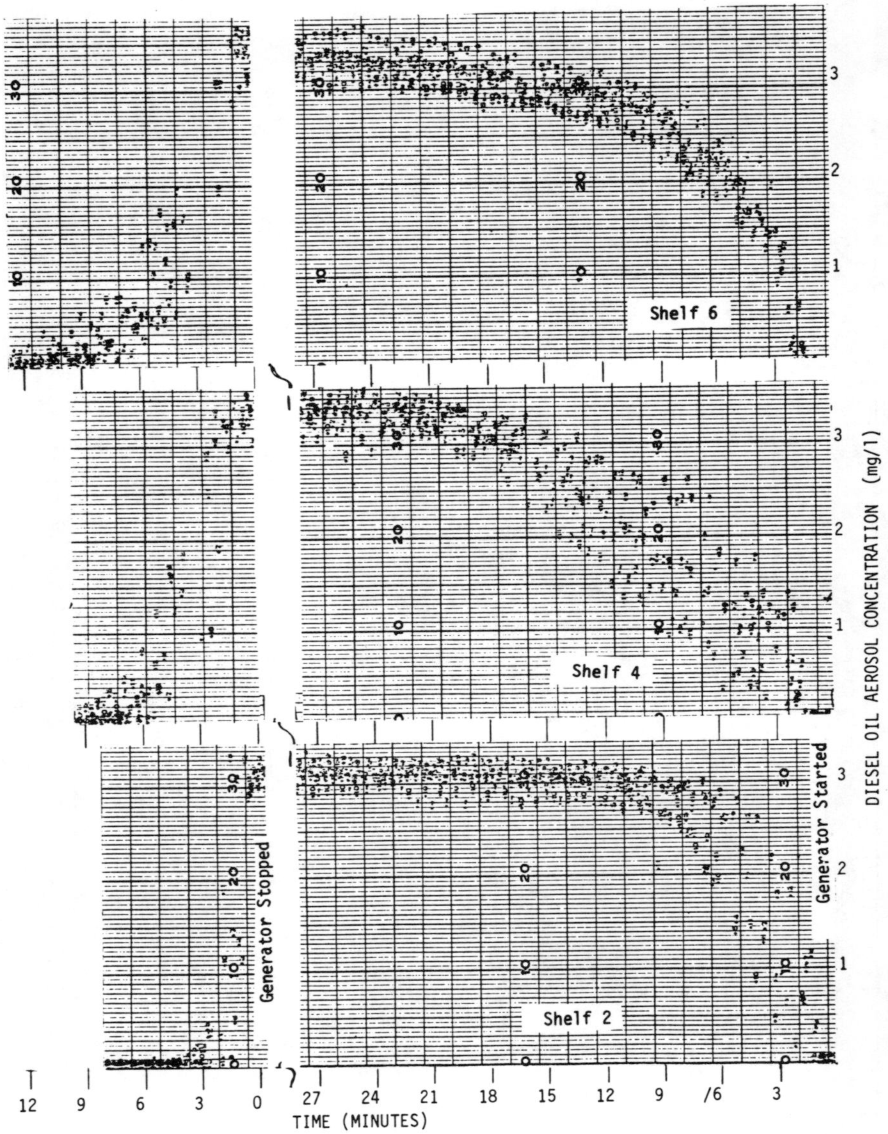

Figure 8. Multipoint Recordings from Six Particle Sensors Arrayed in Horizontal Plane at Three Exposure Shelf Levels.

liquid aerosol is injected into the inner annulus where it is removed from the stream and coalesces to bulk liquid which then flows to a reservoir for subsequent disposal. We have installed somewhat oversized arrays of these filters after each chamber to maintain an acceptable pressure drop. To date they have performed better than anticipated. They remove greater than 99.5% of the aerosol and have yet shown no deterioration with use.

Particle size distributions have been estimated using a Mercer/Lovelace cascade impactor (Mercer, 1962) operating at one liter per minute flow rate. Stage constants have been calculated from measured jet diameters using Stokes parameters determined by Marple (Marple, 1974). Direct weighing of the impactor stages was found to be unreliable. Consequently, we have used a computer assisted, low resolution gas chromatographic technique for estimating the amount of oil collected on each stage. The glass stage plates are immersed in carbon disulfide to dissolve the oil. An aliquot is injected into the GC, operated isothermally with a short column. The entire band of partially resolved hydrocarbon constituents is eluted in three minutes. The output signal of the GC is fed into an analog to digital converter. The resulting spectrum is displayed on a graphic terminal with sufficient resolution to separate the solvent peak from the oil band. The area under the oil band is integrated and quantitated by comparing this area with standardized solutions of the same oil type.

An example at one aerosol concentration plotted on logarithmic probability coordinates is shown in figure 9. Some growth in size occurs from top to bottom of the chamber. This growth at these high aerosol concentrations is consistant with that predicted from simple second order coagulation theory (Green, 1964). The size at the top tier of the chamber (figure 9) does not represent the "initial" size of the aerosol since it has had time to grow before reaching this point. In a separate experiment, sampling the flowing stream 30 cm below the generator, a mass median aerodynamic diameter of 0.4 μm was found.

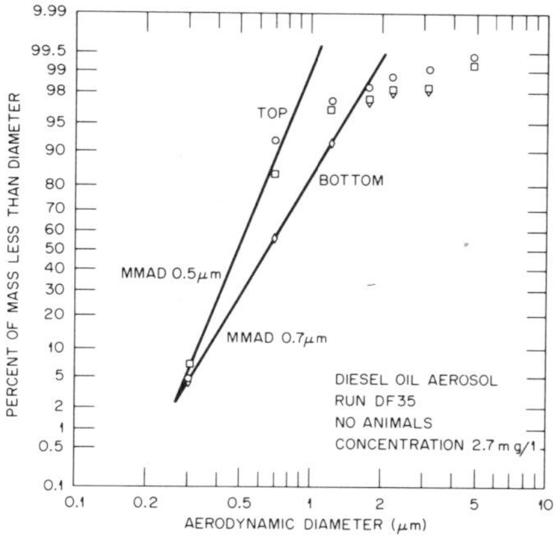

Figure 9. Particle Size as Determined by Cascade Impaction at Top and Bottom of Exposure Chamber.

ACKNOWLEDGEMENT

Research sponsored by the U.S. Department of Defense under Project Order No. 9600, DOE No. 40-1016-79, with the U.S. Department of Energy under contract W-7405-eng-26 with Union Carbide Corporation.

REFERENCES

Gayle, T. M., Higgins, C. E., and Stokely, J. R. (1979). A continuous smoke monitoring device for continuous animal exposure systems. In "Tobacco Smoke Inhalation Bioassay Chemsitry," Oak Ridge National Laboratory report ORNL-5424, p. 63.

Green, H. L. and Lane, W. R. (1964). Particulate Clouds: Dusts, Smokes, and Mists. D. Van Nostrand Co., Inc., Princeton, NJ, 1964, p. 138 ff.

Marple, V. A. and Liu, Y. H. (1974). Characteristics of Laminar Jet Impactors. Env. Sci. & Tech. 8, 1974, 648.

Mercer, T. T., Tillery, M. I., and Ballew, C. W. (1962). A cascade impactor operating at low volumetric flow rates. AEC Research and Development Report LF-5, December 1962. (The impactor used was manufactured by the Sandia Research and Development Co., 1712 Virginia N. E., Albuquerque, New Mexico, 87110.)

An Active Dispersion Inhalation Exposure Chamber

B.K.J. LEONG and D.J. POWELL
Industrial Toxicology and Inhalation Toxicology Laboratories

G.L. POCHYLA and M.G. LUMMIS
Mechanical Engineering

The Upjohn Company
Kalamazoo, Michigan 49001

ABSTRACT

A simple cubical animal exposure chamber was constructed with a wide angle positive pressure air nozzle in the air inlet at one upper corner and an air exhaust at the diagonally opposite lower corner of the chamber. Uniform distribution of aerosols to animals held in cages with excreta collection trays can be acheived when the cages are arranged in a single vertical tier at diagonal-right angle to the direction of the chamber air flow.

INTRODUCTION

Research in inhalation toxicology requires controlled atmospheres containing known concentrations of test contaminants in an exposure chamber for extended periods of time. Animal exposure chambers of various designs are, in general, comprised of an upright, rectangular, stainless steel and glass chamber with pyramidal top and bottom. In operation, air is drawn into the chamber via an air inlet at the top. The test contaminants are introduced into the air stream entering the chamber and are dispersed passively as the air expands under a slightly negative pressure. The chamber atmosphere is then exhausted via an outlet at the bottom of the chamber resulting in a vertical airflow pattern (Fraser et al, 1959; Leach et al, 1959; Hinners et al, 1968). Several disadvantages may be encountered in the operation of these conventional exposure chambers. For examples, the animal exposure cages have to be stacked in 2 or more layers to accommodate the large number of animals which are required per exposure level in a subchronic or chronic inhalation study. Such stacking may result in variation in aerosol concentration between layers due to the filtration of the descending chamber air by the fur of the animals. In addition, the animals at the lower layers are frequently "bombarded" by excreta expelled by animals from above, since excreta collection trays are generally not used. Should trays be used, the vertical airflow pattern would be further disrupted.

Recently, an exposure chamber has been designed to alleviate some of the aforementioned problems. This chamber has "off-center" pyramidal top and bottom, with the exposure cages together with excreta collection trays stacked in "zigzag" layers (Moss, 1979 and 1980). The "odd-shaped" chamber advantageously utilizes a baffle plate at the air entrance and the layers of the trays to create a turbulent vertical airflow pattern for even distribution of aerosols.

Another approach to solving the aerosol distribution and excreta problems can be achieved by using a horizontal airflow pattern. One such exposure chamber has been designed. It consist of four vertical modules which are utilized respectively for air filtration and diffusion, contaminant distribution, animal exposure and effluent collection (Ferin and Leach, 1980). In operation, the four modules are clamped together. Air is drawn through the filter-diffusion module to mix with the test materials in the distribution module. The contaminated atmosphere then flows horizontally across a vertical tier of animal cages to be exhausted via the effluent collection module.

These modified exposure chambers are costly to build and are somewhat difficult to operate. In view of the short comings of the conventional and the modified exposure chambers, there is a need for designing an exposure system which (1) is economical and easy to manufacture; (2) permits exposure of adequate numbers of animals in one tier with excreta collection trays; (3) permits uniform distribution of gaseous, liquid aerosol and dust contaminants; (4) permits the generation of test atmospheres <u>in situ</u> without imposing an inhalation hazard to the investigator; (5) permits the transfer of experimental animals from the exposure chamber to temporary housing unit without subjecting the animal handler to an inhalation hazard; and (6) has a built-in, easy-to-replace filtering system for decontaminating the exhausted air.

THE EXPOSURE SYSTEM

This exposure system has a single unit structure, comprised of a cubical exposure chamber, a test atmosphere generating compartment and an animal housing compartment.

The whole unit is supported on casters for portability purposes (Figure 1).

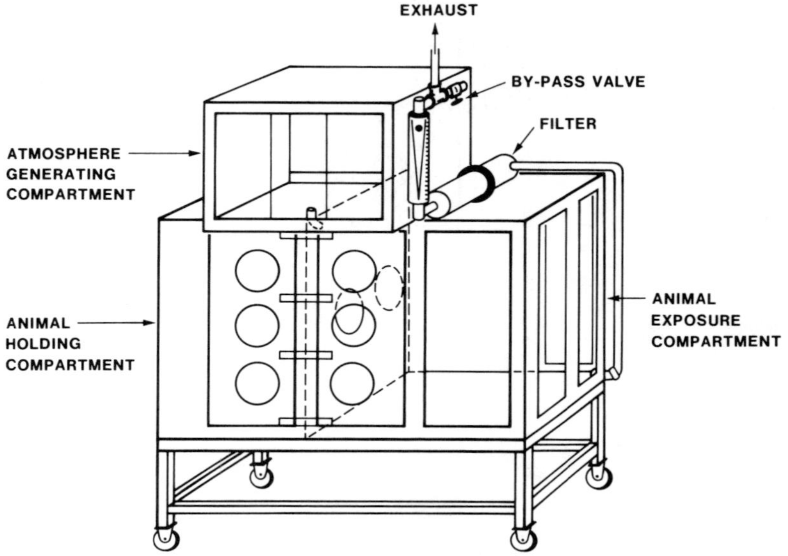

Figure 1. A single unit structured animal exposure system.

There are six unique features in this exposure system.

(1) The air inlet is located at one upper corner of the cubical chamber while the air exhaust is located at the diagonally opposite lower corner. Such an arrangement of air inlet and exhaust advantageously utilizes the three congruent sides of the upper and lower corners of the chamber for creating a laminar airflow pattern. This eliminates the extra work and expense in building the pyramidal top and bottom which are essential for a conventional vertical airflow pattern exposure chamber.

(2) For dispersing the test compound in the chamber atmosphere, a wide angle (72 degrees) positive pressure air nozzle is employed. The nozzle is located, in-line with the chamber air inlet and outlet, at the apex of the upper corner of the chamber (Figure 2). The test compound is metered to the tip of the spray nozzle from the atmosphere generating compartment above and is dispersed by a "cone" of compressed air. This "active" air dispersion method is far more effective than the "passive" dispersion and/or the use of a baffle plate in a conventional exposure chamber, as the baffle plate may retain a large quantity of aerosol particles via impaction. Such an approach has been found to be effective for chambers with dimensions ranging from 20 inches cubed to as large as six feet cubed.

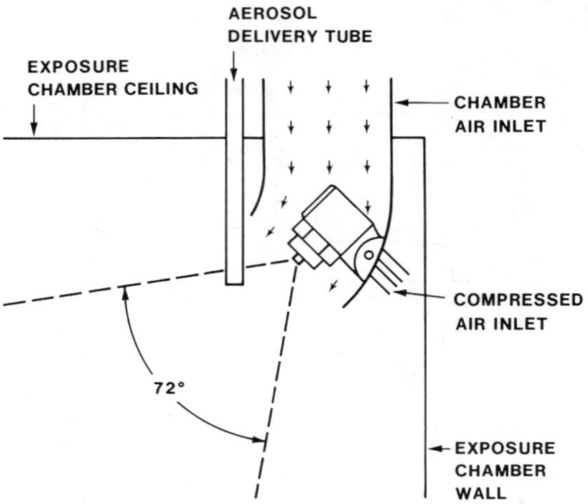

Figure 2. Close-up view of the air spray nozzle assembly.

(3) The animal exposure cages, with built-in excreta collection trays, are situated as one vertical tier at a diagonal-right angle to the direction of the airflow. With such an airflow pattern, the animals held in different locations can be uniformly exposed to the air contaminants with little or no disturbance of the airflow pattern by the excreta trays (Figures 3a and 3b).

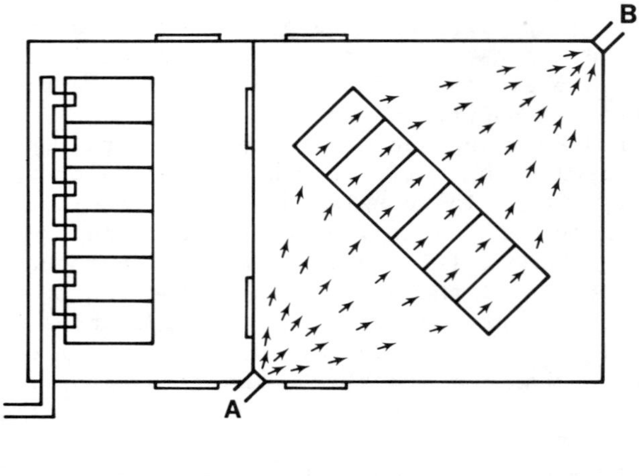

Figure 3a. Top view of animal exposure and holding compartments, and the location of animal exposure cage

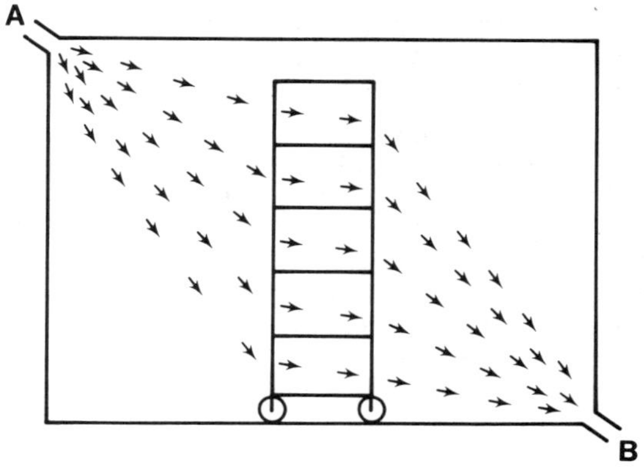

Figure 3b. Side view of exposure chamber on plane A to B, and the location of the exposure cages.

(4) The exposed and contaminated animals can be transferred via a sealable port-hole from the exposure chamber to the animal holding compartment without subjecting the animal handler to an exposure hazard. After the animals are transferred and the port-holes are closed, the exposure chamber can be hosed-down and decontaminated without affecting the animals in the adjacent holding compartment (Figure 4).

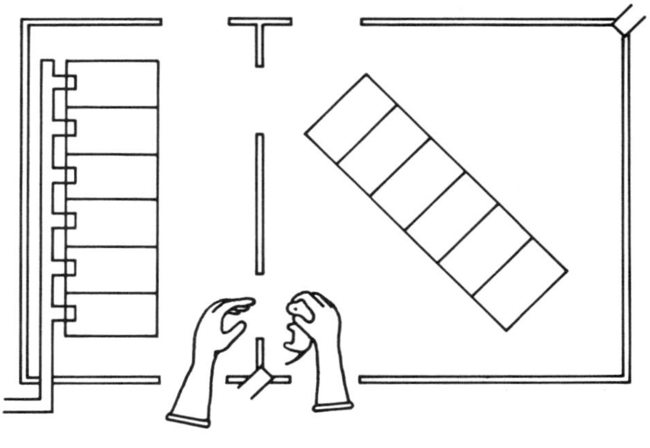

Figure 4. Top view of exposure system and the port-holes for animal transfer.

(5) The atmosphere generating compartment is located advantageously on the flat top of the cubical exposure chamber. This compartment also utilizes the existing chamber air exhaust pump to create a slight negative pressure for preventing possible escape of test materials from its enclosure.

(6) This exposure system has a built-in filter system for decontaminating the test atmosphere exhausted from the chamber. The filter holder permits insertion of a six-inch layer of fiber-glass wool, a commercially available foam filter, a high efficiency particulate air filter (HEPA), and a six-inch layer of activated charcoal in succession. All the filters can be exchanged easily and the duct works can be uncoupled easily for routine maintenance.

OPERATION AND TESTING CONDITIONS

For testing the homogeneity of distribution of dust in such an exposure system, a 150 liter chamber was used. In testing, a constant chamber airflow of 28.3 to 113.2 liters per minute (l/min) was maintained by means of a rotary air vacuum pump located at the exhaust side of the chamber. The rate of total chamber airflow was equal to the sum of (a) air ejected from a dust generator at an average rate of approximately six l/min, (b) air ejected from a positive pressure air spray nozzle (disperser) at the rate of 16 l/min and (c) make-up air at a balancing rate.

Inside the chamber, the animal cage rack was placed at a diagonal-right angle facing the incoming dust laden air.

In determining the distribution of dusts by sedimentation and/or impaction in cages at different locations in the rack, pre-weighed, vasoline coated, filter papers were placed on the floor of the front and rear of each of the 12 cages in the rack. A dust atmosphere of Diatomaceous Earth (DE) having mean optical diameter of three micrometers (3μm), was generated by metering the powder at a constant rate using The Upjohn Dust Generator (Leong et al, this symposium volume). The powder was dispersed by the air from the nozzle to the cages. The filter papers were exposed for one hour and the (DE) deposited on each filter paper was gravimetrically determined (Table 1).

Table 1. Horizontal profile of distribution of (DE) dust in the exposure chamber operated under various airflow conditions.

Experiment Number	Chamber Airflow (l/min)	Nominal Concentration (mg/l)	X ± SD of Sample Weight (mg) Mean Horizontal Profiles Front (F)	Rear (R)	% Variation F vs R
1	28.3	3.37	4.7 ± 0.7[a]	4.4 ± 0.9[a]	6.3
2	28.3	5.07	7.0 ± 1.3	6.9 ± 1.1	1.4
3	56.6	1.71	4.4 ± 0.9	3.6 ± 0.6	18.2
4	56.6	2.21	5.7 ± 0.8	4.7 ± 0.7	17.5
5	84.9	1.23	5.2 ± 0.8	3.7 ± 0.4	28.8
6	84.9	1.51	8.2 ± 4.1	4.8 ± 1.2	41.5
7	113.2	0.99	6.1 ± 3.5	5.3 ± 3.1	13.1
8	113.2	1.00	6.7 ± 4.1	5.9 ± 4.1	11.9

[a] Each entry represents the mean of 12 samples

HORIZONTAL DEPOSITION PROFILE

For determining the horizontal profile of dust deposition, the mean weights for the 12 samples in the front and the 12 samples at the rear of the cages were calculated. The data suggested a biphasic pattern of dust distribution, depending on the rate of the chamber airflow. Indeed, at a relatively low rate of 28.3 l/min. (approximately 18% of the chamber volume), the dust appeared to deposit evenly throughout a cage. As the rate increased from 28.3 to 56.6 and then to 84.9 l/min., the dust appeared to "impact" more heavily on the front than on the rear portion of each cage. With further increase of the rate to 113.2 l/min., the dust initially impacted on the front portion began to be dislodged, and then resettled to the rear portion of the cage or was redispersed by the relatively strong airflow.

VERTICLE DEPOSITION PROFILE

In order to evaluate the verticle profile of dust distribution, the ratios between the weight of (DE) retained on each of the 24 locations (12 front and 12 rear samples) relative to the mean weight were calculated (Table 2). Each experiment was duplicated.

The verticle distribution profile showed deviations of 12.1, 10.1, 24.0 and 48.5% for the four respective chamber airflows from 28.3 to 113.2 l/min. Again, the dust distribution appeared to be more homogeneous at the lower than at the higher airflow rates. It appeared that the "cone" of air ejected from the air nozzle was not affected by the "circumscribing" make-up air and was effectively dispersing the (DE) to all cages. However, at higher chamber airflows, the flow rates of the make-up air greatly increased while the nozzle ejection rate remained constant. The "cone" of air ejected from the nozzle was apparently "collapsed" or "narrowed down" by the "circumscribing" make-up air. Consequently, the dust was more heavily distributed in the central than in the peripheral cages.

The results of the distribution profile studies thus suggested that the optimal chamber airflow for even distribution of dust in a cubical chamber appears to be 18-36% of the chamber volume per minute rather than "the higher the airflow, the better will be the distribution" as it has been believed.

Table 2. Verticle profile of distribution of (DE) dust in the exposure chamber operated under various airflow conditions.

Verticle Profile (Front & Rear)				Chamber Airflow (l/min)	Mean & SD of Equalized Weight*	Percent Variation
0.9*	1.1	1.1	1.1			
1.0	0.9	0.9	1.1	28.3	0.99 ± 0.12	12.1
0.9	0.8	0.9	1.2			
0.9	1.0	1.1	0.9			
1.0	0.9	1.0	1.1	56.6	0.99 ± 0.10	10.1
1.0	0.9	0.9	1.2			
0.8	1.0	1.0	0.7			
1.1	1.4	1.4	1.2	84.9	1.00 ± 0.24	24.0
0.8	0.8	0.8	1.0			
0.7	1.4	1.0	0.6			
0.8	1.3	2.2	1.2	113.2	0.99 ± 0.48	48.5
0.5	0.6	0.7	0.9			

*Equalized Weight: Average weight of front and rear samples in each cage divided by the mean of the averages of the 12 cages.

AIRBORNE DUST CONCENTRATION

In evaluating the homogeneity of distribution of the airborne (DE) particles in the chamber atmosphere, air samples were taken simultaneously at five locations (center and four corner cages) of the cage rack. Open-faced samplers with Millipore® filters were used and the sampling rate was 1.5 l/min. The duration of sampling was one minute. The quantity of (DE) trapped in each filter was weighed. The mean and standard deviation were calculated. The data in Table 3 showed that the average percent of the dispersed (DE) remaining airborne was 48.5, 37.5, 53.6, and 60.4% for chamber airflows of 28.3, 56.6. 84.9 and 113.2 l/min., respectively. This data seems to support the observation that some of the deposited dusts were redispersed at the highest chamber airflow. The distribution pattern at equilibration had average deviations of 12.1, 10.9, 17.9 and 10.0% for the four respective chamber airflows. It appeared that the rate of airflow did not greatly affect the distribution of the airborne particles in the chamber atmosphere.

CONCLUSIONS

A cubical animal exposure chamber with unconventional design of air-inlet with an air nozzle together with a diagonally opposite located air exhaust can provide even distribution of dusts to animal exposure cages with built-in excreta collection trays. The cages are arranged in a single verticle tier in a cage rack. The rack is situated at a right angle to the chamber airflow. Such an arrangement of cages also permits more animals to be exposed as a single layer per unit exposure surface. This type of cubical chamber is relatively compact and easy to construct and install in a laboratory with a regular ceiling height. The flat chamber top permits placement of contaminant generating equipment in an easily reachable enclosure.

Provision is also made for transferring contaminated animals to a built-in animal holding compartment without imposing an exposure hazard to the animal handler.

Other safety features include an easy-to replace filtering system which is an integral part of this unit-structured, portable exposure system.

Table 3. Concentration of Diatomaceous Earth in Air Samples Obtained at 5 Locations of the Exposure Cage Rack in the Chamber Operated Under Various Airflow Conditions

Experiment Number	Chamber Airflow (1/min)	Dust Nominal Concentration (mg/1)	X ± SD Analytical Concentration[a] (mg/1)	Percent Deviation[b]	Percent Recovery[c]
1	28.3	0.49	0.36 ± 0.04	11.1	73.5
2	28.3	2.40	0.64 ± 0.10	15.6	26.7
3	28.3	2.92	1.35 ± 0.13	9.6	46.2
4	56.6	1.75	0.67 ± 0.08	11.9	38.3
5	56.6	2.27	0.80 ± 0.05	6.3	35.2
6	56.6	2.27	0.89 ± 0.13	14.6	39.2
7	84.9	1.33	0.73 ± 0.13	17.0	54.9
8	84.9	1.36	0.57 ± 0.13	22.8	41.9
9	84.9	1.36	0.87 ± 0.12	13.8	63.9
10	113.2	1.00	0.65 ± 0.09	13.8	65.0
11	113.2	1.04	0.65 ± 0.06	9.2	62.5
12	113.2	1.06	0.57 ± 0.04	7.0	53.8

[a]Each entry represents the mean of 5 samples.

[b](Standard deviation/mean) x 100

[c](Analytical concentration/nominal concentration) x 100

REFERENCES

Ferin, J., and Leach, L. J. (1980) Horizontal airflow inhalation exposure chamber. In: Generation of aerosols and facilities for exposure experiments. K. Willike, Ed., Ann Arbor, Science Publishers Inc., pp. 517-523.

Fraser, D. A., Bales, A. E., Lippman, M. and Stockinger, H. (1959) Exposure chambers for Research in Animal Inhalation. Public Health Monograph No. 57, U.S. Government Printing Office.

Leach, L. J., Spiegl, C. J., Wilson, R. H., Sylvester, G. E. and Lauterbach, K. E. (1959) A Multiple Chamber Exposure Unit Designed for Chronic Inhalation Studies. Amer. Ind. Hyg. Assoc. J. 20, 13-22.

Hinners, R. G., Burkhart, J. K. and Punte, C. L. (1968) Animal Inhalation Exposure Chambers. Arch. Environ. Health 16, 194-206.

Moss, O. R. (1979) U. S. Patent No. 4,216,741.

Moss, O. R. (In Press) Can We Design Chambers for Uniform Exposure to Particulates on Several Tiers with Catch-pans? In: Inhalation Chamber Technology. R. T. Drew, Ed. Brookhaven National Laboratory Report.

Novel Chambers for Long Term Inhalation Studies

J.E. DOE and D.J. TINSTON
Inhalation Toxicity Section
Imperial Chemical Industries Limited
Central Toxicology Laboratory
Alderley Park
Macclesfield, Cheshire, UK

ABSTRACT

A long term inhalation toxicity unit has been commissioned containing 26 chambers of a novel design incorporating several labour saving features and other measures designed to ensure even atmosphere distribution. The animals are housed within wire mesh cages hung at six equidistant points around a wheel and the whole of this structure rotates within the chamber. Atmospheres with the desired level of contaminant are drawn in from the top of the chamber at the front and flow around the entire chamber in a cyclonic pattern, concurrent with the rotation of the cages, before exhaust at the top rear. This pattern of cage rotation and air flow ensures uniformity of animal exposure. There is a self cleaning facility for the trays suspended beneath the cages for the collection of animal waste. The animals are retained within the chamber for the duration of the experiment which minimises the risks of cross contamination between groups, cross infection and operator contamination. Distribution of both heavy and light vapours within the chambers is uniform to within 5% throughout the chambers. The chambers may also be used for particulates when the rotation of the cages avoids the shadowing effect of cages at more than one level and minimises the effect of stratification of the particles. The chambers provide a versatile longer term inhalation toxicity facility.

INTRODUCTION

During the design of a new inhalation toxicity facility at ICI Ltd's Central Toxicology Laboratory, the performance criteria for the inhalation chambers were discussed at great length. The following factors emerged as being important for the planning of a long term inhalation facility with as many chambers as possible within the given floor area:

1. The chambers should provide uniform, stable and quantifiable exposure of the test material to the test animals regardless of whether the test material is present as a gas, vapour, aerosol or dust.

2. The chambers should operate with the minimum man-power requirements for both atmosphere analysis/generation and animal husbandry.

3. The animals contained within the chamber should be easily observed during exposure.

4. The animals should remain within the chambers continuously in order to:
   minimise the risk of infection,
   reduce animal housing space,
   reduce the labour requirements for moving animals,
   avoid contamination of the laboratory by the test material during exposure and from the animals after exposure.

5. Simple provision of services to the chamber.

The chamber described in this paper was designed to meet these criteria.

DESCRIPTION OF THE CHAMBER

The chambers were designed in consultation with and manufactured by E Gowrie Ltd, Edwin Road, Phillips Park Road, Manchester, M11 3ER under US Patent No: 4201154, patents applied for in other countries. Their general conformation is shown in Figure 1 and they were described previously by those responsible for their development (Carney, 1979; Carney and Gowrie, 1980).

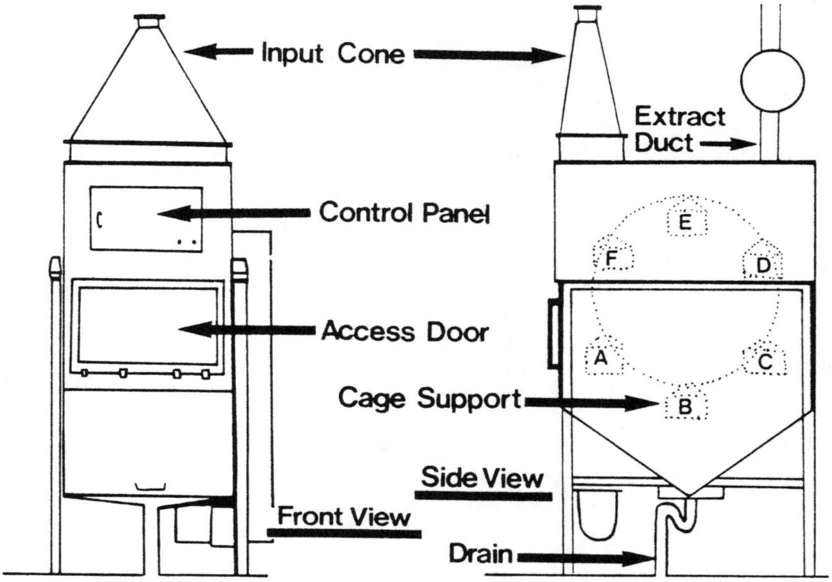

Figure 1. General Conformation of Exposure Chamber

The chambers are made from stainless steel and the test animals (rats, mice or hamsters) are housed in cages hung at six equidistant points around a wheel. The wheel rotates at 0.5 revolutions/min within the chamber. Atmospheres with the desired level of contaminant are drawn in via the distribution cone at the top front and flow around the entire chamber in a cyclonic pattern, concurrent with the rotation of the cages, before exhaust at the top rear, the whole chamber operating under negative pressure. The chambers are supplied with air conditioned to 22°C and 50% RH. Access to the animals is via a glass door at the front of the chamber. There are trays beneath the animal cages to collect animal waste, and these are scraped clean once a cycle by a scraper mechanism. There is also a flushing facility, governed by a time switch, which can be used to wash down both the trays and the bottom of the chamber for a pre-determined period in order to flush the waste to the drain. The internal illumination of the chamber is controlled independently of the external illumination, and can provide a reversed day cycle if considered necessary. Food and water are normally withdrawn during exposure periods and replaced at the end of each exposure. The internal volume of the chamber is 3.4 m^3, which provides capacity for 72 rats or 144 mice. The chamber air flow rates can be regulated from 300-1,000 l/min depending on duration of exposure and supply of test compound.

PERFORMANCE TESTS AND DISCUSSION

This chamber design has allowed most of our performance criteria to be met, as listed below:

1. <u>Uniform, stable atmospheres with gases, vapours and dusts</u>

This is probably the most important criterion of chamber design. The most ergonomically efficient chamber is of little use if the animals are not exposed to uniform, controlled atmospheres. The chamber was designed to allow both good distribution and the functional advantages described in the following sections. The rotating cage design fulfils two purposes which facilitate equal exposure of all the animals. Firstly, the cyclonic paddle-wheel movement of the cages and trays assists the air to flow through the chamber and avoid dead areas. Secondly, each cage receives the same integrated dose of contaminant should the distribution be uneven throughout the chamber. The run-up times, the distribution and the run-down times for gases and aerosols have been examined and the results are shown below:

The first material examined was a halocarbon, molecular weight 86.5, boiling point -41°C. Nineteen sample points were drilled into a chamber in the positions shown in Figure 2.

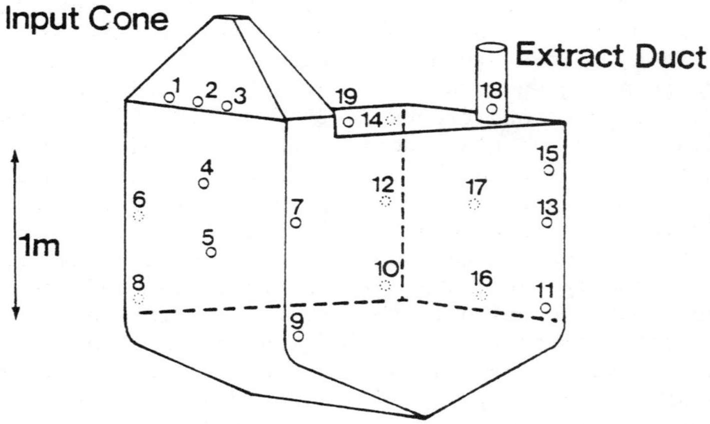

Figure 2. Distribution of Sampling Points.

The build-up and run-down of the halocarbon concentration, as measured in the extract duct (point 18) are shown in Figure 3. The t90, t95 and t99 were determined and were found to be very close to the ideal mixing situation, as described by Silver (1946), in the equation:

$$tx = K \frac{a}{b}$$

tx = time to reach x% of input concentration
K = relevant constant
a = chamber volume
b = input flow rate

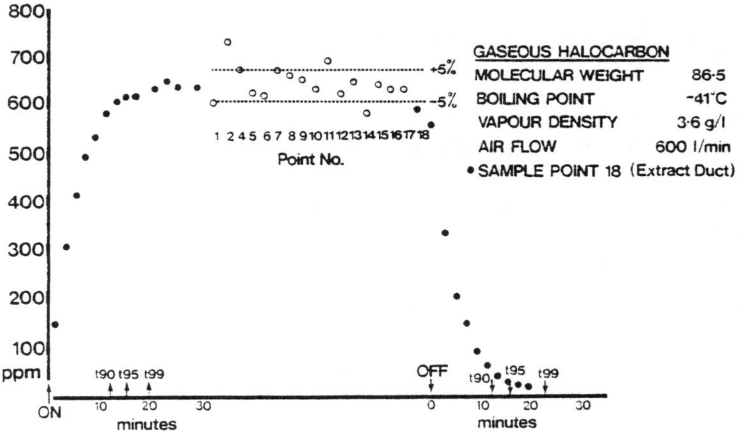

Figure 3. Run-up and run-down as measured at extract duct (point 18) and simultaneous samples at other points with light halocarbon.

The values were similar for both run-up and run-down. Once equilibrium had been reached simultaneous samples were taken from points 1-18. The concentrations at these points were all within ±5% of the nominal equilibrium concentration, except for four points which were within ±10%.

The run-up and run-down concentrations were measured with the same material at a sample point in the middle of the rear of the chamber (point 17). The results are shown in Figure 4.

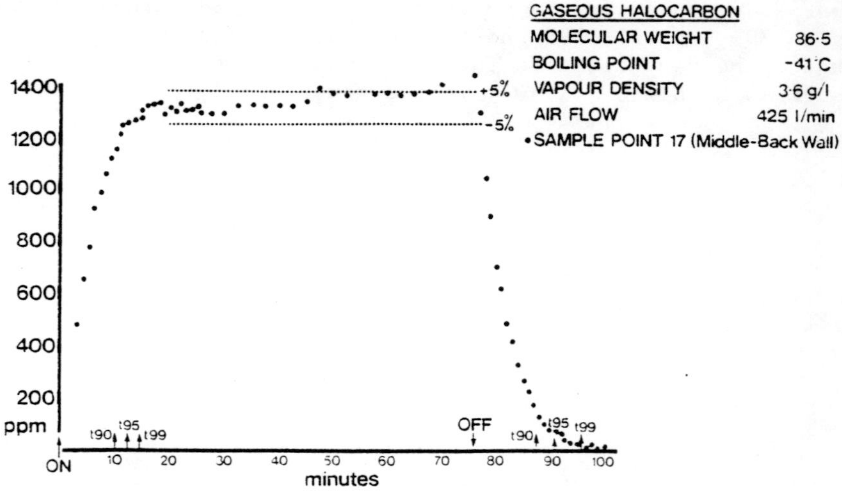

Figure 4. Run-up and run-down at middle of rear of the chamber (point 17) - light halocarbon gas.

The tx values are shown in Table 1 and indicate that for this relatively light gas the chamber behaves in an almost ideal manner.

TABLE 1

GASEOUS HALOCARBON

MOLECULAR WEIGHT 86.5 - BOILING POINT - -41°C - VAPOUR DENSITY 3.6 g/l

Sample Point	Number	Chamber Air Flow	Equilibrium Concentration (ppm)	Run-up Times (minutes)			Run-down Times (minutes)		
				t90	t95	t99	t90	t95	t99
Extract duct	18	600 l/min	635	12 (13)	15 (17)	19.5 (26)	12	15.5	22.5
Middle-back	17	425 l/min	1300	10 (18)	12 (24)	14 (37)	11	15	30

Times in parentheses are calculated values based on perfect mixing.

Since the input and extract ducts are both at the top of the chamber, distribution problems might arise when using a gas of high vapour density. The behaviour of a halocarbon of molecular weight 165.4, boiling point -4°C, vapour density 6.9 g/l, was examined to explore this situation. The run-up and run-down concentrations as measured at the middle of the rear of the chamber (point 17), and the distribution after equilibration are shown in Figure 5.

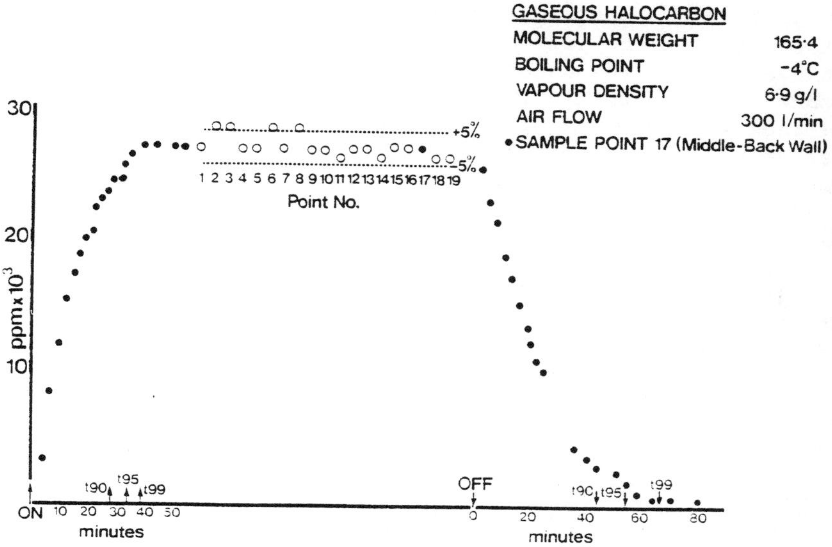

Figure 5. The run-up and run-down at middle of rear of chamber (point 17) with dense halocarbon.

The tx times were faster than ideal for run-up and slower than ideal for the run-down. This indicates non-uniform distribution with some layering of the gas during run-up to and run-down from equilibrium. However, the distribution throughout the chamber at equilibrium was good, with all points within ±5% of the nominal equilibrium concentration. Table 2 shows the tx for two different flow rates and

TABLE 2

GASEOUS HALOCARBON

MOLECULAR WEIGHT 165.4 - BOILING POINT - -4°C - VAPOUR DENSITY 6.9 g/l

Sample Point	Number	Chamber Air Flow	Equilibrium Concentration (ppm)	Run-up Times (minutes)			Run-down Times (minutes)		
				t90	t95	t99	t90	t95	t99
Top-front	2	600 l/min	1910	13.5 (13)	17 (17)	21 (26)	12	20	27
Bottom corner-back	11	300 l/min	29750	36 (26)	41 (34)	53 (52)	87	98	110
Middle-back	17	300 l/min	26750	28 (26)	33 (34)	37 (52)	45	55	66
Extract duct	18	300 l/min	26750	25 (26)	28 (34)	33 (52)	45	77	95
Bottom corner-side	8	300 l/min	30500	33 (26)	38 (34)	?	124	?	?
Middle-port	5	300 l/min	29750	24 (26)	27 (34)	31 (52)	64	69	84

Times in parentheses are calculated values based on perfect mixing.

several points. These data indicate some delayed clearance of the gas from the bottom of the chamber. This problem has been overcome by the use of an air jet at the bottom of the chamber during purging of the gas. These experiments indicate that the chamber is satisfactory for use with both relatively dense and light gases at the relatively low air flow rates (300 l/min) which were used. Low air flow rates minimise the amount of test material to be generated, an important consideration with expensive development compounds.

Similar studies have been undertaken using an aerosol generated from sodium chloride solutions. Particle size distribution data are shown in Figure 6, which shows most particles to be within the respirable range. These determinations were made by a Quartz Crystal Microbalance (C1000A) ten stage cascade impactor, and sampling was from the front of the chamber (point 5).

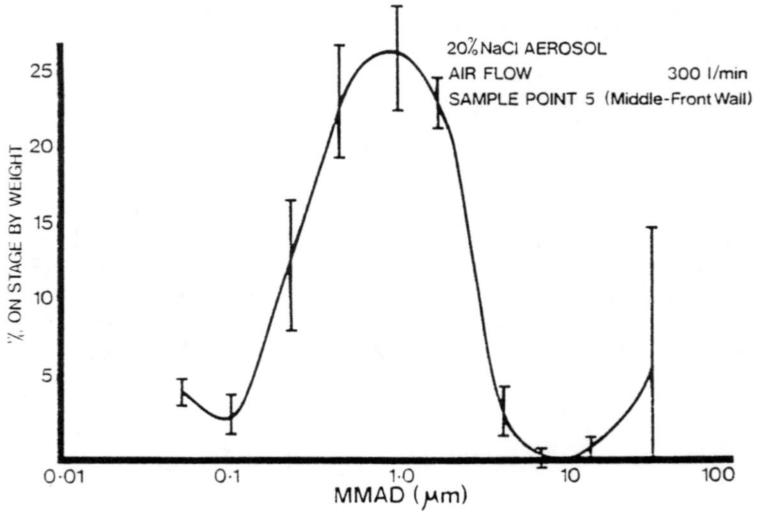

Figure 6. Particle size distribution of aerosol.

The characteristics of the run-up and run-down of the aerosol concentration were determined using a particle size elutriator (SIMSLIN) placed within one of the cages. This instrument measures the mass of respirable (<7μm) particles in the atmosphere. It has a solid state memory which can be interrogated so that the data can be displayed in analogue form. Figure 7 shows the run-up, steady state and run-down at two flow rates. It is possible to determine slight variations (<5%) in concentration during run-up and run-down which are probably due to the rotation of the cage containing the SIMSLIN through different concentrations. However once equilibrium had been reached there was little or no variation. The tx's during run-up were shorter than during run-down, but both sets of values are acceptable.

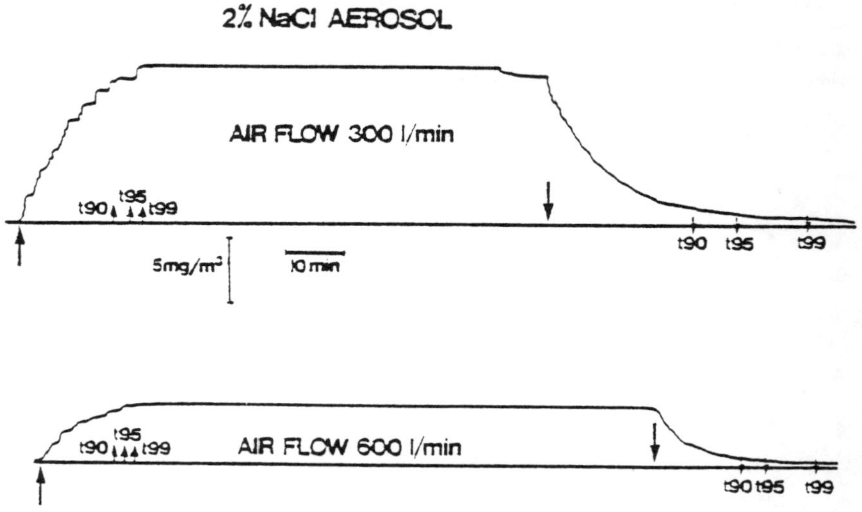

Figure 7. Run-up and run-down at two flow rates, measured inside cage with SIMSLIN with NaCl aerosol.

Figure 8 shows an experiment with two flow rates, which indicates that concentration was proportional to flow rate. During equilibrium the cage containing the SIMSLIN was stopped at each of the positions A-F to enable the concentration at each position to be recorded. It will be noted that the concentrations were within 5% of each other even though the cages were not rotating. The tx's using two different air flow rates and two concentrations of sodium chloride are shown in Table 3. These results indicate that the chamber is suitable for use with a particulate test material.

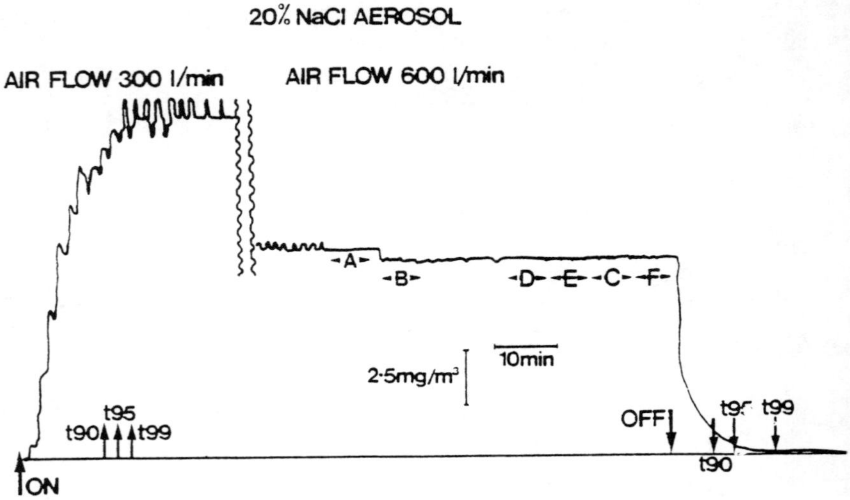

Figure 8. Aerosol concentrations at two flow rates, cage containing SIMSLIN stopped at six positions.

TABLE 3
SODIUM CHLORIDE AEROSOL

Nebuliser Solution	Aerosol Concentration mg/m³	Chamber Air Flow	Run-up Times (minutes)			Run-down Times (minutes)		
			t90	t95	t99	t90	t95	t99
20% NaCl	10.75	600 l/min	10 (13)	13 (17)	16 (26)	12.5	16	22.5
20% NaCl	16.25	300 l/min	16 (26)	17 (34)	22 (52)	22.5	31	43
2% NaCl	5.00	600 l/min	12 (13)	13 (17)	14.5 (26)	13	17	25
2% NaCl	13.00	300 l/min	15 (26)	18 (34)	19 (52)	31	38	49

Times in parentheses are calculated values based on perfect mixing.

2. Minimised Manpower Requirements

Generation and analysis: The top of each chamber and the inlet ducting are contained within a vented cupboard, operating at negative pressure, inside which the appropriate generation apparatus is placed. This cupboard is easily reached by a raised walkway at the rear of the chambers. This arrangement allows the generation equipment to be adjusted easily and safely if required.

The analysis of the test atmosphere can be achieved via sampling ports. These can be connected to a centralised gas chromatograph by sampling lines for analysis if appropriate. The use of a microprocessor controlled multiport sampler allows the atmospheres to be sampled and analysed automatically. This arrangement allows the minimum of time to be spent on analysis and processing results.

Animal Husbandry: The self cleaning mechanism of the cage trays and chamber reduces the necessary animal husbandry time. Animal husbandry time can thus be concentrated on observation of the state of health of the animals. Each pair of cages can be rotated to the front door and can be easily reached by animal attendants.

3 and 4. Observation of the Animals and Retention of the Animals

The arrangement discussed above allows for the easy observation of all the animals in the chamber, as each cage comes to the front window once every two minutes. This is a major advantage over conventional chambers, where animals caged at the back of the chamber may not be observed easily. The self-cleaning arrangement of the cage trays allows the animals to be housed within the chamber continuously, with the consequent advantages as described in the design criteria.

5. Simple provision of services to the chamber

There are three major services to the chamber: electrical power for light and rotation of the cages, water and drains for cleaning, and a conditioned air supply. In order to avoid complex plumbing the water is supplied and removed from the base of the chamber. The air is supplied to and extracted from the chamber via a main supply duct and a common extract duct which run along and above the chambers. Electricity supply is more easily ducted and is provided by spurs from a ring main from above each chamber.

CONCLUSION

The new chamber has been shown to fulfil its design criteria, as defined in the Introduction. The chambers present significant reductions in the manpower required to operate them, when compared with other conventional chambers, they enable better observation of the animals and they are suitable for use with both gases and particulates.

ACKNOWLEDGEMENTS

It is a pleasure to thank Mr I P Bennett, Mr S Millward, Mr R A Riley and Mr D Woodcock for their expertise in performing the distribution and dynamic studies on the chambers.

REFERENCES

Carney I F, (1979). Biological Problems in Defining Hygiene Standards for Particulates. Ann Occup Hyg 22, 163-173.

Carney I F and Gowrie E, (1980). A new exposure chamber for long-term inhalation studies. Tox appl Pharmac 52, A40.

Silver S D, (1946). Constant flow gassing chambers: Principles influencing design and operation. J Lab Clin med 31, 1153-1161.

A Method for Chronic Nose-Only Exposures of Laboratory Animals to Inhaled Fibrous Aerosols*

DAVID M. SMITH, LAWRENCE W. ORTIZ, RUBEN F. ARCHULETA, JOHN F. SPALDING, MARVIN I. TILLERY, HARRY J. ETTINGER, and ROBERT G. THOMAS
Toxicology Group
Life Sciences Division and Industrial Hygiene Group
Health Division
University of California
Los Alamos National Laboratory
Los Alamos, NM, 87545 USA

ABSTRACT

A study is being conducted at our laboratory to determine any biological effects when rats and hamsters inhale man-made mineral fibers (MMMFs). MMMF's to be tested include glass fibers, mineral wool, and ceramic fibers, with crocidolite asbestos serving as a positive control aerosol material. A prime objective of this study is to expose animals to high airborne concentrations of long thin fibers ($\leq$ 3 μm diam x > 10 μm in length). Animal exposures are currently being conducted with a 0.45 μm mean diameter glass microfiber material and the standard UICC crocidolite. Aerosols are produced from bulk materials using a modified Timbrell type fibrous aerosol generator and a controlled density infusion plug packing procedure.

A specialized method of restraining rats and hamsters for inhalation exposure was also developed providing for aerosol exposure only to the nose and a small fraction of the animal's head. This method eliminates external contamination and prevents animals from burying their noses in their fur to filter out aerosolized particles. Stainless steel chambers have been modified by placing two metal insert panels in place of doors, each containing 45 insert ports for Syrian hamsters or 32 for rats. Animals are loaded into tapered polycarbonate holding tubes and the tubes placed in the panel inserts for exposure. Body weights, rectal temperatures, clinical chemistry profiles, complete blood counts, and plasma corticosterone levels clearly indicate that this technique does not produce measureable stress in the animals.

*Funded by the U.S. Thermal Insulation Manufacturer's Association (TIMA) and the U.S. Department of Energy (DOE).

INTRODUCTION

In our program to assess the potential long-term effects in laboratory animals of inhaled man-made mineral fibers, the whole-body exposure systems were not considered because, in our experience: 1) animals often pile-up together or hide their faces in their axillary spaces, using body hair as a filter, reducing the amount and quality of aerosol actually inhaled; 2) the aerosolized material is deposited cutaneously, resulting in increased gastro-intestinal tract deposition from grooming and the potential for personnel working with the animals to be exposed during handling; 3) some have large chamber volumes that require large amounts of aerosol to be generated; 4) some require many chambers to expose large numbers of animals; and 5) loading and unloading animals can cause undue trauma to the animals, including injury and even amputation of limbs.

Consequently, an inhalation exposure system was needed that would: 1) be able to expose relatively large numbers of Osborne-Mendel (O-M) rats and Syrian golden hamsters 6 hours a day, 5 days a week for periods up to 24 months; 2) minimize trauma and stress to animals; 3) minimize potential exposure to the aerosolized materials by personnel handling the animals; and 4) have small chamber volumes so that only minimal amounts of aerosol need be generated while the quality and distribution of the aerosol would be optimal.

Described in this presentation are an MMMF aerosol generation system and a method we developed for long-term nose-only exposure of laboratory rats and hamsters to fibrous aerosols.

METHODS

Inhalation Exposure Chamber and Animal Restraining Tubes

Chambers originally designed for whole-body inhalation exposures (Hinners _et al_, 1968) were purchased from Unifab Corp., Kalamazoo, MI. The two glass doors, internal shelving and cages were removed and two inserts placed into the openings created by removal of the doors. These inserts were made of 5 mm thick dural (6061-T6, Kaiser Aluminum Corp., Los Angeles, CA). The portions extending into the chambers (Figure 1) measured 33.5 cm high x 56.5 cm wide and 22.0 cm deep. Trilaminar plates consisting of 1/4 inch thick pieces of Silastic® (Dow Corning Corp., Midland, MI) laminated between two plates of 5 mm thick dural are held in place on the internally extended chamber inserts by 7 cm long suitcase hinges (Figure 1). These trilaminar plates contain multiple circular ports which hold the animal restraining tubes in place. The holes have a 5.2 cm diameter for the tubes used with rats and a 4.7 cm diameter for those used with hamsters. Thus, one plate and insert panel will hold either 32 rats or 45 hamsters. The trilaminar plates are held together by 1/8 inch-32 socket-head screws located between each tube port opening. They are tightened so that the Silastic® is forced slightly into the port openings, forming occlusive seals when the animal restraining tubes are in place. The Los Alamos National Laboratory Plastics Shop made the animal restraining tubes of polycarbonate by an extrusion process. Their dimensions are as follows:

RATS (used with female O-M and female and male Fischer-344's)
- Inside Diamter: 4.8 cm
- Thickness: 2.5 mm
- Length: 22.5 cm
- Nasal Orifice: 1.7 cm diameter
- Taper: 63° beginning 3.0 cm from nasal end

SYRIAN HAMSTERS
- Inside Diameter: 4.4 cm
- Thickness: 2.0 mm
- Length: 17.0 cm
- Nasal Orifice: 1.5 cm diameter
- Taper: 63° beginning 2.5 cm from nasal end

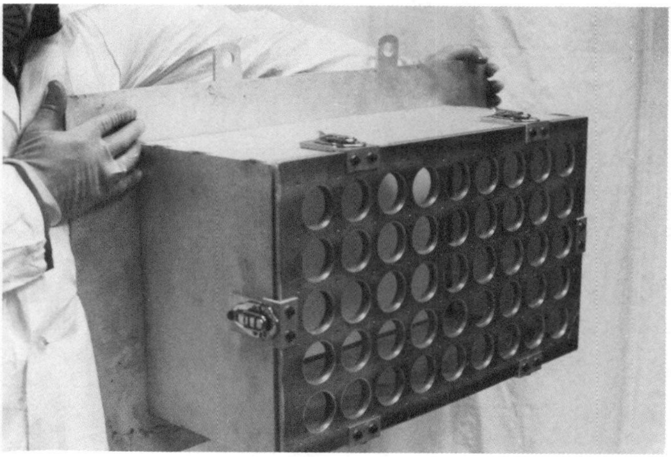

Figure 1. Chamber insert panel with plate containing 45 ports for polycarbonate hamster holding tubes.

To maintain hermetic integrity and prevent the aerosols from getting around the animals and leaking out into the room, a polyethylene cap with a centrally located 1.0 cm diameter hold, which allows the rats' tails to protroude, is used to cover the end of the tube. A seal is then obtained and the rat's tail supported by placing one of the hamster tubes whose tapered end has been left sealed in the cap, as demonstrated in Figure 2. Tubes used to contain the Syrian hamsters are sealed with polyethylene caps.

After each 6 hour exposure, the tubes and caps are washed thoroughly in a disinfectant detergent and rinsed.

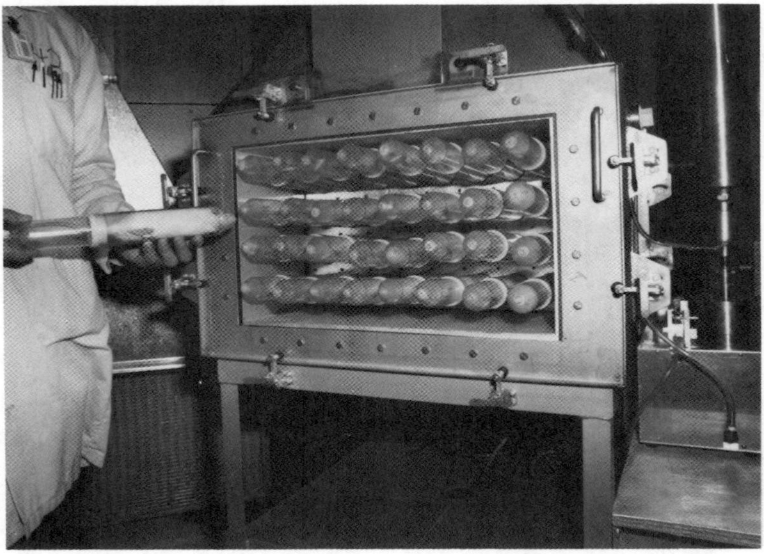

Figure 2. Insert panel in place in exposure chamber. The ports are filled with polycarbonate restraining tubes.

AEROSOL PRODUCTION

The device used to generate our fibrous aerosols is schematically illustrated in Figure 3. This generator, described in detail elsewhere (Ortiz _et al_, 1977) was modeled after one developed by Timbrell _et al_ (1968b). The operating principle of this device is based on the controlled feeding of a fixed density, fibrous plug compact, into a rotating blade assembly to produce the aerosol. Fibers are shaved from the end of the advancing plug by the blades and a stream of air exhausts the airborne fibers from the generator chamber.

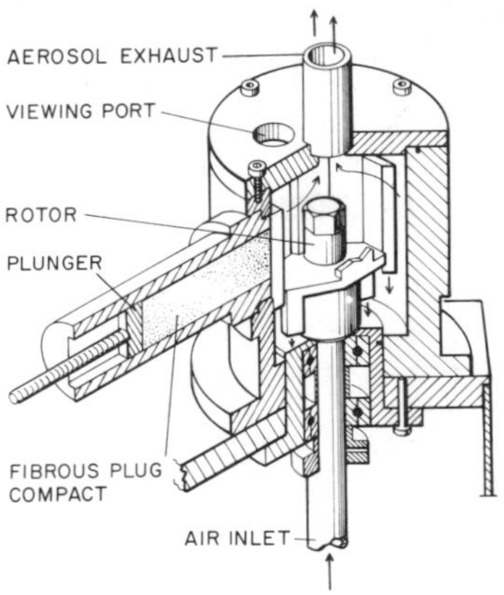

Figure 3. Schematic diagram of generator used to aerosolize fibrous materials. The plug compact is slowly advanced into the rotating blade assembly, shearing off fibers produced as an aerosol.

Figure 4 illustrates the aerosol generator exposure chamber hookup arrangement. The aerosol leaves the generator, travels through an intermediate dilution device where

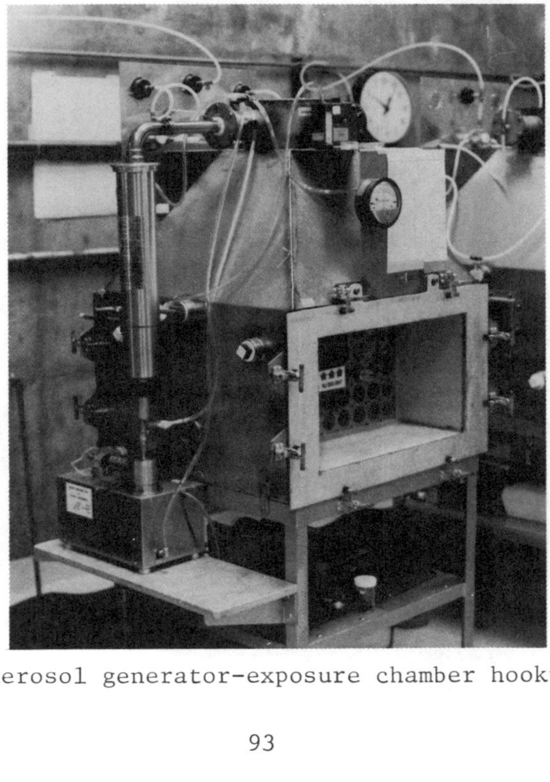

Figure 4. Aerosol generator-exposure chamber hookup.

additional clean air is mixed with the aerosol, then the diluted aerosol is passed through a 10 mCi Krypton 85 aerosol deionization source (Thermo Systems, St. Paul, MN) and into the top of the animal exposure chamber. Aerosol flow in the chamber is from top to bottom. Total airflow rate into the exposure chamber was ∿30 l/min (15 l/min primary aerosol carrier air and 15 l/min clean dilution air). Generator feed plug infusion rate was set at 20 μm/min with rotor speed fixed at ∿1000 RPM for these aerosol uniformity tests.

Figure 5 illustrates the sampling arrangement used for obtaining gravimetric filter samples. These samplers are 6.3 mm I.D. copper tubing probes, fitted with Gelman, 25 mm in-line filter holders (Gelman Instrument Co., Ann Arbor, MI), which have been adapted to shortened animal holding tubes for positive seal support (Figure 6). These adapted sampling probes are placed in vacant animal exposure ports for aerosol collection and are designed to simulate "breathing zone" samples of the rodents undergoing exposure. This aerosol monitoring arrangement also minimizes the possibility of human exposure to the aerosol as both collection filter and holder are located outside the exposure chamber.

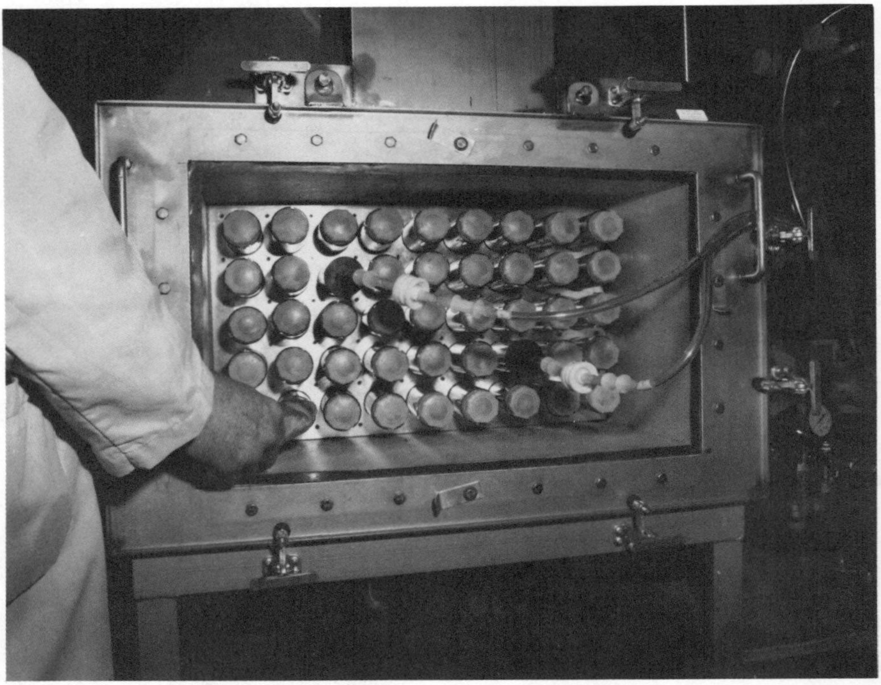

Figure 5. Two sampling probes in place in exposure chamber during sampling operation.

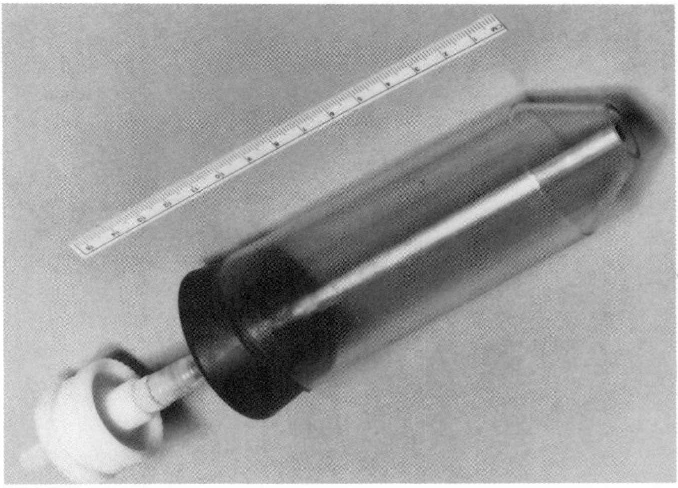

Figure 6. Polycarbonate restraining tube modified to form sampling probe.

Animal Experiments

Female O-M rats were obtained from Camm Research Laboratory Animals, Wayne, NJ, and male Syrian golden hamsters from Engle Laboratory Animals, Hammond, IN. All animals were housed in Class-100 laminar flow clean rooms (Hazleton Systems, Inc., Cornwell Heights, PA), two to a polycarbonate cage containing low-dust-factor aspen shavings. The cages were suspended on aluminum shelves and covered with spun polyester filters (DuPont #22 Spinbonded Polyester Filter, E. I. DuPont Co., Wilmington, DE). Cages were changed twice a week. The rats were fed Teklad Rat and Mouse Diet® and the hamsters, Teklad Hamster Diet® (Teklad Mills, Winfield, IA). All animals were given chlorinated water *ad libitum*.

Stress Analysis

A study was initiated to examine any stress associated with nose-only exposures compared to whole-body exposures. One hundred days-old female O-M rats were randomized to 1 of 3 groups: 1) caged controls that received no experimental manipulation; 2) a group that was exposed to atmospheric air in the chamber nose only 6 hours a day, 5 days a week; and 3) a group that was exposed to atmospheric air in the chambers in the traditional whole-body mode, 6 hours a day, 5 days a week. After either 1, 10 or 30 exposures, 10 animals each from the nose-only and whole-body groups were sacrificed by decapitation and blood samples taken for complete blood counts (CBC's), clinical chemistry profiles (SMAC-20's, New Mexico Medical Reference Laboratory, Santa Fe, NM) and plasma corticosterone assays using a modification of the method of Foster and Dunn (1974). These last assays were performed by Dr. J. Standefur, Department of Pathology, University of New Mexico Medical School, Albuquerque, NM. All experimental and control animals were treated as much alike as possible, i.e., housed in same room, cages changed at same time, etc., so not to introduce extraneous stress in one group compared to another.

Other parameters monitored included measurements of body weights and body (rectal) temperatures.

RESULTS

Aerosol Characterization

Aerosol distribution data presented are limited to that obtained against two fibrous aerosols currently being used in our ongoing study: 1) a glass aerosol produced from a bulk material having a ∿0.45 μm nominal fiber diameter and 2) an asbestos aerosol produced from UICC (International Union Against Cancer) crocidolite (Timbrell et al, 1968a). Figure 7 is an example illustrating aerosol mass output as a function of generator operating time obtained during a single aerosol generation consistency test. Each mass concentration measurement reported is the average result obtained from five separate gross filter samples simultaneously collected from the aerosol exposure chamber. For this particular test, the generator system was allowed to operate undisturbed for 1 hour for equilibration purposes prior to initiating sampling. Thereafter, aerosol mass concentration was determined by collecting gross filter samples on preweighed Gelman DM-800 membrane filters. Five simultaneous samples were collected from opposite sides (3 samples on one side, 2 on opposite) of the chamber every hour for 15-min sampling intervals at a flow rate of 1.0 l/min. There were no animals in the chamber during this test. Total generator running time for this test was 10 hours of uninterrupted operation. A total of 10 separate sets of filter samples were collected during this test (5 samples per set). The maximum port to port variation observed during this test was ±17% as measured simultaneously from 5 separate ports for each point. The average coefficient of variation for simultaneous samples taken at 50 different sampling locations within the containment chamber was +10%. The fibrous aerosol mass concentration variation observed during this test ranged from a minimum of 1.8 mg/m to a maximum of 2.4 mg/m^3 with the mean concentration being 2.0 ± 0.2 mg/m^3. These data demonstrate that aerosol mass concentrations in the chamber, at port level, were relatively constant and uniform throughout this glass microfiber aerosol consistency test.

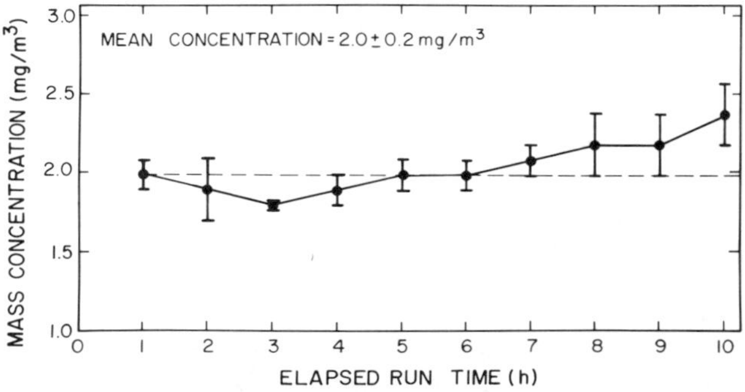

Figure 7. Aerosol mass concentration versus time output for microfiber aerosol.

Figure 8 is an optical photomicrograph of collected glass microfiber aerosol illustrating the polydisperse (multidiameter, multilength) characteristics of the fibrous material currently being used for animal exposure studies.

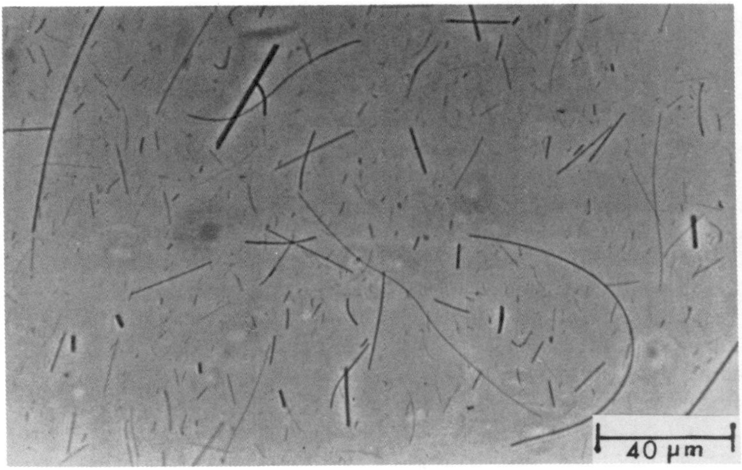

Figure 8. Optical photomicrograph of glass fiber aerosol (1000x).

Figure 9 is a Scanning Election Micrograph (SEM) of the same collected aerosol illustrating a more detailed microscopic view of this glass microfiber exposure aerosol. This SEM appear to enhance the proportion of short fibers contained in the aerosol as compared to photomicrograph obtained at similar magnifications using traditional phase contrast optical microscopy. This phenomenon is related to enhanced contrast and imaging properties of all collected particulates when viewed by SEM versus optical microscopy, as samples for SEM are collected on smooth surfaced, 0.22 μm pore Nucleopore® filters (Nucleopore Corp., Pleasanton, CA). All fiber sizing data being accumulated in our study are being done via SEM.

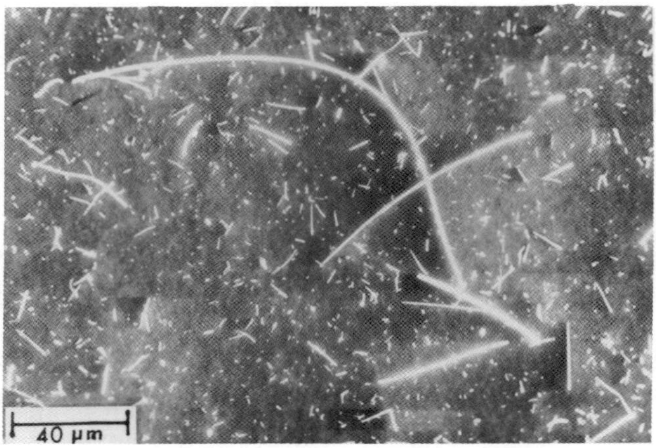

Figure 9. Scanning electron photomicrograph of glass fiber aerosol (1000x). Note enhancement of "short" fibers in this micrograph compared to optical photomicrographs in Figure 8.

A scanning electron micrograph illustrating our UICC crocidolite exposure aerosol appear as Figure 10. Similar aerosol mass concentration data obtained against this material is summarized in Figure 11. Again, each plotted point is the mean gravimetric value obtained from five simultaneous samples taken from said modified exposure chamber. The sampling interval was once every hour with 20 minute samples simultaneously collected from opposite chamber sides at a flow rate of 2.5 l/min. The maximum port-to-port variation observed for any of the 5 simultaneous samples taken per set for this aerosol was ±12%. The mean aerosol mass concentration was 6.0 ± 0.4 mg/m^3 for the entire 9 hr test period. The coefficient of variation for all 40 samples taken from 40 different ports was ±7%.

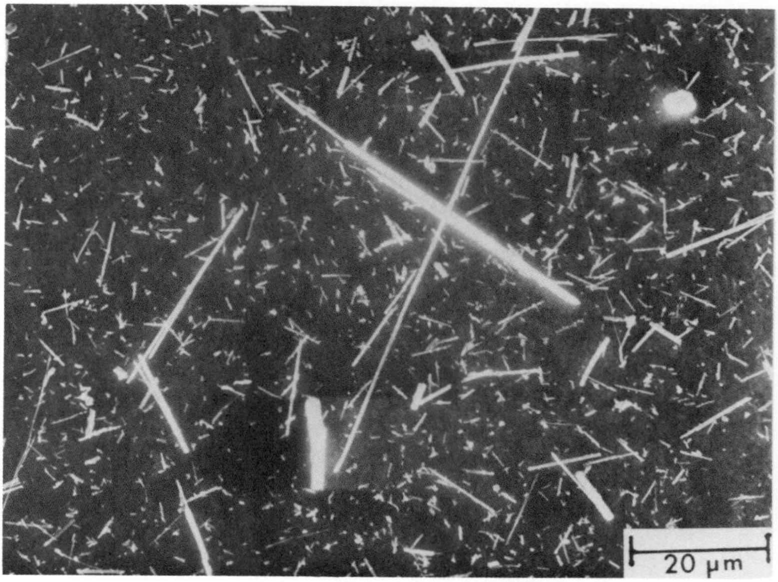

Figure 10. Scanning electron photomicrograph (2000x) of crocidolite asbestos aerosol.

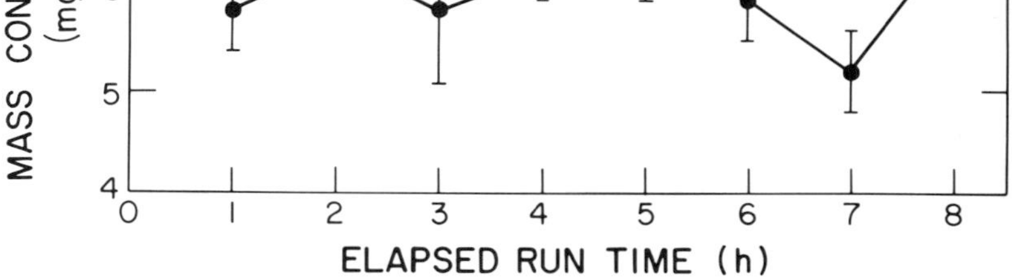

Figure 11. Aerosol mass output time for crocidolite asbestos aerosol.

Animal Observations

Fischer-344 and O-M rats and Syrian hamsters have been exposed to several particulate aerosols using this system, 6 hours a day, 5 days a week, for periods up to 24 months. No apparent clinical differences were observed between sham control animals exposed nose-only and their caged control counterparts. Sham control rats and hamsters routinely outlive caged unmanipulated controls--some groups have up to 50% longer mean life-spans. The longer life spans may be a result of the nose-only exposed animals being handled at least twice a day when being loaded and unloaded from the tubes.

Body weights for sham control and caged control female O-M rats and male Syrian hamsters up to 14 months of exposure, 6 hours a day, 5 days a week, are given in Table I. No significant differences emerged in body weights between sham controls and caged controls at either 5, 8, 11, or 14 months into the exposure regimen.

TABLE I
BODY WEIGHTS (g) I S.D.

Female O-M Rats	Cage Controls	Sham Controls
Initiation	272 ± 9	242 ± 12
5 Months	281 ± 9	289 ± 12
8 Months	285 ± 11	290 ± 17
11 Months	331 ± 13	338 ± 22
14 Months	333 ± 12	340 ± 20
Male Syrian Hamsters		
Initiation	137 ± 23	129 ± 10
5 Months	150 ± 12	142 ± 9
8 Months	152 ± 17	153 ± 13
11 Months	208 ± 14	192 ± 18
14 Months	209 ± 15	195 ± 12

Body (rectal) temperatures did not increase in either rats or hamsters while they were in the restraining tubes in the chambers as long as the number of air changes in the chambers was kept greater than 10/hour. When the number of air changes was lower than 6, hyperthermia inversely proportional to the number of changes resulted.

In the stress assessment study, no significant differences were seen between nose-only versus whole-body after 1, 10 or 30 exposures (6 hours a day, 5 days a week), or unmanipulated caged controls, measuring the following parameters: body weights, complete blood counts (white blood cell count, red blood cell count, hemoglobin, hematocrit, mean corpuscular volume, mean corpuscular hemoglobin, mean corpuscular hemoglobin concentration and differential white blood cell count) and clinical chemistry profiles (glucose, blood urea nitrogen, creatinine, uric acid, calcium, phosphorus, sodium chloride, carbon dioxide, electrolyte balance, blood urea nitrogen: creatinine ratio, cholesterol, triglycerides, total bilirubin, direct bilirubin, serum glutamic oxaloacetic transminase, alkaline phosphatase, lactic acid dehydrogenase, total protein, albumin and globulins).

Plasma corticosterone levels are given in Table II. These data indicate that nose-only exposure is no more stressful, or perhaps even less stressful, than whole-body exposure.

TABLE II
PLASMA CORTICOSTERONE LEVELS
(μg/dl) I S.E.

	Number of Exposures[A]			
	10	1	10	30
Untreated Cage controls (30 animals)	54 ± 4	-	-	-
Nose-only (10 animals/point)	-	49 ± 5	48 ± 4	56 ± 6
Whole-body (10 animals/point)	-	49 ± 7	74 ± 3[B]	64 ± 5[C]

[A] 6 hrs a day, 5 days a week

[B] $P<0.001$ vs. Nose-only (10 exposures) or untreated cage controls

[C] $P<0.005$ vs. untreated cage controls

DISCUSSION/CONCLUSIONS

Aerosol distribution data obtained against two different fibrous aerosols demonstrate that both aerosol mass concentration, and aerosol mass distribution within these modified exposure chambers are relatively consistent and uniform at the animal "breathing zone" under exposure conditions currently being employed. Laboratory animals have been exposed to particulate aerosols via nose-only systems for many years. Large test tubes (Cohn et al, 1956; Willard et al, 1958; Casarett, 1964), baby feeding bottles (Djuric et al, 1962) and plastic restrainers (Snider et al, 1973) have all been used to hold animals. With these types of apparatus, the animals in their holders were then placed in aerosol chambers for the exposures. More recent techniques have used special restraining tubes that were plugged into aerosol chambers so that only the noses of the animals came in contact with the aerosol (Evans et al, 1973; Raabe et al, 1973; Wehner et al, 1977; Thomas and Smith, 1979; Phalen et al, 1980). However, all of these systems were used only for a single or a relatively few exposures. Problems preventing long-term use that arose included over-restraining the animals in their tubes by pushing them forward with forceful plunger devices, resulting in excessive anxiety and stress and death in some cases. This is not a problem with our method because the animals are not forced forward; instead, they appear to be quite comfortable and extend their noses into the chamber environments as demonstrated in Figure 12.

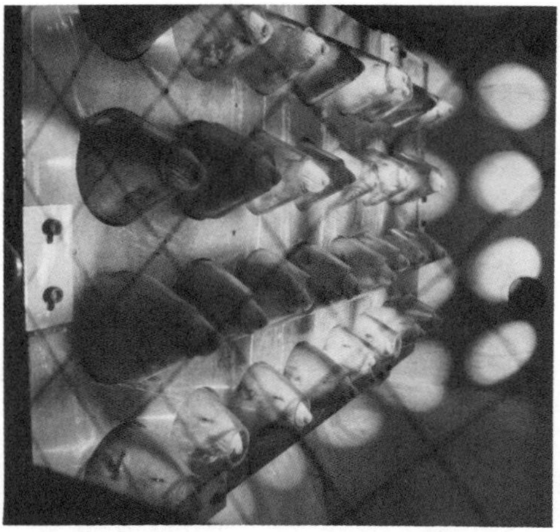

Figure 12. View of inside of exposure chamber with male Fischer-344 rats contained in polycarbonate tubes.

Another problem previously was that the animals chewed through the plastic tubes requiring either that the tubes be changed more frequently or that the nasal end of the tubes be made of a more durable, expensive material, such as machined aluminum. This was overcome in our approach by using polycarbonate tubes, which have useable life-spans of over one year. A third drawback in some systems was that the angle of the nasal end taper was too acute causing traumatic keratitis and panthalmitis with long-term use.

The described nose-only method in our laboratory has proven itself to be a very satisfactory means of exposing relatively large numbers of laboratory rats and hamsters in a limited space for 6 hours a day, 5 days a week for long periods. Analysis of CBC, clinical chemistry profile and adrenal cortical function data has shown that this nose-only exposure system is no more stressful or perhaps even less stressful than some whole-body exposure systems.

ACKNOWLEDGEMENTS

The authors are grateful for the invaluable contributions of Bonnie Isom who was responsible for the electron microscopy, Joe Martinez who assisted with the aerosol mass distribution determination, Cheryl Greenaugh who assisted in the animal exposures, Jerry London and Glessie Drake who collected and prepared blood samples for stress analysis, Joe Gonzales, Arthur Knight and John Elliot of the Health Research Laboratory Shops Department who fabricated the inhalation chamber inserts, Rosco Faussone of the Chemistry-Materials Science Division for casting the Silastic® sheets, and Carolyn Stafford and Marla Griffith for editorial assistance in preparing this manuscript.

BIBLIOGRAPHY

Casarett, L.J. (1964). Distribution and excretion of polonium-210. Radiat. Res., Supp. 5: 148-165.

Cohn, S.J., Lane, W.B., Gong, J.K., Sherwin, J.D., Fuller, R.K., Wiltshire, L.L. and Milne, W.L. (1956). Uptake, distribution and retension of fission products in tissues of mice exposed to a simulant of fallout from a nuclear detonation. AMA Arch. Ind. Health 14: 333-340.

Djuric, D., Thomas, R.G. and Lie, R. (1962). The distribution and excretion of trivalent antimony in the rat following inhalation. Int. Arch. for Gewerbepathologie und Gewerbehygiene 19: 529-545.

Evans, J.C., Evans, R.J., Holmes, A., Hounam, R.F., Jones, D.M., Morgan, A. and Walsh, M. (1973). Studies on the deposition of inhaled fibrous material in the respiratory tract of the rat and its subsequent clearance using radioactive tracer techniques. I. UICC crocidolite asbestos. Environ. Res. 6: 180-201.

Foster, L.B. and Dunn, R.T. (1974). Single-antibody technique for radio-immuno-assay of cortisol in unextracted serum or plasma. Clin. Chem. 20: 365-370.

Hinners, R., Burkart, J.K. and Puente, C.L. (1968). Animal inhalation exposure chambers. Arch. Environ. Health 16: 194-206.

Ortiz, L.W., Black, H.E. and Coulter, J.R. (1977). A modified fibrous aerosol generator. Ann. Occup. Hyg. 20: 25-37.

Phalen, R.F., Kenoyer, J.L., Crocker, T.T. and McClure, T.R. (1980). Effects of sulfate aerosols in combination with ozone on elimination of tracer particles inhaled by rats. J. Toxicol. Environ. Health 6: 797-810.

Raabe, O.G., Bennick, J.E., Light, M.E., Hobbs, C.H., Tillery, M.I. and Thomas, R.L. (1973). An improved apparatus for acute inhalation exposure of rodents to radioactive aerosols. Toxicol. Appl. Pharmacol. 26: 264-273.

Snider, G.L., Hayes, J.A., Korthy, A.L. and Lewis, G.P. (1973). Centrilobular emphysema experimentally induced by cadmium chloride aerosol. Am. Review Respir. Disease 108: 40-48.

Thomas, R.G. and Smith, D.M. (1979). Lung tumors from PuO_2-ZnO_2 aerosol particles in Syrian hamsters. Int. J. Cancer 24: 594-599.

Timbrell, V., Glison, J.C. and Webster, I. (1968a). UICC standard reference samples of asbestos. In. J. Cancer 3: 406-408.

Timbrell, V., Hyett, A.W. and Skidmore, J.W. (1968b): A simple dispenser for generating dust clouds from standard reference samples of asbestos. Ann. Occup. Hyg. 11: 273-281.

Wehner, A.P., Busch, R.H., Olson, R.J. and Craig, D.K. (1977). Chronic inhalation of cobalt oxide and cigarette smoke by hamsters. Am. Ind. Hyg. Assoc. J. 38: 338-346.

Willard, D.H., Bair, W.J. and Temple, L.A. (1958). Techniques for exposure of mice to aerosols of radioactive particles. HW-52368, Hanford Atomic Products Operation, Richland, WA.

AEROSOL TECHNOLOGY

Criteria for Size-Selective Aerosol Sampling in Inhalation Exposure Studies

MORTON LIPPMANN
Institute of Environmental Medicine
New York University Medical Center
New York, New York

ABSTRACT

Size-selective sampling criteria have been established which relate human inhalation hazards to the mass concentrations of aerosols within specified aerodynamic size ranges. These include "respirable dust", which was defined as dust penetrating to non-ciliated terminal air spaces of the lungs by the 1959 Pneumoconiosis Conference in Johannesburg, by the U.S. Atomic Energy Commission in 1960, and by the ACGIH Threshold Limits Committee in 1968. However, the numerical definitions of all three differ. In 1979, the U.S. EPA proposed that "inhalable dust" be defined as the aerosol capable of penetrating the upper respiratory tract and entering the trachea. In 1980, an ad hoc working group of the International Standards Organization (ISO) defined criteria for subdividing an aerosol into a series of fractions, including non-inspirable, extra-thoracic (deposition within the airways of the head), tracheobronchial, and alveolar ("respirable"). This paper discusses the applicability of such size-selective sampling criteria to the design of inhalation exposure studies.

INTRODUCTION

During this morning's session, I noted that the concepts of "respirable" dust and "inhalable" dust are misunderstood by some of the people attending this symposium. It is particularly important that these terms be properly defined so as to avoid unnecessary confusion within the field of inhalation toxicology especially, and to the general scientific community as well. The Health Effects Research Lab of EPA has recently recommended a sampler cut-size at 15 μm, with the undersize fraction called "inhalable" dust

(Miller et al. 1979). Unfortunately, some people in EPA have referred to that fraction as "respirable". They appear to be unaware that "respirable" dust has had a clear and definite meaning to occupational health professionals for many years (Orenstein, 1960; Lippmann, 1970), and that the "respirable" dust cut-size is much smaller.

I hope that this presentation will clarify the origins of these concepts, how the various criteria are defined, the extent to which they've been used in the occupational health field, and how they relate to the field of inhalation toxicology.

An assumption implicit in this discussion is that experimental animals have similar regional deposition patterns to humans. While this assumption is not completely true, it is to some extent a reasonable first approximation. The animal deposition data, limited as they are, do show similar penetration to, and deposition in, the pulmonary or alveolar regions of the lung as do humans (Lippmann, 1977; McMahon et al. 1977). At the same time, there are some important differences. Also, there aren't enough animal data to precisely describe regional deposition in any one species, let alone a series of them. Regional deposition data for humans are much more plentiful, but many have been found to have serious deficiencies. Consequently, this paper summarizes only the more reliable human data which are available. These will serve, as indicated previously, as a first approximation for deposition in animals used in toxicology studies.

EXPERIMENTAL DEPOSITION DATA

Total Respiratory Tract Deposition

Figure 1 is a summary of a total respiratory tract deposition during mouth breathing. Since few animals breathe through the mouth, these data do not provide a good representation of total deposition in animals for the larger particles. Nose breathing data for humans would be closer to the animal model, but since the human nose is not as good a filter as most animal's noses, would still underestimate total deposition in animals. On the other hand, most of the human deposition data we have comes from mouth breathing experiments. For such exposures, we can see that for aerodynamic diameters on the order of 5 μm or greater, there is nearly total deposition somewhere in the respiratory tract. Between 0.1 and 1 μm, total deposition is down around 20%, and it's nearly independent of particle size. This occurs because the intrinsic mobility of the particle makes very little difference in this particle size range. For such particles, deposition probability is determined by the extent of the exchange of tidal air with residual air. In any case,

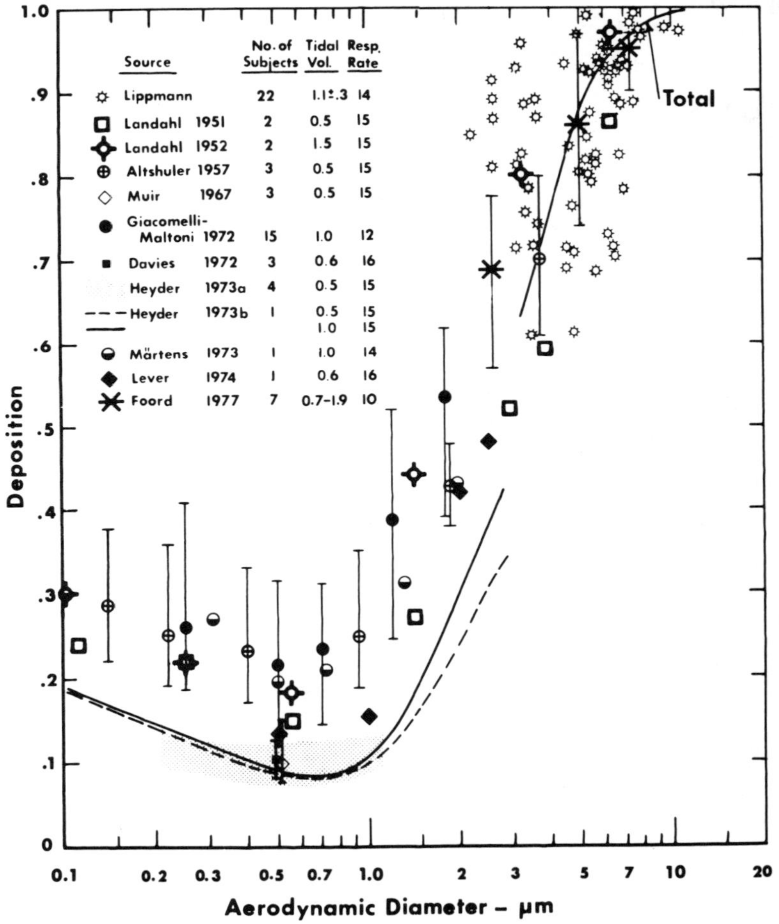

FIGURE 1 Total respiratory tract deposition vs. particle size during mouth breathing for a variety of experimental studies - from Lippmann (1977).

most of these particles will be exhaled unless they change in size. Particles which take up water vapor in the warm and humid respiratory tract will grow and become dilute water droplets.

In any case, total respiratory tract deposition isn't a very useful parameter in most toxicological investigations, because the effective toxic doses are determined by the extent of the particle deposition in the more sensitive parts of the respiratory tract.

Tracheobronchial Deposition

Figure 2 shows recent data on tracheobronchial deposition

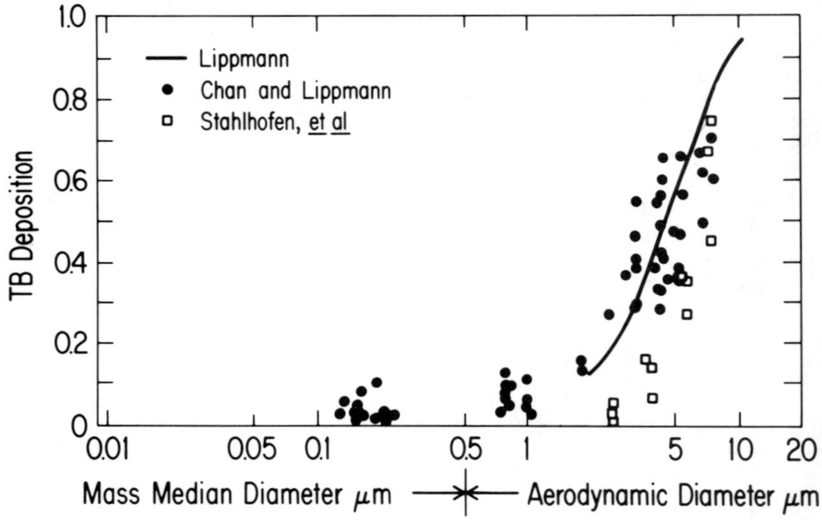

FIGURE 2 Tracheobronchial deposition as a function of particle size for the aerosol entering the trachea.

primarily from data from Tai Chan's thesis work in my laboratory (Chan and Lippmann, 1980). He used γ-tagged monodisperse insoluble aerosols, and external measurements of their retention as a function of time after inhalation. The particle clearance from the thorax within the first day represents the particles deposited on the tracheobronchial airways. His data confirmed the work we did previously for the larger particle size range, and extended it into the smaller particle size range.

Tracheobronchial deposition is very low for particles smaller than ∿ 2 μm, where they are too small for effective operation of the impaction and sedimentation mechanisms. All of these data are for non-smokers. Tracheobronchial deposition is, on average, greater in cigarette smokers because the smoke is bronchoconstrictive (Lippmann, 1977). This acts to increase the bronchial deposition at the expense of the alveolar deposition, since these are sequential regions in a multi-stage collection system.

Alveolar Deposition

Figure 3 shows more of the data from Chan's thesis,

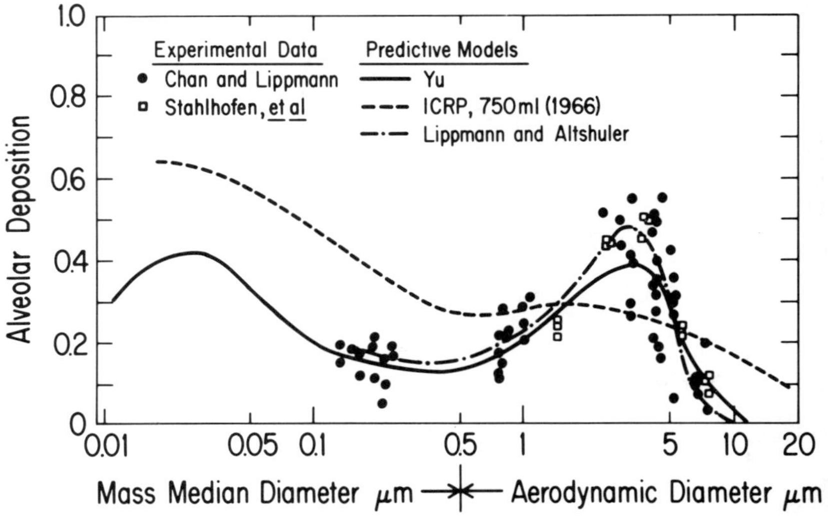

FIGURE 3 Alveolar deposition as a function of particle size during mouth breathing.

specifically data on alveolar deposition in mouth breathing. The solid circles are Chan's data, and are in reasonably good agreement with data of Stahlhofen, et al. (1980). These are the only other body of data on regional deposition measured with tagged aerosols.

Alveolar deposition falls off for large particles because they don't get there. They're removed in the head or bronchial tree. Deposition efficiency also falls off for the small particles, because they can remain suspended in the air and be exhaled. The alveolar deposition for the smaller particles is almost equivalent to total deposition.

Figure 4 summarizes average alveolar deposition in

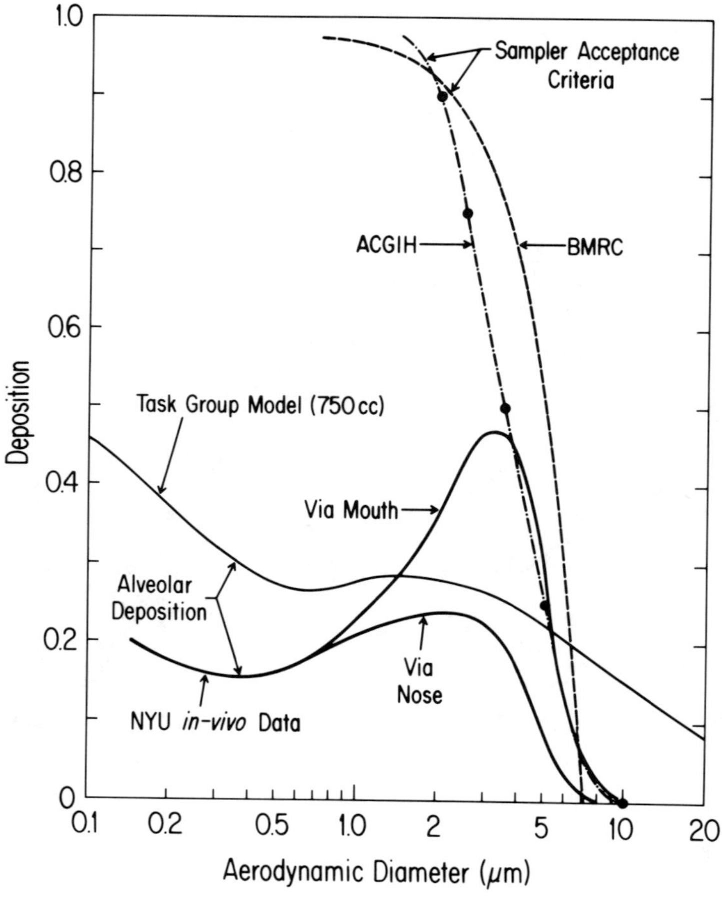

FIGURE 4 Comparison of alveolar deposition as a function of particle size with sampler acceptance criteria of ACGIH and BMRC, and with the Task Group Model (1966).

non-smokers, and shows the effect of the route of entry. It includes a curve for nose breathing, the nose curve is based on a correction of the mouth breathing data according to the difference between head deposition in nose breathing and mouth breathing (Lippmann, 1977). For nose breathing, alveolar deposition is about 20% all the way from ∿ 0.1 μm to ∿ 4 μm, because of the enhanced removal of the larger particles in the nasal air passages.

For other groups, such as cigarette smokers who are healthy, there is a shift in deposition. There is less alveolar and more bronchial deposition. For people with clinical disease, the shift is even greater. While cigarette smoking may not pertain directly to deposition in animals, it was considered in the establishment of some of the models which I'll be discussing later, which make a distinction between healthy people and people who may be a special risk.

REVIEW OF SIZE-SELECTIVE SAMPLING CRITERIA

For healthy workers, Figure 4 shows the basic viability of the currently accepted criteria for "respirable dust". In 1952 the British Medical Research Council (BMRC) defined "respirable" dust as those particles which penetrated through the conductive airways into the pulmonary spaces. In effect they decided that only those particles which could deposit in the non-ciliated alveolar spaces were of interest in terms of the pathogenesis of coal workers' pneumoconiosis, which can only result from dust particles which deposit on the alveoli. They based their criteria on the 1950 paper on regional deposition by Brown, Cook, Ney and Hatch (1950) from the University of Pittsburgh. In 1960, the U.S. Atomic Energy Commission (AEC) applied the same rationale to the uranium milling industry, and their criteria were also based upon the University of Pittsburgh deposition data. The AEC criteria were later modified slightly and adopted by ACGIH for coal mine dust in 1968, and in later years ACGIH extended these criteria to TLV's for other pneumoconiosis producing dusts.

Size-Selective Criteria for Sampling of Respirable Dust

While both BMRC and AEC-ACGIH utilized the same University of Pittsburgh deposition data, they derived different shaped cut-off criteria. The BMRC selected the horizontal elutriator as the sampling instrument of choice, which determined the shape of the cut-off curve. The characteristic elutriator curve was then positioned to lie as close as possible to the deposition data. The later AEC-ACGIH criteria followed the deposition data more closely. It is fortunate that the newer human deposition data match both of these widely used criteria reasonably well. Thus, they continue to represent reasonable approximations for healthy workers in terms of screening out the large particles which tend to dominate the mass concentration of an aerosol when they are present. Currently, the mass concentration of "respirable" dust is the index of choice for occupational health exposure evaluations for pneumoconiosis producing dusts. The agreed definition of "respirable" dust in the field of occupational health is that it's the dust which penetrates to and is available for deposition in the alveolar region.

Size-Selective Criteria for Sampling Dust Affecting the Conductive Airways

"Respirable" dust is not the only possibly hazardous dust. If we are interested in human diseases such as bronchitis, or bronchial cancer, we must also be interested in some of the particles we discard when we are measuring "respirable" dust.

EPA, in preparing its new particulate matter criteria document, has attempted to recognize the possible hazard of the particles which deposit on the conductive airways of the lungs. They have tentatively selected a 15 μm 50% cut as appropriate for the exclusion of the particles which would be removed in the airways of the head, and have called the $<$ 15 μm particles "inhalable". They selected this name to distinguish this cut from the "respirable" dust cut. It should be noted 15 μm was not selected as a mid-point for penetration through the head. The point of reference was the NYU head deposition data (Lippmann, 1977), which indicated that 10-15% of 15 μm particles penetrate through the larynx in mouth breathing, and can enter the lower respiratory tract. Deposition in the head is excluded as non-inhalable. While the selection of the word "inhalable" was a poor choice for general applications, it can be defended as being reasonable for air pollution exposures, where we don't know of any health effects that might result from deposition in the head of particles other than pollens (EPA declines to accept any control responsibility for aeroallergens of natural origin). The 15 μm cut-size may not have been an optimal choice, but a cut somewhere in that range was needed, and 15 was selected to provide a conservative indication of potential lung exposures. Unfortunately, their position paper (Miller et al., 1979) didn't adequately describe this rationale. While the "inhalable" cut is not yet part of any standard EPA sampling protocols, several groups within EPA are using it in their sampling programs designed to gather background data.

The EPA has also encouraged and supported research studies which utilize a second, smaller, cut-size at 2.5 μm. EPA groups concerned primarily with atmospheric characterization prefer such a cut-size because, as shown in Figure 5,

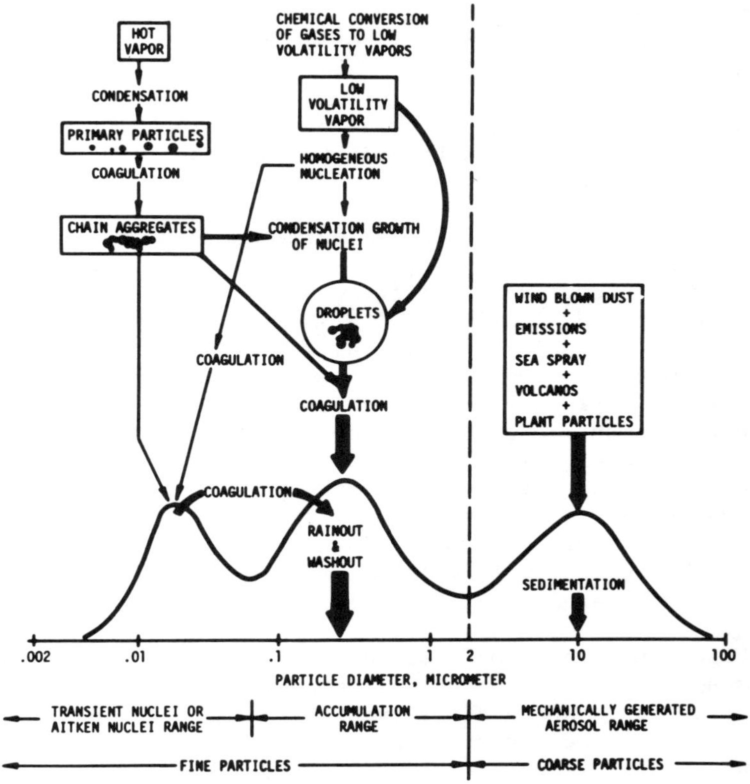

Figure 5 Trimodal distribution of aerosol surface, showing principal modes, main sources of mass in each mode, the principal processes involved in generating the mass in each mode, and the principal removal mechanisms - from Airborne Particles, National Research Council, 1979.

the composition of the coarse mode aerosol larger than 2.5 μm is very different from the composition of the < 2.5 μm fine mode aerosol. The mostly irregular coarse mode solid particles are basic, whereas the smaller accumulation mode and Aitken nuclei mode particles, which together make up the fine aerosol, appear to be acidic. When collected together, the coarse and fine mode particles tend to neutralize each other. Also, their elemental compositions are different, and these differences can be used to relate the atmospheric aerosols to their source materials when they can be collected separately.

The saddle point of the volume or mass distribution of the atmospheric aerosol is about 2½ μm on an aerodynamic basis. Furthermore, EPA would like to have a limited number of cuts for monitoring purposes. They maintain that measurements of composition in any larger number of size-graded fractions is impractical.

Size-Selective Sampling Criteria for Occupational and Environmental Aerosols Developed by an International Standards Organization Working Group

A recommendation on size-selective aerosol sampling which may not be known by more than a few people at this Symposium was developed earlier this year by an ad hoc working group appointed by Committee TC #146 of the International Standards Organization (ISO). The group was formed to prepare recommendations on a size-selective sampling standard for both the workplace and the ambient air. It would be used in the future as a preamble to any standard method. Thus, they wanted something which would have general applicability. The working group completed its report in September of 1980. As I understand it, the members of the TC #146 committee will vote on acceptance of the sampling recommendations by mail ballot. If accepted, it will become an official recommendation of the International Standards Organization early in 1981.

Figure 6 is a summary based on the ISO Working Groups recommendations for size-selective sampling criteria. The curves are based on recently available human regional deposition data in the various regions of the respiratory tract. As indicated previously, it is intended to be general, i.e., to be useful for both occupational health and air pollution applications. The first cut therefore, includes the large particles which deposit in the nose and which, in furniture manufacturing operations, have been reported to cause nasal cancers. The name "inspirable" was proposed for this first cut-off. "Inhalable" might have been a good English word, but EPA has already used it to describe a different cut-size. Therefore, "inspirable" was selected as a suitable word that would not contribute to the confusion.

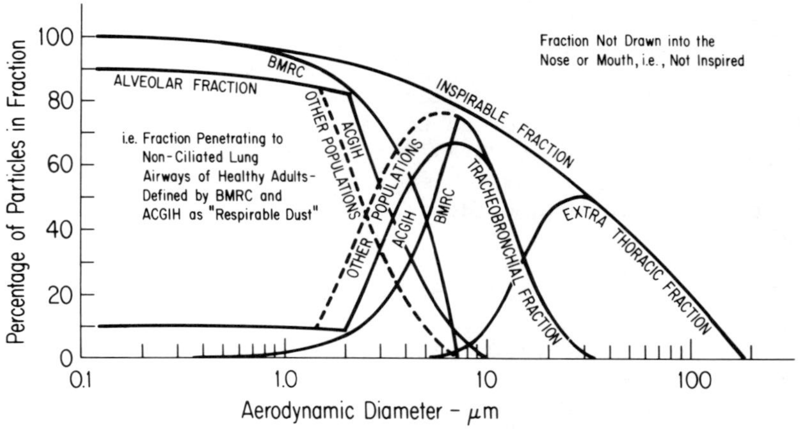

FIGURE 6 Recommended boundaries of size-cuts for occupational health and air pollution sampling of an ad hoc Working Group appointed by Committee TC #146 of the International Standards Organization (ISO).

The "inspirable" dust envelope includes particles that can deposit anywhere in the respiratory tract. As the size increases, fewer of the particles can be aspirated in by the suction exerted by the nose or mouth. The "inspirable" curve is based on recent British and German data, which are internally consistent. The "inspirable" aerosol can be subdivided into the various anatomic classifications that we're already familiar with. The ICRP Task Group on Lung Dynamics (TGLD) (1966) chose to call deposition within the head "nasopharyngeal". This was a particularly unfortunate choice of label, because the head includes several sub-regions which generally have more particle deposition than does the nasopharnyx. The ISO Working Group decided to call the head deposition "extrathoracic", i.e., outside the thorax, but within the respiratory tract.

The next region is tracheobronchial, which I think

everybody agrees extends from the larynx down to the terminal ciliated airways. It represents the conductive airways, also known as the anatomic dead space of the lungs.

The thoracic region includes both the tracheobronchial and the alveolar region. The latter is also known as the pulmonary region and is the region distal to the terminal bronchioles. By long established usage, the dust which penetrates to this region is called "respirable". In particular, we have both the British Medical Research Council (BMRC) definition, and the American Conference of Governmental Industrial Hygienists (ACGIH) definition, both of which are illustrated in Figure 4. Based on the large variability among people which was evident in the data in previously cited figures, one criterion is about as good as the other for the purpose. Thus, the recommendation of the ISO Working Group was that long established national usage should prevail. Those who want to use the ACGIH criterion can use it, while those who prefer the BMRC criterion can use that. As shown in Figure 6, when you use one you get one tracheobronchial envelope and a corresponding alveolar envelope. If you use the other, you get slightly different envelopes.

For occupational exposure considerations you can't be consistently conservative. In a generalized model, where we are concerned about diseases of both the tracheobronchial region and the alveolar region, there's no way to be conservative. If more of the aerosol is collected in one bucket, there will be less collected in the other. On the other hand, in terms of air pollution one can take a different point of view, i.e. to protect the sensitive individual. The population now not only includes reasonably healthy adults, but also young children, infants, old and sick people.

Our experimental regional deposition data indicates that people having narrowed airways, which is a characteristic of bronchitis and congestive airway disease, have a shift in regional deposition so that there's more bronchial and less alveolar deposition. In view of this, the ISO Working Group concluded that for the sensitive populations of general interest with respect to air pollution health effects, the 50% cut-size should be reduced to 2½ μm. This represented somewhat of a practical compromise to conform to what's being done anyway for other reasons, but, at the same time, a reasonable one in terms of what we know about deposition in such people.

CONCLUSION

These size-selective sampling criteria should be considered by inhalation toxicologists when they decide which sizes of particles to generate for inhalation studies. While there are no government regulations or specifications yet on the size distribution of inhalation atmospheres, I think you all will want to try to anticipate what the trends are. Applications of size-distribution models will tend to be established on a more generalized basis, rather than being restricted to pneumoconiosis producing dusts. Such models are likely to become more widely used in industrial hygiene and air pollution sampling specifications, and in inhalation toxicology protocols.

REFERENCES

Brown, J.H., Cook, K.M., Ney, F.G. and Hatch T. (1950) Influence of particle size upon the retention of particulate matter in the human lung. Amer. J. Public Health 40:450-458, 480.

Chan, T.L. and Lippmann, M. (1980) Experimental measurements and empirical modelling of the regional deposition of inhaled particles in humans. Amer. Ind. Hyg. Assoc. J. 41:399-409.

Lippmann, M. (1977) Regional deposition of particles in the human respiratory tract, pp. 213-232, in: Handbook of Physiology - Section 9: Reactions to Environmental Agents, Edited by D.H.K. Lee, H.L. Falk and S.D. Murphy, Bethesda, Md., American Physiological Society.

Lippmann, M. (1970) "Respirable" dust sampling. Amer. Ind. Hyg. Assoc. J. 31:138-159.

McMahon, T.A., Brain, J.D. and Lemott, S. (1977) Species differences in aerosol deposition, pp. 23-32, in: Inhaled Particles IV, Edited by W.H. Walton, London Pergamon.

Miller, F.J., Gardner, D.E., Graham, J.A., Lee, R.E., Jr., Wilson, W.E. and Bachmann, J.D. (1979) Size considerations for establishing a standard for inhalable particles. J. Air Poll. Cont. Assoc. 29:610-615.

Orenstein, A.J. (1960) Proceedings of the Pneumoconiosis Conference, Johannesburg, 1959, J. & A. Churchill, Ltd., London.

Stahlhofen, W., Gebhart, J. and Heyder, J. Experimental determination of the regional deposition of aerosol particles in the human respiratory tract. Amer. Ind. Hyg. Assoc. J. 41:385-398a.

Subcommittee on Airborne Particles, MBEEP Comm., National Research Council. (1979) Airborne Particles, Baltimore, Univ. Park Press.

Task Group on Lung Dynamics (Committee II-ICRP) (1966) Deposition and retention models for internal dosimetry of the human respiratory tract. Health Physics 12:173-207.

Liquid Aerosol Generation for Inhalation Toxicology Studies

J.L. MILLER
Stauffer Chemical Company
Richmond Toxicology Laboratory
Richmond, CA

B.O. STUART
Stauffer Chemical Company
Environmental Health Center
Farmington, CT

H.S. DEFORD and O.R. MOSS
Department of Biology
Battelle
Pacific Northwest Laboratories
Richland, WA

ABSTRACT

Several techniques have recently been developed to generate high concentrations of liquid aerosols for acute inhalation toxicity testing. The inhalation chamber aerosol concentrations of a representative test material were found to increase linearly with increased air pressure (10-60 psi) for the Solo-Sphere® (0.44-5.5 mg/l), Ball-jet® (0.7-2.4 mg/l) and Retec® (0.1-1.7 mg/l) nebulizers. Higher concentrations were produced using auxiliary air (5-40 l/min) to the Solo-Sphere (5.1-10.4 mg/l) and Ball-jet (2.2-3.1 mg/l) nebulizers; output of the Retec nebulizer was not improved. Aerosol particle size distributions were altered by nebulizer air pressure but not by auxiliary air flow. Using the Solo-Sphere, chamber concentrations of $\geq$5 mg/l can be produced in a 450 liter chamber operated at 15 air changes/hr. During 4-hour tests, variability in chamber aerosol concentrations, and in particle size distribution parameters were maintained at $\leq$30%. Determinations of particle size distributions indicated that >95% of aerosol droplets were smaller than 10 um (mass median aerodynamic diameter) for all test materials. Actual chamber air concentrations measured by chemical analysis and/or gravimetric methods were 2-8 fold lower than calculated "nominal" values, demonstrating the fallacy of relying upon nominal values to characterize exposure conditions.

Reliable methods for consistent generation of aerosols from solutions without change in aerosol output or particle size distribution have been achieved using a modified Retec nebulizer employing a secondary bulk solution reservoir.

I. Introduction

The most recent proposed EPA guidelines for acute inhalation toxicity testing specify that an exposure atmosphere containing up to 5 grams per cubic meter ($5g/m^3$) of test material must be presented to the test animals for up to 4 hours. The exposure chamber atmosphere must be sampled repeatedly and must be adjusted as required to minimize variability in mean chamber aerosol concentration. Test aerosols must contain at least 20% of the particles smaller that 10 um (micrometers) aerodynamic diameter. If inhalation testing as described with at least 5 animals per sex shows that the LC_{50} is greater than $5g/m^3$, no further testing is required. If data indicate that the lethal concentration to 50% of the rats, (the LC_{50}) is less than $5g/m^3$, additional exposures are required to establish the LC_{50}. This acute inhalation toxicity information is used by the Environmental Protection Agency as the basis for a number of regulatory decisions including: issuing a rebuttable presumption against registration (RPAR), requirements for special packaging, and container warnings (Fed. Reg. 1978).

Although the scientific literature contains many descriptions of aerosol generators (Lauterbach _et al_, 1956; Dautreband _et al_, 1958; Mercer _et al_, 1968; Raabe, 1976) and inhalation exposure systems (Hinners _et al_, 1968; Drew and Laskin, 1973; Sachsse _et al_, 1974; Phalen, 1976; Raabe _et al_, 1979), special procedures and equipment are required for the generation, containment and characterization of the toxicity of the highly concentrated inhalation test atmospheres required by the EPA acute inhalation toxicity protocol.

This report describes the equipment and procedures we have used to conduct EPA acute inhalation tests on over 25 liquid test materials belonging to several use classes, including herbicide technicals and formulations, solvents, flame retardants, plasticizers, lubricants and industrial chemicals.

II. Inhalation Exposure System

A schematic of the inhalation generation system used in acute inhalation studies is shown in Figure 1. Oil-free compressed air is supplied to a generation air panel containing a pressure regulator, an ultra filter, and calibrated rotameters. The rotameters control air flow to the compressed air nebulizers where the test material is aerosolized. If desired, the concentrated aerosol can be diluted using an inline dilutor-mixer before delivery into a krypton-85 aerosol discharger (10mCi).

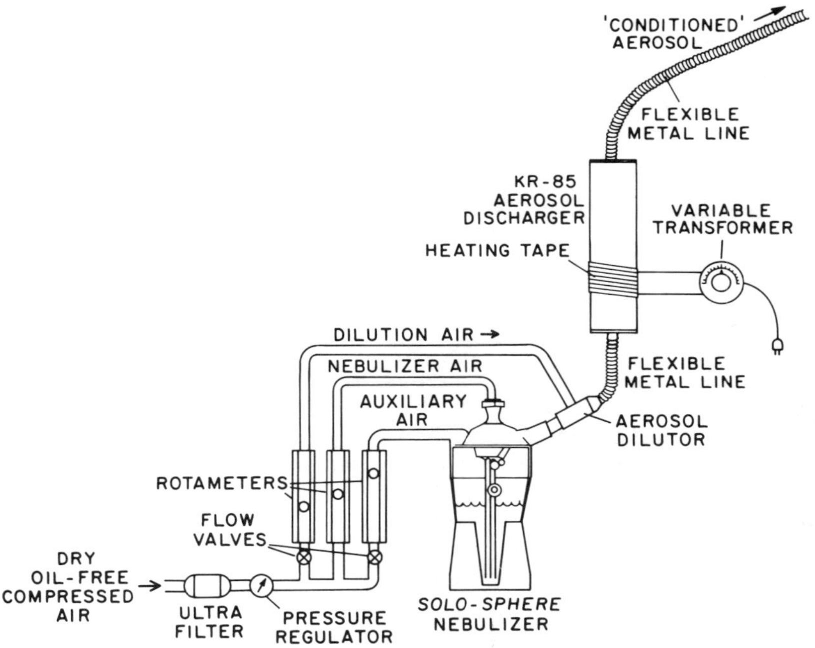

Figure 1 - Aerosol Generation System for Liquid Materials. Typical aerosol generation system using purified air and aerosol discharging unit with Solo-Sphere® Nebulizer. Other high output liquid aerosol generators may be used.

The inhalation exposure system is shown in Figure 2. A damper controls the chamber pressure which is maintained at negative 0.5 inches of water and is monitored using a magnehelic gauge. The test aerosol is delivered to the mixing plenum of the chamber using stainless steel flexible tubing with an inside diameter of one (1) inch. At this point, conditioned and filtered room air mixes with the aerosol and forms the test atmosphere that is presented to the individually housed test animals. The "used" aerosol leaves the chamber through a calibrated orifice meter system that provides a continuous reading of chamber flow rate. The exposure chamber flow is controlled by a stainless steel globe valve and is maintained at a flow of 110 l/min which is equivalent to 15 air changes per hour. The chamber exhaust enters flexible stainless steel exhaust lines of four (4) inch inside diameter that allow removal of much of the aerosol by settling. The exhaust is filtered prior to venting into the atmosphere. Studies in our laboratory have shown that with an animal loading of 2% of chamber volume, a chamber flow of 15 air changes per hour is adequate to provide good aerosol distribution to both tiers of test animals and to maintain oxygen concentrations of at least 19%. Stable temperature and humidity readings are also easily maintained at this flow rate.

III. Liquid Aerosol Generation

A. Approach

High output aerosol generators are required to produce the very high concentrations of liquid aerosols required by the described inhalation protocol. We have evaluated the performance of several experimental and commercial nebulizers. Desirable performance characteristics of nebulizers for acute inhalation studies are as follows:

- *The nebulizer must produce high output of respirable aerosols.
- *The particle size distribution of the test aerosol should be stable and reproducible.
- *Aerosol output should be adjustable to provide a range of chamber aerosol concentrations.
- *Other considerations in nebulizer selection are ease of operation, chemical resistance and availability.

In nebulizer evaluation studies, the test liquid used was a commercial liquid with a density of 1.01 grams per ml, a viscosity of 2.5 centipoises, and a vapor pressure of 13 u Hg at 25°C.

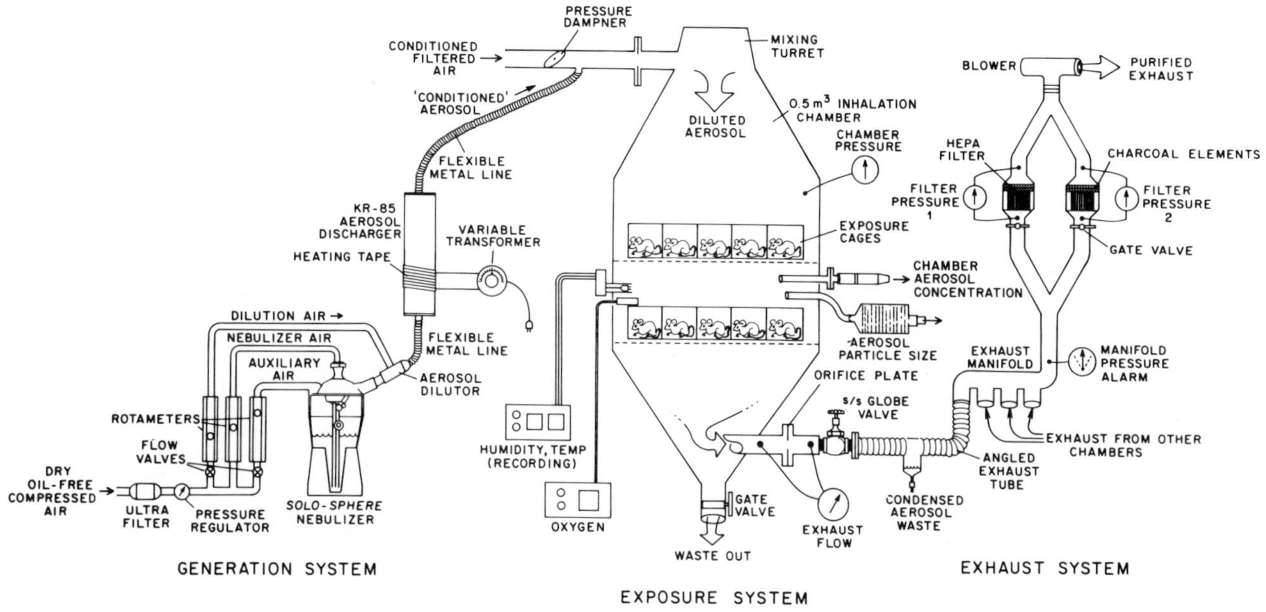

Figure 2 - Inhalation Exposure System for Liquid Aerosols.
This system uses a high output liquid aerosol generator with a continuous flow inhalation exposure chamber capable of exposing 10 male and 10 female rats for a period of 1 to 4 hours. Chamber aerosol concentrations and particle size distributions are monitored directly from chamber atmospheres.

Chamber aerosol concentrations and aerosol particle size were determined by sampling the chamber atmosphere using Gelman Type A-E filters and a 7 stage cascade impactor, respectively. Isokinetic sampling conditions were maintained in all sampling procedures. The amounts of test material on filters and impactor stages were determined by gas-liquid chromatography. A graphical method, described by Raabe was used to describe the aerosol particle size distributions. Values are reported in mass mean aerodynamic resistance diameters (MMAD) and geometric standard deviations (σg) of the distributions.

B. Results of Comparative Studies Using the Solo-Sphere, Ohio and Retec Nebulizers

The performance evaluations indicated that three nebulizers had desirable operating characteristics for acute inhalation studies. The Ohio Ball-jet, the Retec and the Solo-Sphere nebulizers are shown in Figure 3 as they were received.

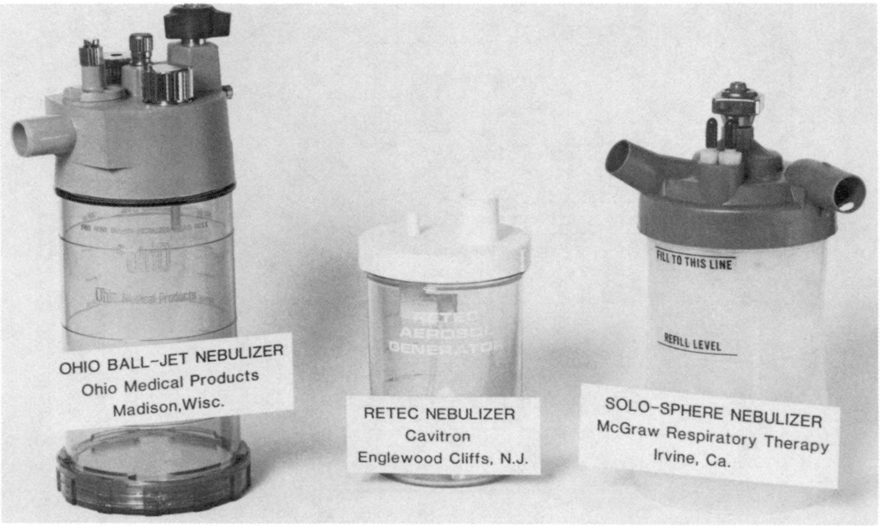

Figure 3 - Three high output liquid aerosol generators as received from the manufacturers. The particular liquid test material to be generated must be tested for compatibility with the reservoirs.

These nebulizers are typically used for humidification of hospital oxygen tents. For convenience, nebulizers were fitted with one-way flow air fittings. The Retec and the Ohio Ball-jet nebulizers produce aerosols by entraining the test material in an air stream and forcing the stream through a small orifice against a baffle. The Solo-Sphere utilizes the patented Babington system for aerosol generation (Raabe, 1976).

1. Test using the Solo-Sphere Nebulizer

The principle of operation of the Solo-Sphere is shown in Figure 4. Air enters the Solo-Sphere via the gas inlet and continues down the manifold tube to the aerosol generator. A small portion of the air by-passes the aerosol generator and continues to the bubble pump plug where the pressure is substantially reduced. The low pressure air continues down the tube until it reaches the bottom where bubbles are formed moving the test material into the upper reservoir. The test material flows by gravity over the surface of a hollow glass sphere containing a small orifice. The test material forms a continuous film over the sphere.

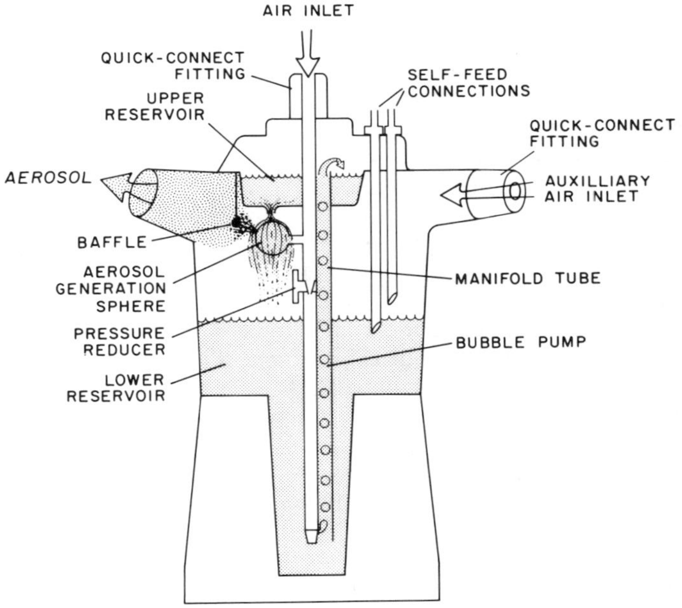

Figure 4 - Schematic representation of the operation of the Solo-Sphere® Nebulizer based on the Babington principal. An uninterrupted flow of liquid test material over the aerosol generation sphere must be maintained.

Air at sonic velocity exits through the jet, shattering the film and forming primary aerosol. The larger aerosol particle impact against a baffle, forming additional fine droplets.

The air flow and aerosol exiting from the nebulizer creates a negative pressure at that side of the nebulizer. Auxiliary air added to the nebulizer can increase aerosol output, possibly by providing more rapid removal of aerosol droplets as they are formed. This results in an increased volumetric output of aerosol. The Ohio Ball-jet nebulizer also is designed to incorporate auxiliary air flow into normal operation. In our modification, for safety, the auxiliary air vent was sealed and air was metered into the opening using a rotameter. The performance of the Solo-Sphere nebulizer is shown in Figure 5. The chamber aerosol concentration in milligrams per liter is shown by the solid line. Each point is the mean of two determinations. At operating pressures of 10 to 60 psi, a linear increase in chamber aerosol concentration was observed. The maximum chamber aerosol concentration achieved was 5.5 milligrams per liter (5500 mg/m^3). At operating pressures of 10 to 30 psi, aerosol particle size (MMAD) was decreased from about 5 um at 10 psi to 4.4 um at 30 psi. However, at operating pressures of 30 to 60 psi, the aerosol particle size distribution remained constant with a MMAD of 4.3 um and σg of 1.5.

The Solo-Sphere nebulizer was operated at 60 psi and auxiliary air was metered into the nebulizer. Chamber aerosol concentrations increased linearly with the addition of auxiliary air, as shown in Figure 6. At 40 liters per minute of auxiliary air, a maximum chamber aerosol concentration of 10.2 milligrams per liter, (10,200 mg/m^3), was achieved. At auxiliary air flows greater than 50 liters per minute chamber aerosol concentrations became variable. Throughout the range of auxiliary air flow, median aerosol particle size remained essentially constant at 4.2 um. A σg of about 1.6 was maintained throughout the range of auxiliary air flows.

2. Tests using the Ohio Ball-Jet Nebulizer

The performance of the Ohio Ball-jet nebulizer is shown in Figure 7. As with the Solo-Sphere, chamber aerosol concentrations for the Ohio nebulizer were increased in a linear manner at operating pressures of 10 to 60 psi. The maximum chamber aerosol concentration measured at an operating pressure of 60 psi was 2.5 milligrams per liter.

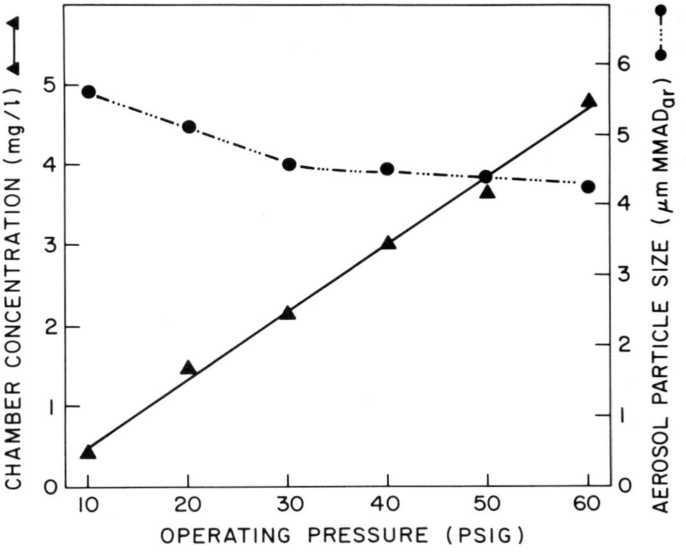

Figure 5 - Performance of the Solo-Sphere® Nebulizer as a function of operating pressure of air supplied to the nebulizer. Pressures in excess of 60 psig are not recommended.

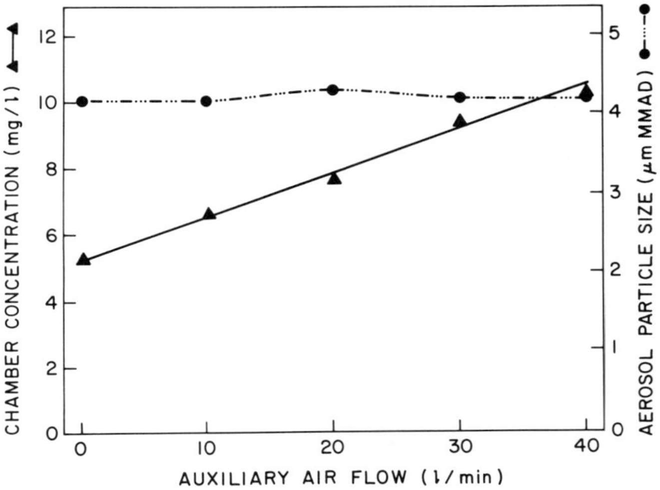

Figure 6 - Performance of the Solo-Sphere® Nebulizer as a function of auxiliary airflow supplied to the nebulizer. Operating characteristics will change with different liquid test materials.

This concentration is about one-half of that achieved by the Solo-Sphere operated at the same pressure. Median particle size was relatively constant at about 4.5 um for operating pressures of 10 to 40 psi. However, at the higher operating pressures a trend of decreased particle size is evident. Throughout the range of operating pressures, σg's were relatively constant at 1.6 to 1.8.

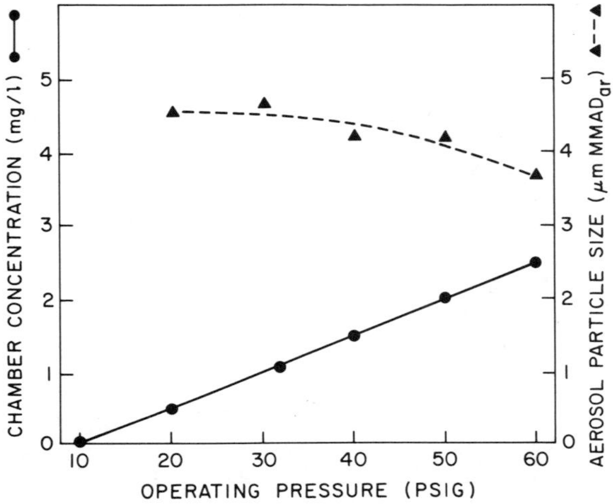

Figure 7 - Performance of the Ohio Ball-jet® Nebulizer as a function of operating pressure of air supplied to the nebulizer. Supplied air pressure of greater than 60 psig are not recommended.

Aerosol concentrations were increased to a maximum of about 3 mg/l as auxiliary flow was increased to 30 liters per minute (Figure 8). Addition of auxiliary air at flow rates greater than 30 l/min was not effective in increasing chamber aerosol concentration. Aerosol particle size remained very constant throughout the range of auxiliary flows with a MMAD of 3.9 and a σg of 1.5.

3. Tests using the Retec Nebulizer

Figure 9 shows the performance of the Retec nebulizer. At operating pressures of 10 to 40 psi a linear increase in chamber aerosol concentration was achieved to a maximum of 2.5 milligrams per liter. At these pressures, aerosol particle size distribution is stable with an MMAD of about 3.8 um and a σg of about 1.5. At operating pressures of 50 to 60 psi, both chamber aerosol concentration and aerosol particle size were decreased.

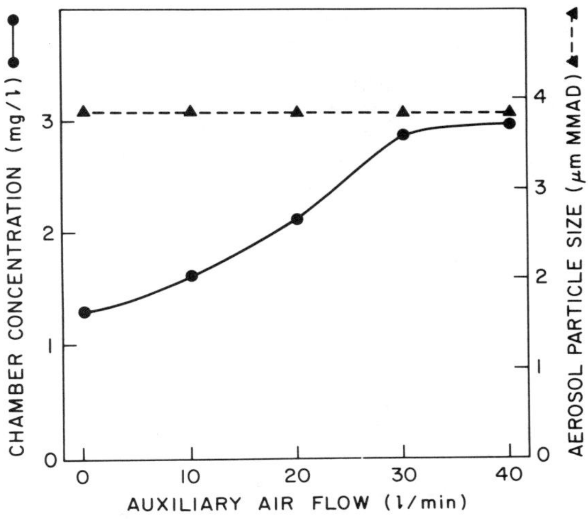

Figure 8 - Performance of the Ohio Ball-jet® Nebulizer as a function of the auxiliary airflow supplied to the nebulizer.

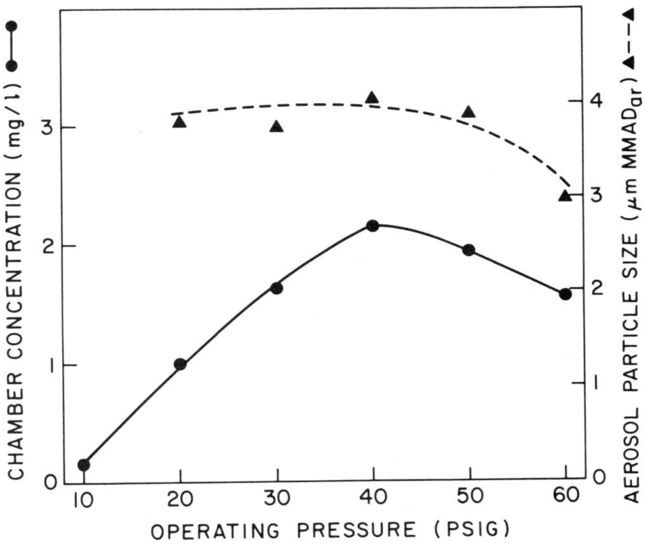

Figure 9 - Performance of the Retec® Nebulizer as a function of operating air pressure supplied to the nebulizer. Output of the nebulizer as indicated by measured chamber concentration tends to decrease at supplied air pressures above 40 psig.

4. Comparative Summary of Results

The performance of the three nebulizers is summarized in Table 1. The Solo-Sphere nebulizer has the highest aerosol output. Aerosol output can be altered linearly by increases in pressure or auxiliary air flow. The range of chamber aerosol concentrations produced in this study was 0.4-10.4 mg/l, or a 20-fold range. The MMAD's of aerosol particle size distribution, ranged from 5.6 to 4.3 um, but were stable at operating pressures above 30 psi. Under all operating conditions, the σg's were stable at 1.5. The nebulizer is easy to disassemble and clean, and all components have good chemical resistance to organics. Parts are readily available.

The Ohio nebulizer has an aerosol output that can be attenuated by both pressure and auxiliary flow. Chamber aerosol concentrations ranged from 0.7 to 3.1 mg/l, a 5-fold range. The median aerosol particle size ranged from 3.8 to 4.5 um and σg's ranged from 1.5 to 1.8. The nebulizer reservoir can be degraded by some organics. We have found it necessary to machine new reservoirs from Teflon® or polypropylene. Parts are somewhat difficult to obtain.

The Retec nebulizer has relatively low output. Output can be attenuated by pressure to 40 psi. However, the nebulizer is not designed to accommodate auxiliary air. The range of chamber aerosol concentrations produced was 0.2 to 1.7 mg/l, a 9-fold range. Median aerosol particle size was decreased from 3.8 um to 3.1 um at operating pressures greater than 40 psi; σg's were constant at about 1.5. Chemical resistance to organics is very poor for components except the aerosol generation jet assembly. For use with organics, the generator components can be constructed out of poly-propylene.

Using the Solo-Sphere nebulizer, more than 25 commercial liquids have been tested as described by the EPA protocol. These liquid test materials belonged to several use classes including: herbicide technicals and formulations, flame retardants, plasticizers and industrial chemicals. The physical properties of the test materials varied widely. Densities ranged from 0.9 mg/l to 3.2 mg/l. Viscosities ranged from 2 to about 150 centipoises. We have found that the efficiency of the Solo-Sphere is decreased for test materials with viscosities greater than about 300 centipoises.

Table 1

Summary of Nebulizer Performance

Nebulizer Type	Aerosol Output	Range of Chamber Aerosol Concentrations (mg/1)	Attentuate Output		Efficiency mg aerosol / 1 nebulizer air	Resistance to Organics
			Pressure	Aux. Flow		
Solo-Sphere	Very High	0.4-10.4 (20)	Yes	Yes	27 (60 psi)	Good
Ohio	Medium	0.7-3.1 (5)	Yes	Yes (limited)	5 (50 psi)	Fair
Retec	Low	0.2-1.7 (9)	Yes (limited)	No	6 (40 psi)	Poor

Nominal concentrations were calculated by dividing the amount of test material lost from the nebulizer by the total air flow through the exposure system. The ratio of the nominal concentration divided by the actual chamber aerosol concentration ranged from 1.2 to greater than 8. The factor was not correlated with any operating parameter of the exposure chamber or nebulizer or any physical property of the test material. These data indicate that the calculated nominal concentration may over-estimate the actual chamber concentration by as much as 800%. In addition, this factor cannot be predicted from exposure system operating conditions.

For all test materials, the aerosol particle size determinations indicated that more than 95% of the aerosol droplets were smaller than 10 um in aerodynamic diameter. For all test materials aerosol particle size determinations performed at 1 and 3 hours during the 4 hour exposure period were essentially identical. These data indicate that aerosols produced by the Solo-Sphere nebulizer have very stable aerosol size distributions and that two determinations are adequate to monitor aerosol particle size, provided that the exposure system is accurately calibrated and closely monitored.

C. A Modification of the Retec Nebulizer to Produce a Stable Generator for Liquid Aerosols Derived from Solutions.

Pneumatic nebulizers such as those described above can also be used to aerosolize solutions. The size of liquid particles generated by nebulization of solutions rather than homogenous test materials is determined by volume and concentration of the original liquid particle droplet. Thus, aerosol median particle size can be altered by changing the air pressure used to operate the nebulizer, effecting particle volume, or by changing the concentration of the nebulized solution, which effects droplet concentration. The disadvantage of this type of nebulizer as a liquid aerosol source is the instability of its output. Solvent evaporates from the solution reservoir into the driving air, causing the solution to become increasingly more concentrated; there is then a corresponding increase in the size of particle generated.

Methods attempted in the past to reduce such effects have included presaturation of the incoming air with solvent (Lauterbach et al, 1956), and by supplying fresh solution to the atomizer from another reservoir (Liu and Lee, 1975). These methods have proved complicated and somewhat cumbersome.

Deford and Moss have modified a Retec pneumatic nebulizer by adding a unique reservoir system. The added modifications were found to stabilize the output of the nebulizer by isolating the effects of solvent evaporation to a small replaced volume of the parent solution. The modified nebulizer is shown in Figure 10. The unit combines a Retec pneumatic nebulizer with a double reservoir configuration. The base of the Retec nebulizer has been removed and its reservoir and with its tube extended to form an aspirating reservoir that is open at the base. A one hole stopper inserted into the open end of the reservoir allows entry of fresh solution from a second reservoir, but minimizes mixing of the solutions. This assembly is placed in one liter filtering flask, which acts as a bulk solution reservoir. There is also a vent tube which is open to the atmosphere at one end and extends into the bulk solution on the other. A vacuum source is fitted to the hose nipple on the filtering flask to provide a vacuum above the bulk solution. The vacuum draws solution from the aspirating reservoir and the vent tube until air bubbles in from the vent tube. The vent tube fixes the position of the aspirating solution level by limiting the vacuum head above the bulk solution. The position of the lower end of the vent tube fixes the height of the solution in the aspirating

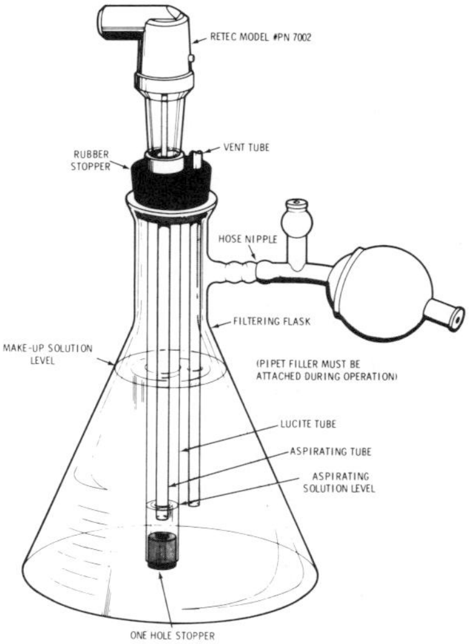

Figure 10 - Retec® Liquid Aerosol Generator for use with solutions. A unique large volume glass reservoir has replaced the reservoir initially provided by the manufacturer. (Courtesy of American Industrial Hygiene Association JOURNAL)

reservoir. As solution is drawn from the aspirating reservoir it is replaced from the bulk reservoir. The solution leaving from the primary reservoir is replaced by air entering from the vent tube. The air incoming through the vent tube maintains the vacuum balance necessary to hold the solution in the aspirating reservoir to a constant level. The concentrating effects of solvent evaporation are confined to the much smaller solution volume of the aspirating reservoir in this system. Thus, in this aspirating reservoir, evaporative pressure from the nebulizer is countered by the continuous influx of fresh solution and rapidly reaches and equilibrium concentration.

A method developed by DeFord and Moss to increase generator output is shown in Figure 11. This figure shows a configuration allowing a single reservoir to supply solution to several aspirating assemblies. This system works in essentially the same way as the case of the single nebulizer. The bulk fluid reservoir is stoppered as before and a vent tube extends through the stopper into the solution. In this configuration, tubing carries solution from the bottom of the bulk reservoir to the bottom of aspirating assemblies that are positioned beside it rather than within it. The application of vacuum to the bulk fluid container and proper positioning of the vent tube again insures a fixed solution level and stable solution concentration with each aspirating volume of each nebulizer. This arrangement allows several nebulizers to be remotely positioned from a single parent solution source, and can linearly increase aerosol output as a function of the number of nebulizers.

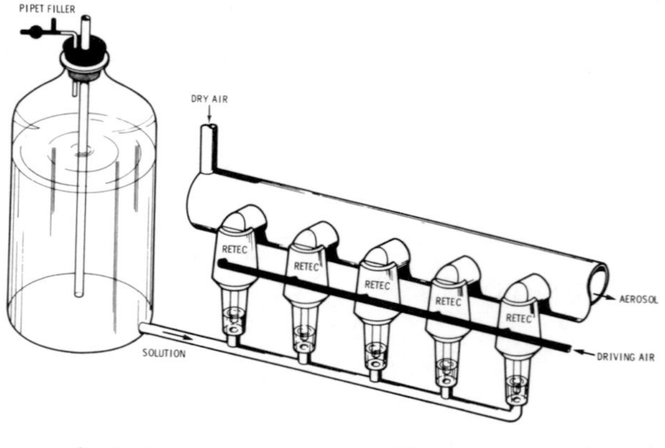

Figure 11 - A multiple generator configuration that allows a single reservoir to provide solution to several aspirating assemblies for higher aerosol output. (Courtesy of American Industrial Hygiene Association JOURNAL)

The performance of the Retec nebulizer with the reservoir system described above was compared to the performance of one modified to have the same total reservoir volume while retaining the conventional single reservoir configuration.

Solution concentrations were monitored measuring the conductivity of a 1 mg/ml NaCl in water solution from the operating generators. Solution was pumped from the reservoirs, through a conducting meter probe, and back to the reservoir. A 14% increase in conductivity occurred when the standard nebulizer was operated at 20 psi from a starting volume of 500 ml solution. This change in conductivity represents a 35% increase in the concentration of the solution. When the modified nebulizer was operated at the same pressure and starting volume, there was a slight increase (<5%) in the conductivity of the aspirating solution during the first hour, but no significant change during the next three hours. There was no corresponding increase in output found when the aerosol output from this generator was monitored. The conductivity of the bulk solution remained stable throughout the 4 hour period.

The output from each nebulizer was continuously monitored for an 11 hour period by a RAM-1® aerosol monitor and recorded on a chart record. The generators were filled with 800 ml of a 2 mg/ml NaCl in water solution and operated at 20 psi. The aerosol was measured at the exhaust end of an aging or drying chamber where the water evaporated, leaving NaCl particles. Figure 12 shows the output from the double reservoir nebulizer. There was no significant change in aerosol output over the 11 hour period. On the other hand,

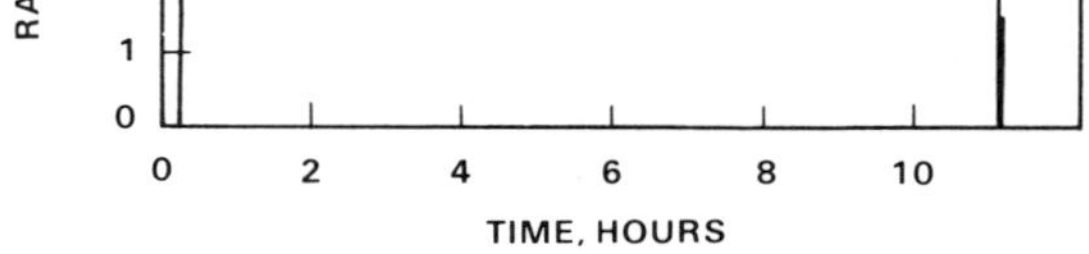

Figure 12 - The output from a RAM-1® aerosol monitor measured at the exhaust end of an aging chamber. No significant change in aerosol production occurred over the extended period of the test. (Courtesy of American Industrial Hygiene Association JOURNAL)

the output from the standard nebulizer increased @ 1.2% per hour for a total increase of 13% for the 11 hour period, demonstrating the greatly increased stability of the modified nebulizer. Such double reservoir nebulizers are currently in use in daily studies requiring inhalation exposures of rodents.

REFERENCES

Dautrebande, L., Beckman, H. and Walkenhorst, W., (1958) New Studies on Aerosols. III. Production of Solid Small-Sized Aerosols. Arch. Int. Pharmacodyn. 66:170-186

Drew, R.T. and Laskin, S., (1973) Environmental Inhalation Chambers. In: Methods of Experimentation. Vol. IV, Academic Press Inc., New York, pp. 1-41

Hazard Evaluation: Humans and Domestic Animals in the Environmental Protection Agency Proposed Guidelines for Registering Pesticides in the United States. Fed. Reg. 43:37331-37402 (1978).

Hinners, R.G., Burhart, J.K. and Punte, C.L., (1968) Animal Inhalation Exposure Chambers. Arch. Environ. Health. 16:194-206

Lauterbach, K.E., Hayes, A.D. and Coelho, M.A, (1956) An Improved Aerosol Generator. AMA Arch. Ind. Health. 13:156-160

Liu, B. Y. H. and Lee, K. W., (1975) An Aerosol Generator of High Stability. Amer. Ind. Hyg. Assoc. J. 36:861-872

Mercer, T.T., Tillery, M.I. and Chow, H.Y., (1968) Operating Characteristics of Some Compress Air Nebulizers. Amer. Ind. Hyg. Assoc. J. 20:66

Phalen, R. F., (1976) Inhalation Exposure of Animals. Environ. Health Perspect. 16:17-24

Raabe, O.G., (1976) The Generation of Aerosols of Fine Particles. In: Fine Particles: Aerosol Measurement, Sampling and Analysis. B.Y.H. Liu, ed., Academic Press, Inc., New York. pp. 129-143

Raabe, O.G., MacFarland, K.D. and Tarkington, B.K., (1979) Generation of Respirable Aerosols of Power Plant Fly Ash for Inhalation Studies with Experimental Animals. Env. Sci. Technol. 13:836-840

Sachsse, K., Ullmann, L., Voss., G. and Hess, R., (1974) Measurement of Inhalation Toxicity of Aerosols in Small Laboratory Animals. In: Preceedings of the European Society for the Study of Drug Toxicity. Vol. XV, American Elsevier Publishing Co., New York, pp. 239-251

Dust Sampling, Characterization and Concentration Monitoring in Toxicity Studies

ROBERT L. CARPENTER
Lovelace Inhalation Toxicology Research Institute
Albuquerque, NM

JOHN A. PICKRELL
Lovelace Inhalation Toxicology Research Institute
Albuquerque, NM

ABSTRACT

Inhalation toxicity studies using toxic dusts present unique particle dispersal and inhalation exposure monitoring problems often not associated with liquid or water soluble toxicants. When the dust being aerosolized is composed of fibrous particles, additional analytical difficulties arise. Relationships between the parameters used to characterize aerosols (size distribution, mass concentration and particle number concentration) may be readily established for compact, nearly spherical particles because the volume of a sphere is related to the diameter cubed. For fibers approximating right circular cylinders, particle volume depends on the diameter squared and the length. Thus, two parameters must be measured for each particle to determine the fiber volume distribution; determination of average fiber length and average fiber diameter are not adequate to determine average fiber volume.

The methods described here were employed to control a 19-day inhalation exposure and characterize the fiber aerosol used as a toxicant. Simultaneous fiber length and diameter determinations were used to classify fibers in a length/diameter matrix. Median fiber length was 11.4 micrometers and average fiber diameter was 0.16 micrometers. From this classification, fiber volume distribution could be determined allowing total fiber number and fiber number greater than 20 micrometers to be calculated. The exposure fiber aerosol contained 42000-61000 fibers/cc of which 6-8% were longer than 20 micrometers. Feedstock characterization of material from a single manufacturer suggests a relationship between observed fiber length and diameter which, if generally valid, could materially reduce fiber sizing requirements.

INTRODUCTION

Inhalation toxicity studies using dust aerosols present a unique set of experimental difficulties in comparison to similar studies using liquids or water soluble toxicants. These differences become more significant when the dust under consideration is composed of fibrous particles instead of spherical (or nearly spherical), compactly shaped particles. When aerosolized, soluble or liquid toxicant particle size is usually controlled by the apparatus used to generate the aerosol. In contrast, aerosolization by dust dispersal cannot produce an aerosol having particles smaller than those present in the feedstock material. Thus, feedstock characterization becomes an important preliminary step in determining achievable aerosol particle sizes.

Inhalation toxicity studies require aerosol sampling and characterization efforts for two distinct but often overlapping purposes. During the daily exposure period, measurement of one or more aerosol parameter (particle size distribution, particle number concentration or aerosol mass concentration) must be carried out on a nearly real-time basis to provide the information necessary to control the aerosol generator and chamber ventilation apparatus. Although practice varies widely, these measurements are made either by continuously reading instruments (nephelometers or optical particle size analyzers) or repeatedly using grab sampling techniques (Snellings, 1981). Additional aerosol characterization measurements are often made to further define the aerosol size distribution parameters and the aerosol chemical composition. The data obtained in turn establish the quantity and nature of the inhaled toxicant dose and subsequent biological fate. These measurements need not be made on a near real-time basis. Aerosol size distribution, number concentration, mass concentration and chemical composition may be measured by a variety of instruments for compact particles. Their use and limitations have been recently reviewed along with current practice in inhalation toxicology and aerosol generation (Willeke, 1980).

Although the need to control dust inhalation exposures and characterize the aerosolized particles remains when the dusts used are composed of fibrous particles, the equipment available for the task is more limited. Fiber aerosol mass may be measured using filters as in the compact particle case. In principle, fiber number concentration may be measured with the Fibrous Aerosol Monitor that has recently become available (GCA Corporation, Bedford, MA). However, this instrument, intended primarily a fiber monitor for workplace exposures, is limited to low fiber count rates (20 fibers/cc) (Lilienfield, 1977). Many investigators exposing animals to fibers have only been able to report fiber mass concentration, relying on the use of reference materials such as UICC asbestos to define the physical size distribution of this fiber aerosol (Timbrell, 1968; Hounam, 1970).

Continued research has indicated that fiber toxicity for both asbestos and glass fibers is related to fiber size (Ki, 1979; Stanton, 1977; Morgan, 1978; Timbrell, 1971). The recognition of these size effects resulted from examination of aerosolized and instilled fiber preparations by optical and electron microscopy. Average fiber diameter and average fiber length have been the parameters reported. However, it is important to recognize that the conversion from aerosolized fiber mass to fiber number concentration requires a knowledge of the average fiber volume which cannot be obtained from a knowledge of average fiber dimensions alone.

We wish to report the use of a method of classifying fibers by length and diameter which allows conversion from fiber mass to fiber number concentration. This method requires minimal additional sampling during an inhalation exposure but does involve considerable additional fiber sizing effort. Length/diameter fiber classification further allows one to apply length and diameter criteria to the observed fiber population and determine fiber number within a defined subpopulation. During a 19-day inhalation exposure of rats to an experimental microfiber, the exposure was controlled on the basis of fiber concenrtration from filter samples taken during the exposure. Additional samples were taken with a sampling electrostatic precipitator for sizing from scanning electron micrographs. We also wish to report that fiber feedstock examination suggests the presence of three subpopulations of fibers in insulation produced by a single manufacturer. In the case of these insulation fiber preparations, evidence exists for a length/diameter relationship which, if validated would substantially reduce the fiber sizing effort required to characterize the exposure aerosol.

MATERIALS AND METHODS

Glass fiber household insulation from a commercial source and two microfiber insulation materials were characterized as potential source materials for inhalation exposures. These materials were prepared for light and scanning electron microscopic examination as well as aerosolization by embedding the insulation material in polyethylene glycol (Carbowax) blocks, microtoming the blocks, washing the fibers with distilled water and separating the fibers by centrifugation from the water soluble carbowax (Pickrell, 1978). Fibers were dispersed using an amyl nitrate and cellulase acetate suspension medium. Drops of the fiber suspension were smeared onto glass slides for microscopic examination. Sample preparation for scanning electron microscopy (SEM) required fiber dispersion in a eutectic mixture of camphor and napthalen. After dispersion, the eutectic mixture was smeared onto a carbon sample substrate. The camphor napthalene mixture was removed by freeze drying. During animal exposures, fiber samples were collected directly from the exposure chamber using a point-to-plane electrostatic precipitator originally described by Morrow and Mercer (1964) (In-Tox Products, Albuquerque, NM). The electrostatic precipitator was operated on a current of 3 microamperes and a flow of 100 cc/min. (Cheng, 1981). Fibers collected in this manner were deposited directly on the SEM carbon sample substrate. A drop of ethanol was used to lay the fibers flat on the substrate surface before placing the fibers in the microscope (See Results). From SEM photomicrographs, length and diameter of each fiber were measured in randomly selected fields. SEM photomicrographs were taken at 1000X magnification. These measurements were classified into a length/diameter matrix (Table I) using cells of 5-10 micrometers (length class interval) and 0.05-0.1 micrometers (diameter class interval). The classification of fibers by both length and diameter allowed calculation of not only count median diameter (CMD) and length (CML) but also average fiber volume, average fiber mass and the number of fibers associated with a given mass sample. Average fiber volume was computed from fiber CMD and CML as well as being determined from the fiber volume distribution based on individual fiber volumes.

Fischer-344 rats were exposed to aerosolized glass microfibers using the system illustrated in Figure 1. Aerosols of prepared fibers were generated for 5-6 hours per day, 5 days per week, for 19 days to create an exposure atmosphere in a modified 27-inch Laskin type chamber. Two fluidized bed aerosol generators were used to aerosolize the fibers (Carpenter, 1980a; Carpenter, 1980b). A 2 to 5%

Table I. Composite Fiber Dimensions, Length/Diameter Matrix

D (μm) L (μm)	5	5-10	10-15	15-20	20-25	25-30	30-40	40	a	cf[b]
0.05	46	24	14	5	5	1	0	0	95	0.25
0.05-0.10	41	27	10	5	1	1	0	2	87	0.48
0.10-0.15	32	25	5	1	0	1	2	1	67	0.66
0.15-0.20	13	25	5	1	0	1	0	1	47	0.78
0.20-0.25	13	11	5	2	2	0	1	0	34	0.87
0.25-0.30	1	6	3	2	1	0	0	0	13	0.90
0.30-0.40	4	9	4	3	0	1	0	0	21	0.96
0.40	0	6	3	3	2	0	0	0	14	CMD = 0.11 μm
cf	0.40	0.75	0.88	0.94	0.97	0.98	CML = 6.47 mm			

[a]Total number of fibers within the indicated interval.

[b]Cumulative fiber fraction of total fibers counted.

NOTE: Diameter class interval: 0.05 μm, Length class interval: 10 μm. Fibers are summed by both length (horizontal rows) and by diameter (vertical rows) to obtain data for cumulative length and cumulative diameter distributions.

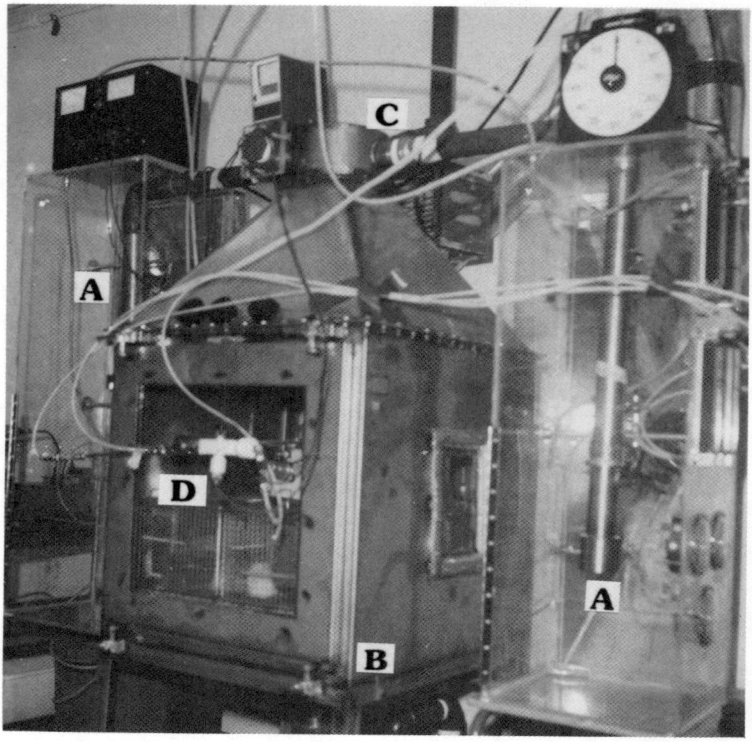

FIGURE 1 Photograph of inhalation exposure apparatus for glass fibers. A. Fluid Bed Aerosol Generators; B. Exposure Chamber; C. Aerosol inlet ducts; D. Sampling filters and electrostatic precipitor.

slurry of distilled water and 1 g of the microfiber preparation were sonicated and added to 200 ml of bed material. The wetted material was mixed and dried overnight. This preparation was repeated to supply adequate material for each aerosol generator as needed. Each aerosol generator operated with 35 liters per minute (LPM) air flow and employed an ^{85}Kr discharger (Teague, 1978). Generators contained 200 ml of the bed material/glass fiber mixture. The generators were emptied and refilled with a fresh bed material mixture every 2 hours. The system was operated by alternately refilling each generator at one-hour intervals.

Open-face filter samples of the aerosolized fibers were collected for exposure mass concentration measurement. These filters were weighed immediately and aerosolized fiber mass concentration calculated. The results were used to control the aerosol generators. A Medical Research Council (MRC) horizontal elutriator (Casella, London, England) was operated at different positions within the chamber for 1 to 3 hours to estimate respirable fiber mass concentration. Samples collected by the horizontal elutriator could not be analyzed until after each daily exposure was completed. At specified intervals during the exposure, electrostatic precipitator (ESP) samples were collected for SEM photomicrographic analysis of fiber length and diameter.

RESULTS

The fiber aerosols produced by the inhalation exposure system are single fiber aerosols (Figure 2). However, examination of steroscopic scanning electron micrographs revealed a considerable number of fibers collected by a point-to-plane electrostatic precipitator lie at varying angles to

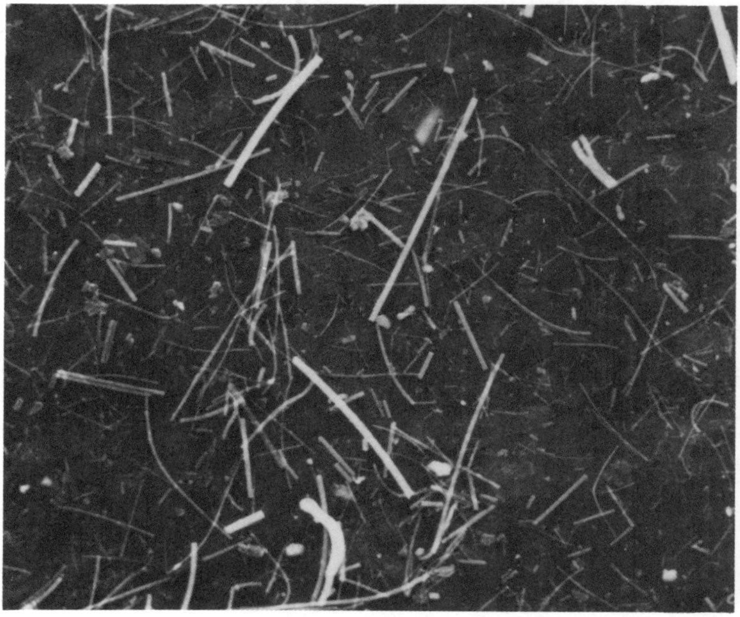

FIGURE 2 Scanning electron micrograph of aerosolized fibers

the plane of the carbon substrate (Gray, 1980). Placing a drop of ethanol on the substrate surface when viewed in the same manner. Figure 3 shows the alteration of median fiber dimensions as a result of this treatment.

Inhalation exposures were carried out for 19 days. During each exposure day the fiber mass concentration fluctuated due to the alternate refilling of the aerosol

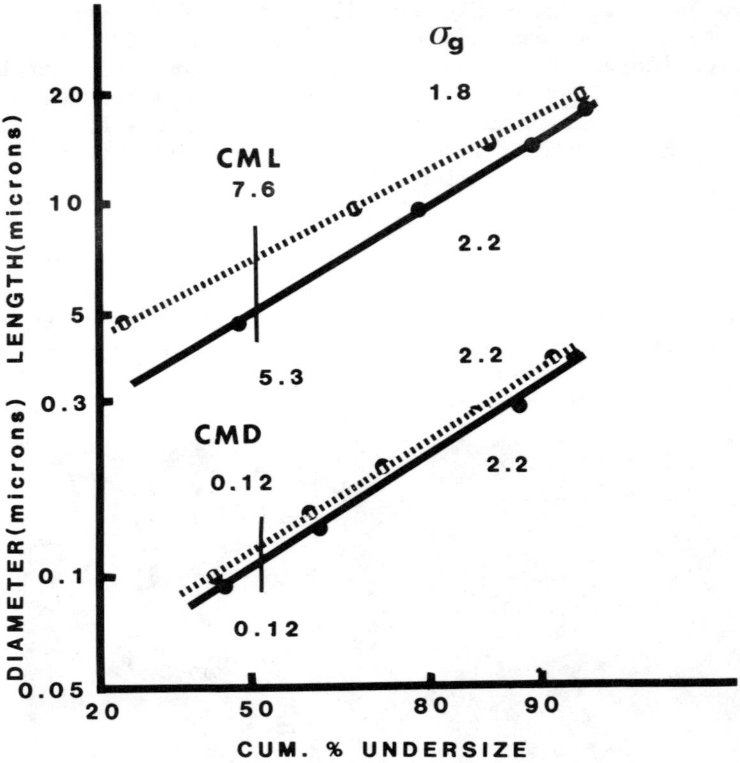

FIGURE 3 Effects of ethanol treatment on observed fiber population dimensions after collection by electrostatic precipitation. Dashed line represents fiber population after treatment and solid line represents that before treatment.

generators. Figure 4 shows the daily fiber mass concentrations observed during the exposure period. Peak mass concentrations were those observed immediately after changing an aerosol generator bed. Integrated average concentrations were obtained from an open face filter operated throughout the exposure day. "Respirable particles" refer to the fiber mass concentration obtained from the MRE elutriator.

Fiber dimensions were obtained from SEM micrographs and classified in length/diameter matrices as described. From these data, cumulative plots of fiber length and diameter were obtained. Figure 5 summarizes the three weekly averages obtained. The fiber CML was 11.4 micrometers and fiber CMD was 0.16 micrometers. Average fiber volume was 3.1 x 10^{-13} cc corresponding to 0.77 pg average mass/fiber. These

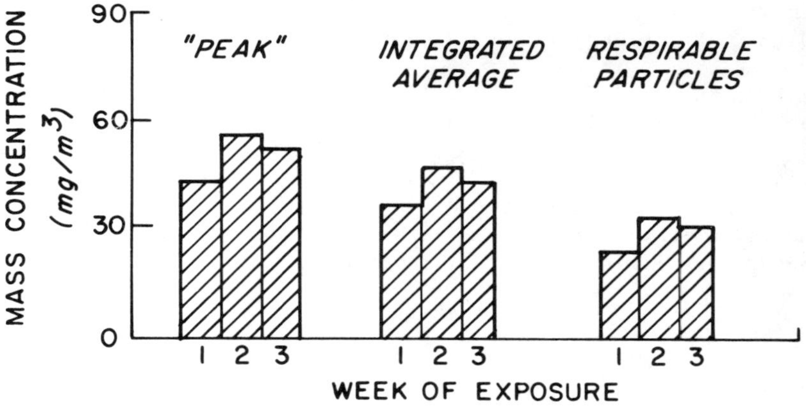

FIGURE 4 Average daily fiber mass concentration during rat inhalation exposure studies. Respirable fiber mass is determined by the MRC Horizontal Elutriator (Aerodynamic Diameter)

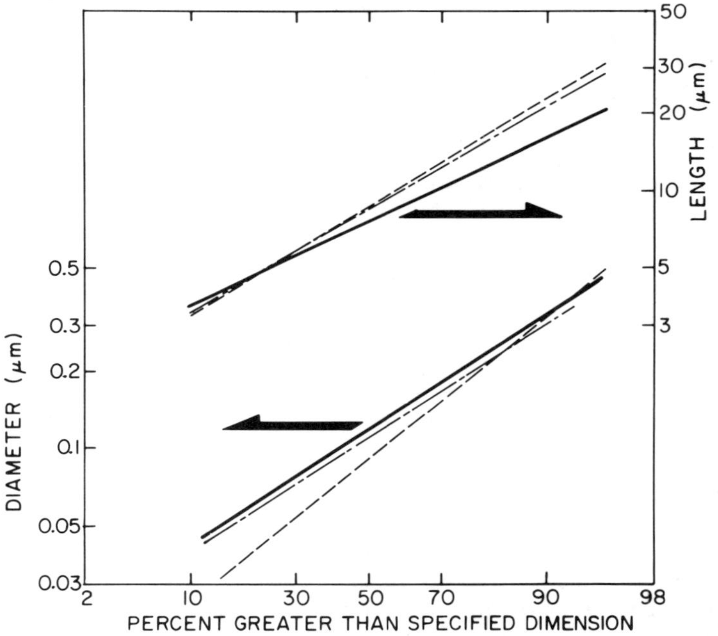

FIGURE 5 Aerosolized fiber length and diameter as a function of percent less than stated dimension

mass and concentration data correspond to 42000-61000 fibers/cc in the exposure chamber. Of these fibers, 6-8% or from 2500 to 5100 fibers/cc were longer than 20 micrometers.

Examination of fiber feedstock material with SEM indicates that fiber diameters are not log-normally distributed (Figure 6). The data for experimental microfiber two may be resolved into a mixture of two log-normal distributions, 33% of the fibers belonging to a population having a modal diameter of 1.3 micrometers (σ_g = 1.7) and 67% belonging to a population having a modal diameter of 0.2 micrometers (σ_g = 2.1).

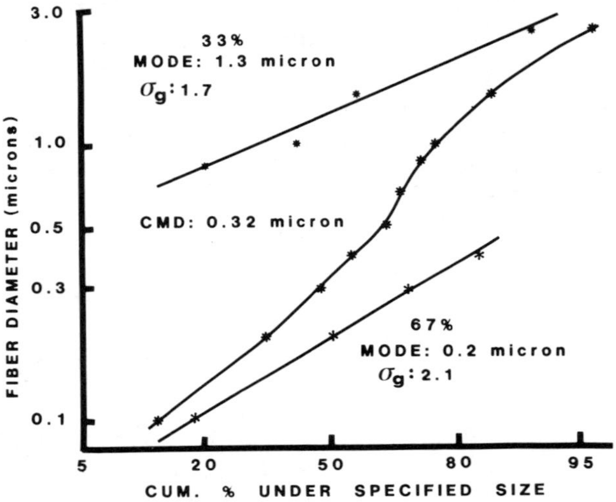

FIGURE 6 Cumulative size distribution of experimental microfiber two. The fiber diameter distribution may be proportioned between two log-normal distributions, indicating that 33% of the fibers have a CMD of 1.3 μm and 67% have a CMD of 0.2 μm.

DISCUSSION

The combined use of fiber mass concentration measurement and fiber size determination from photomicrographs offers several advantages over mass concentration measurements alone for characterizing fiber inhalation exposures. During the course of an inhalation exposure, exposure control must be based on the measurement of some readily available parameter. Inhalation studies using compact particles may be controlled on the basis of particle concentration, size or composition. Monitoring instrumentation to measure these parameters on a real-time or near real-time basis is available in many instances. Mass concentration is, however, the only readily available parameter for exposure control if the toxicant aerosol is fibrous. Considerable additional information is available if length and diameter measurements are made on samples of the exposure aerosol. The use of a sampling electrostatic precipitator allows one to examine the aerosol with a minimum of sample preparation, allowing observations concerning the presence or absence of aggregates in the exposure aerosol. The problems associated with fiber collection at an angle with the ESP may be eliminated by using ethanol to lay the fibers over. The data in Figure 4 provide some insight into the nature of this collection phenomena. Neither CMD nor $_D\sigma_g$ (geometric standard deviation of diameter distribution) of the observed fiber population is changed by the ethanol treatment, suggesting that essentially identical populations were counted before and after the ethanol treatment. However, CML increased following ethanol treatment while the $_L\sigma_g$ (geometric standard deviation of length distribution) was reduced, suggesting that shorter fibers were collected at more variable angles than were long fibers. The mechanisms responsible for this phenomena require additional elucidation.

When length and diameter measurements are made on the same fiber and the fibers are classified in a length/diameter matrix, the volume distribution of the aerosolized fibers may be computed. If fiber density is known, the fiber mass distribution may be estimated. Average fiber dimensions taken from independent fiber length and diameter measurements cannot be used to estimate average fiber mass because these average fiber population parameters bear an unknown relationship to the fiber volume distribution. Data from our exposures indicate that the use of average dimensions will underestimate the average fiber mass of the fiber aerosol. The mass of a right circular cylinder 11.4 micrometers long and 0.16 micrometers in diameter and having a density of 2.5 g/cm^3 is 0.57 pg. The average fiber mass of the exposure aerosol having the above average dimensions was 0.77 pg based on the observed fiber volume distribution.

The fiber aerosol to which Fischer-344 rats were exposed was log-normally distributed with respect to length and diameter (Figure 5). The aerosol had a CMD of approximately 0.1 micrometers and a CML approximately 11 micrometers yielding an aspect ratio of approximately 100, clearly exceeding the generally accepted fiber criteria of a 3:1 aspect ratio. This aspect ratio was variable making mass/diameter relationships complex and variable. Further investigation of these relationships is under way at ITRI. Clearly, they are not well enough defined at this point to be used as a major criteria of fiber aerosol characteristics, although fiber aspect ratios do reflect the shape of aerosolized fibers.

Length/diameter characterization may also be applied to fiber feedstock materials for aerosolization. We have compared median length and diameter characteristics of the fibers prepared by microtoming with those observed in the workplace by a number of investigators (Figure 7) (Fowler, 1971; Corn, 1976; Esmen, 1978; Esmen, 1981). From the available data, it is apparent that this laboratory preparation procedure yields fibers similar in length and diameter to those found in the workplace. Whether or not the fiber aspect ratios are similar is unknown.

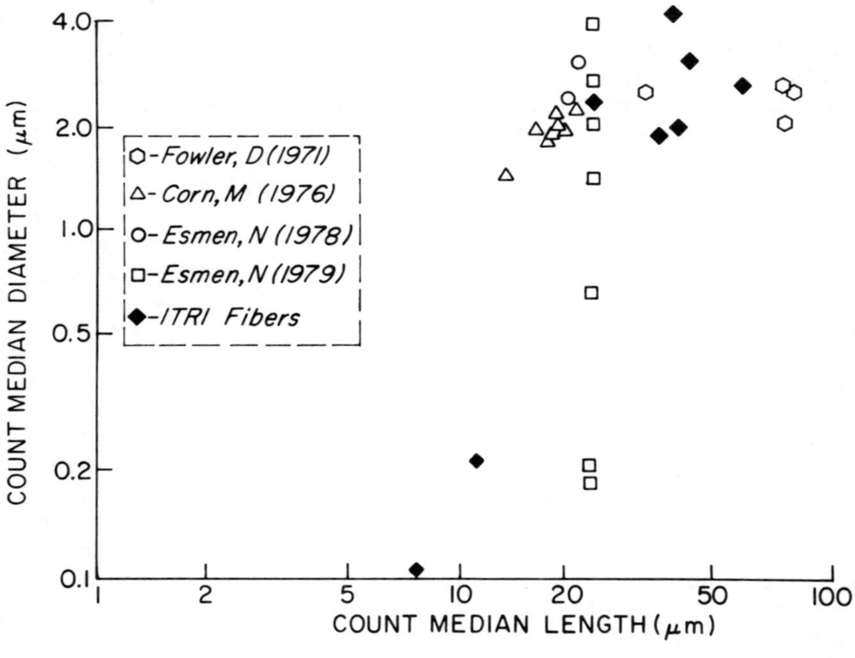

FIGURE 7 Comparison of fibers sampled in the workplace and fibers prepared at ITRI from commercial material.

Fiber feedstock characterization reveals that the exposure aerosol contained fibers from two discernible fiber populations. No more than 67% by number of the fibers placed in the FBG were from the small diameter population of primary interest from an inhalation toxicity standpoint.

Similar characteristics have been observed for the other insulation materials examined as potential aerosol feedstocks. These fiber preparations not only had more than one distribution of fiber sizes, but that these distributions could be grouped into small (modal diameter 0.1-0.2 micrometers), medium (modal diameters 1-1.3 micrometers) and large (modal diameter 2-4 micrometers). Figure 8 summarizes these data. Although these data are from a limited number of insulation materials, they suggest that as the median diameter of insulation materials decreases from that used today (2-4 micrometers) to smaller, more thermally efficient fibers (0.1 to 0.3 micrometers), the relative amounts of medium and small fibers may increase. Since Stanton et al. (1977) believe that these may be dangerous if long enough (8 micrometers), an inhalation hazard may exist if widespread use is made of microfiber insulation material.

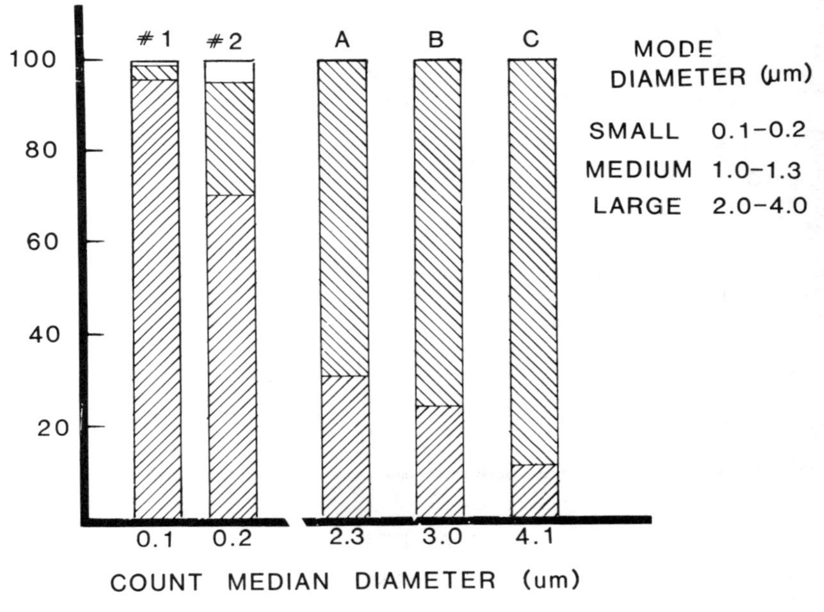

FIGURE 8 Size distribution components in fiber preparations. [hatched box] Small Diameter [hatched box] Medium Diameter [open box] Large Diameter

Examination of feedstock materials prepared from insulation materials produced by one manufacturer also suggests that the fibers in these preparations may show a correlation between length and diameter which extends not only to microfibers but also to household (commercial insulation fibers) of much larger diameter (Figure 9). If this correlation is present among the aerosolized fibers, the use of either fiber length or diameter distributions would be sufficient to describe the fiber aerosol. The numerical constants of the correlation equation could be used to define the fiber aspect ratios in the aerosol. Such a relationship would also define fiber mass as a function of diameter, greatly simplifying fiber characterization.

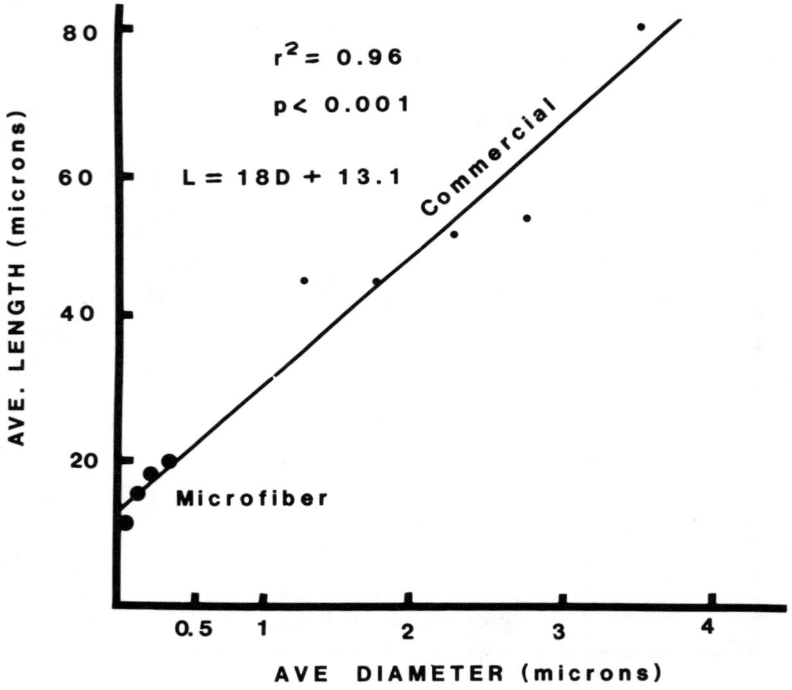

FIGURE 9 Correlation between fiber length and fiber diameter

In conclusion, it should be pointed out that control and characterization of fiber aerosol inhalation exposures is complicated by a lack of real-time monitoring equipment and by the fact that fiber mass determination requires determination of two parameters for each particle rather than a single parameter (diameter in case of spherical particles). Concurrent mass and size distribution samples allow extensive fiber aerosol characterization if length and diameter measurements are made on the same fibers and they are classified by length and diameter.

ACKNOWLEDGEMENTS

The authors gratefully acknowledge the helpful advice of their colleagues, Drs. H. C. Yeh, B. V. Mokler and G. M. Kanapilly. We also wish to express our appreciation to Drs. C. H. Hobbs and R. O. McClellan for their support. We are indebted to Ms C. S. Sass and Ms F. C. Strauss for their patience in sizing glass fibers, and Mr. K. L. Yerkes for his assistance in setting up and operating the experiment. Research supported under U. S. Department of Energy Contract No. DE-AC04-76EV01013.

REFERENCES

Carpenter, R. L. and Yerkes, K. L. (1980a) Relationship between fluid bed aerosol generator operation and the aerosol produced. Am. Ind. Hyg. Assoc. J. 41;888-894.

Carpenter, R. L., Pickrell, J. A., Mokler, B. A., Yeh, H. C., DeNee, P. B. (1980b) Behavior of a fluid bed aerosol generator as a source of aerosolized fibers. Inhalation Toxicology Research Institute Annual Report, LMF-84, p 501 (available from NTIS, U.S. Department of Commerce, Springfield, VA 22161).

Cheng, Y. S. and Yeh, H. C. (1981) Collection efficiencies of a point-to-plane electrostatic precipitator. Am. Ind. Hyg. Assoc. J. (submitted).

Corn, M., Hammad, Y., Whittier, D. and Kotsko, N. (1976) Employee exposure to airborne fiber and total particulate matter in two mineral wool facilities. Environ. Res. 12: 59-74.

Esmen, N., Hammad, Y. Y., Corn, M., Whittier, D., Kotsko, N., Haller, M. and Kahn, R. A. (1978) Exposure of employees to man-made mineral fibers: Mineral wool production. Environ. Res. 15: 262-277.

Esmen, N., Corn, M., Hammad, Y., Whittier, D. and Kotsko, N. (1981) Results of measurement of employee exposure to airborne dust and fiber in sixteen facilities producing man-made mineral fibers. Am. Ind. Hyg. Assoc. J. (in press).

Fowler, D. P., Balzer, J. L. and Cooper, W. C. (1971) Exposure of insulation workers to airborne fibrous glass. Am. Ind. Hyg. Assoc. J. 32: 86-91.

Gray, R. H., Kanapilly, G. M., DeNee, P. B., Cheng, Y. S. and Wolff, R. K. (1980) Stereographic analysis of aggregate aerosols. Inhalation Toxicology Research Institute Annual Report, LMF-84, p 416 (available from NTIS, U.S. Department of Commerce, Springfield, VA 22161).

Haunam, R. K. F. (1970) The konimiser-A dispender for the continuous generation of dust clouds from milligram quantities of asbestos. Ann. Occup. Hyg. 14: 329-355.

Ki, P. Lee, Barras, C. E., Griffith, F. D. and Warity, R. S. (1979) Pulmonary response to glass fiber by inhalation exposure. Lab. Invest. 40: 123-133.

Lilienfield, P. (1977) Development and fabrication of a prototype fibrous aerosol monitor. DHEW (NIOSH) Publication No. 78-125 (available from NTIS, U. S. Department of Commerce, Springfield, VA 22161.

Mercer, T. T. and Morrow, P. E. (1964) A point-to-plane electrostatic precipitator for particle size sampling. Am. Ind. Hyg. Assoc. J. 25: 8-14.

Morgan, A., Talbot, R. J. and Holmes, A. (1978) Significance of fibre length in the clearance of asbestos fibers from the lung. Br. J. Ind. Med. 35: 153.

Pickrell, J. A., Mokler, B. V., Villa, D. A., Sass, K. S., Hobbs, C. H. and DeNee, P. B. (1978) Preparation and characterization of commercial insulation fibers for use in inhalation studies. Inhalation Toxicology Research Institute Annual Report, LF-60, p 463 (available from NTIS, U.S. Department of Commerce, Springfield, VA 22161).

Snellings, W. M. (1981) Everything you always wanted to know about chronic inhalation testing but were afraid to ask. In Inhalation Chamber Technology, Brookhaven National Laboratory Report (in press).

Stanton, M. F., Layard, M., Tegeris, A., Miller, E., May, M. and Kent, E. (1977) Carcinogenicity of fibrous glass: Pleural response in the rat in relation to fiber dimension. J. Natl. Cancer Inst. 58: 587-603.

Teague, S. V., Yeh, H. C. and Newton, G. J. (1978) Fabrication and use of krypton-85 aerosol discharge devices. Health Phys. 35: 392-395.

Timbrell, V., Hyett, A. W. and Skidmore, J. W. (1968) A simple dispenser for generating dust clouds from standard reference samples of asbestos. Ann. Occup. Hyg. 11: 273-281.

Timbrell, V. and Skidmore, J. (1971) The effect of shape on particle penetration and retention in animals lungs. In Inhaled Particles and Vapors III, Vol. 1, (W. H. Walton, ed.) Gresham Press, Surrey, England, pp 48-57.

Willeke, K. (1980) Generation of aerosols and facilities for exposure experiments. Ann Arbor Science Publishers, Ann Arbor, MI.

A New Dust Generator for Inhalation Toxicological Studies

B.K.J. LEONG and D.J. POWELL
Industrial Toxicology and Inhalation Toxicology Laboratories

G.L. POCHYLA
Mechanical Engineering

The Upjohn Company
Kalamazoo, Michigan 49001

ABSTRACT

A dust generator capable of dispersing a variety of powders of different flow capabilities in air for inhalation toxicological studies has been developed. This dust generator consists of a horizontal rotating disk for transporting the powders from a pressurized reservoir to a "blow-hole" where the powder is discharged in puffs as a deagglomerated dust atmosphere.

INTRODUCTION

In dust inhalation toxicological studies, the experimental animals have to be exposed to a controlled dust atmosphere in an exposure chamber for an extended period of time. In order to generate and maintain a constant level of the dust in the test atmosphere, a dust generator capable of metering and dispersing a defined quantity of powder per unit time into the chamber airflow is required.

Powdery materials may be arbitrarily classified in accordance with their flow properties into "free-flowing", "non-free-flowing" and a whole spectrum of flowability in-between. A free-flowing powder is likely to be hydrophobic, granular, smooth surfaced and relatively monodispersed in particle size, whereas a non-free-flowing powder is likely to be hydrophilic, fiberous, rough-surfaced and polydispersed in particle size (Carr, 1965 a and b). The free-flowing powders are also likely to be more easily dispersed in air to form a dust atmosphere than the non-free-flowing powders.

Many devices have been developed for metering and dispersing free-flowing powders. One device, a commonly used laboratory dust feed apparatus, operates by allowing a powder to flow from a vibrating hopper onto a rotating turntable. A stationary blade then scrapes the powders into a uniform powder "ribbon". As the front of the ribbon passes under the suction head of a compressed air aspirator-ejector, the powders are sucked into the air stream and dispersed upon leaving the ejector nozzle (Silverman, 1956). Another device, called the NBS dust generator, which is commercially available, allows the powder to flow from a hopper into calibrated grooves of a rotating gear. The powder is than aspirated and dispersed by a compressed air ejector (Dill, 1938).

Both aforementioned devices suffer from the following deficiencies: (a) lack of powder containment structure for preventing the powder from spreading and contaminating the whole apparatus; (b) require a high airflow rate for aspirating and dispersing the powders into dust atmosphere; (c) lack precision in delivering small quantity of powder per unit time; and (d) do not work well for non-free-flowing powders.

For generating dust atmospheres from non-free-flowing powders, the most widely used generator is the Wright Dust Feed (Wright, 1949,1950). It is operated by pre-packing a powder manually or with a hydraulic press into a feed cylinder. The surface of the powder cake is then mechanically scraped off at a controlled rate into loose powder again for dispersion by a stream of high velocity compressed air. This apparatus works well for a variety of packable fine powders but not for the coarse and non-packable powders. It is not workable for hygroscopic materials. The dust output is very small in comparison to those of the turntable and the NBS generators.

Another technique for aerosolizing powders is by the use of a TSI fluidized-bed aerosol generator (Marple, 1978). In operation, the powder is fed at a constant rate via a chain conveyor from a reservoir into a fluidized bed of bronze beads where the powders are deagglomerated and aerosolized. In the process, the fine particles are segregated from the larger particles resulting in a change in particle size distribution and perhaps a change in the composition of a test material. It takes about 3.5 hours for the fluidized bed to achieve constant output following the initial introduction of powder from the reservoir. The maximum concentration of dust atmosphere exiting the generator is approximately 0.175 mg/l which is much too low a concentration to meet the requirements of most inhalation toxicity studies.

Most recently, a dust generator (IRDC dust generator) has been tested and proven to be suitable for generating high dust concentrations for toxicological studies (Leong, 1979). This dust generator consists essentially of a rotating disk with calibrated "holes" for transporting a consistent amount of powder per unit time from a reservoir to a "blow-hole". At the "blow-hole" the powder in the hole is dispersed by a jet of pressurized air. For generating dust atmosphere from free-flowing powders, this apparatus can be operated with little or no maintenance for several hours. For dispersing non-free-flowing powders, some attention is needed to ensure the stirring mechanism in the reservoir keeps filling the holes properly. Because of the many sealed shaft bearings and ball bearings which are essential for supporting the drive shafts of the rotating disc and the stirring mechanism, some attention in cleaning the bearings and freeing the shafts are needed during or at the end of a run of several hours.

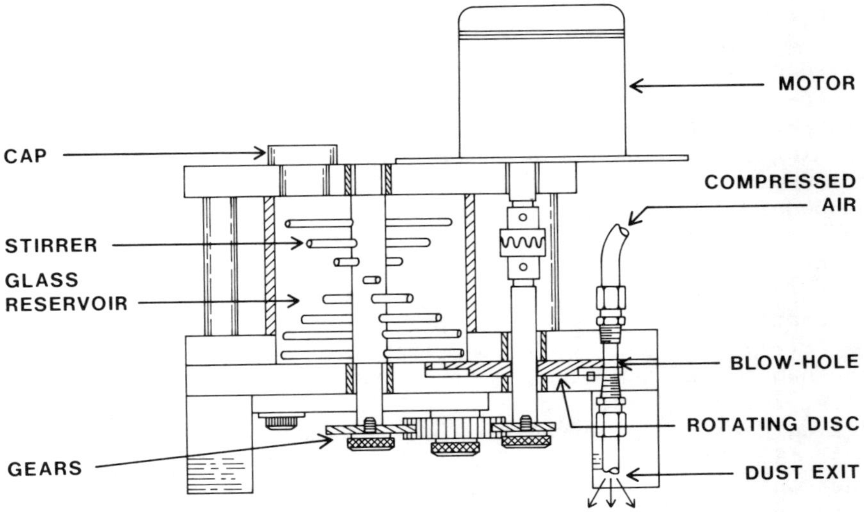

Figure 1. Diagram of the IRDC dust generator.

In view of the shortcomings of the aforementioned dust generators, there is a need for designing a dust generator which (1) is economical and easy to manufacture; (2) permits the generation of dust atmospheres from free-flowing and non-free-flowing powders; (3) is capable of operating for a long period of time with minimal maintenance requirements; and (4) can generate dust atmospheres at a wide range of concentration.

THE NEW DUST GENERATOR

The new dust generator consists of a base plate having a horizontal and circular recess which houses a rotatable circular disk. This disk has eight or more transverse openings which circumvent coaxially with the disk. A cover plate partially covers the disk and has a screw mount for any type of screw cap bottle with a 2" opening. The bottle and the circular recess together form an air tight compartment with the powder in direct contact with the disk. A pair of coaxial openings are provided through the cover and the base plates for successive alignment with the transverse openings as the disk rotates. These two openings are in communication with a compressed air source. A leakage space is provided between the disk and the cover plate so that compressed air can pass through the space into the powder container when the transverse opening is not in alignment with the coaxial openings. The powder is thereby agitated and loaded into the transverse openings as the bottle is being pressurized. When a powder-laden transverse opening moves into alignment with the coaxial openings, the powder is discharged as a "puff" of deagglomerated dust (Figure 2).

There are several useful features in this new dust generator.

(1) The rate of dust dissemination is regulated by the number and the size of the transverse openings in the disk, the gear ratio between the disk gear and the motor driven gear, and the speed of the driving motor.

(2) For loading a wide variety of powders, free-flowing and non-free-flowing, into the calibrated transverse openings, an air vibrator can be mounted on the powder reservoir. The loading efficiency can be adjusted by sliding the vibrator up or down the cylindrical bottle, and by regulating the rate of air flowing through the air vibrator and hence the frequency of the vibration.

(3) The powder reservoir is mounted on the top of the rotating disk allowing the use of a bottle of any size and shape as long as it has the same screw thread as that of the mounting plate.

(4) Any unused powder can be returned to the bottle by

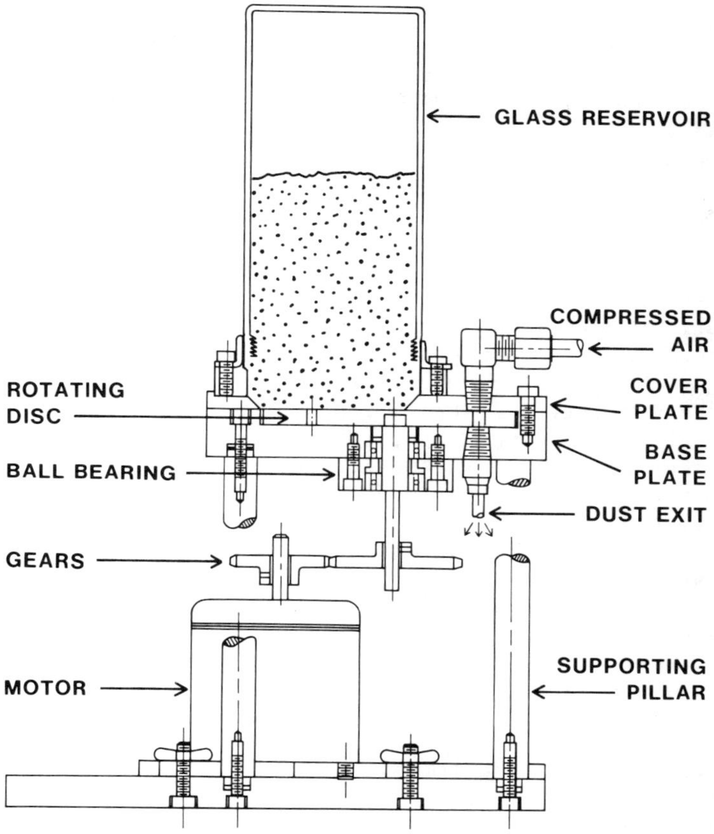

Figure 2. Diagram of the new dust generator.

inverting the dust generator without the need of dissembling the dust generator. Thus, a total containment of a toxic powder can be achieved.

(5) The reservoir (glass bottle) can be pressurized and depressurized to help agitate the powder up-and-down for better loading of the powder into the transverse openings.

(6) The driving motor is easily dismounted for ease of changing motor and gears.

(7) The gear train is simple in design and requires only one shaft and one bearing. The entire assembly is located in such a way that there is no direct contact with the powder in the reservoir. Consequently, the problem of shaft and gear jamming is minimal.

(8) This dust generator is simple and relatively economical to manufacture.

OPERATION AND TESTINGS

In operation, an air vibrator mounted on the base of the reservoir was used to aid the packing of powder into the transverse openings of the rotating disk. The speed of the disk was regulated at 18 puffs per minute. The air pressure within the reservoir was approximately two pounds per square inch gauge value (PSIG) and the resultant rate of air flow emerging from the generator was approximately six liters per minute (l/min). Each puff of powder was delivered to the air inlet of a 150 liter animal exposure chamber of new design (Leong et al, this symposium volume). At the air inlet, each puff of powder was further dispersed by a "cone" of air ejecting from a 72 degree air nozzle at an airflow rate of 16 l/min. The total chamber airflow was set at 28.3 l/min. In this manner, even distribution of the dust in the chamber atmosphere was observed. The concentration of the dust in the chamber atmosphere was monitored at approximately five minute intervals for a period of 60 minutes. For sampling the dust, two open-faced samplers with pre-weighed Millipore® filters were used at each time interval. One sampler was placed at a short distance from the chamber air inlet and the other from the chamber exhaust. The two air samples were taken simultaneously at a sampling rate of 1.5 l/min for one minute. Thereafter, the weight of powder retained by each filter was gravimetrically determined.

MODERATELY FREE-FLOWING POWDER

For testing the stability of the dust generator in disseminating a moderately free-flowing powder, a mixture of two parts talcum powder and one part diatomaceous earth was used. This experiment was conducted four times and the results are summarized in Table 1. The results indicated that this new dust generator was able to deliver a moderately free-flowing powder at an acceptably consistent rate over a period of one hour. The average variation in concentration of the dust in the chamber atmosphere, which reflects the delivery rate of powder by the generator, was approximately 11% for the inlet side and 12% for the exhaust side. It appeared that there was no significant difference in dust concentration between the inlet and exhaust side of the chamber. In examining the dust concentration buildup with respect to time, it can be seen that the dust concentration reached equilibrium within approximately 10 minutes.

Table 1. Analytical chamber dust concentrations of a moderately free-flowing powder[a] dispersed by the Upjohn Dust Generator

Sampling Time Intervals (min)	Concentration, $\bar{X}$±S.D.(mg/l)		Deviation (%)	
	Inlet Side[c]	Exhaust side[c]	Inlet Side[c]	Exhaust Side[c]
5	1.03±0.09[b]	0.94±0.12	9	13
10	1.25±0.08	1.22±0.13	6	11
15	1.45±0.33	1.40±0.18	23	13
20	1.37±0.09	1.37±0.07	7	5
25	1.24±0.11	1.30±0.20	9	15
30	1.07±0.19	1.07±0.12	18	11
45	1.15±0.14	1.22±0.10	2	8
59	1.07±0.14	1.09±0.21	13	19
Average	1.19±0.20	1.20±0.20	17	17

Footnotes:

[a] = a mixture of 2 parts talcum powder and 1 part diatomaceous earth

[b] = each entry represents the mean of 4 values obtained in 4 separate experiments

[c] = sampling locations

MODERATELY NON-FREE-FLOWING POWDER

A similar set of experiments was conducted to study the ability of the dust generator to deliver a moderately non-free-flowing powder. A mixture of two parts diatomaceous earth and one part talcum powder was used. Samples of the chamber atmosphere were taken only at the exhaust side of the chamber since the results obtained in the first set of experiments indicated that there was no significant difference between the inlet and exhaust sides. The results are presented in Table 2. The data indicated that this dust generator was equally suitable for delivering moderately non-free-flowing powder at an acceptably consistent rate. The average variation in dust concentration over a period of one hour was approximately 14%.

COMMENTS ON CHAMBER DUST CONCENTRATION EQUILIBRATION

One important finding from the studies on the chamber dust concentration was the observation of the rapid build-up of dust to plateau (p) concentration within the new "active dispersion" exposure chamber (Leong et al, this symposium volume). The dust concentration apparently reached equilibrium in five to ten minutes (Tables 1 & 2) instead of 24.4 minutes as calculated based on the classical t_{99} equation (Silver, 1946) where

$$t_{99} = 4.605 \times \frac{150\ \text{l (chamber volume)}}{28.3\ \text{l/min (chamber airflow)}} = 24.4\ \text{min}$$

The t_{99} equation is applicable to the situation when an airborne contaminant is continuously mixing with the chamber air until it reaches an equilibrium. However, if the airflow pattern through a chamber is laminary, there will be minimal mixing between the front of the advancing airborne contaminant and the receding chamber air. The clean chamber air will be essentially "pushed" en masse towards the exhaust side of the chamber. In this situation, the time required to complete one "air change" will be equal to the quotient of the volume of the chamber divided by the flow rate of the contaminant entering the chamber, i.e.,

$$t_{(p)} = \frac{150\ \text{l (chamber volume)}}{28.3\ \text{l/min (chamber airflow)}} = 5.3\ \text{min}$$

Based upon this rationale, it is reasonable to suggest that the wide angle (72 degrees) air nozzle installed at the air inlet of the new "active dispersion" chamber, may help to create a laminar airflow pattern and facilitated the even distribution of the dust particles in the chamber atmosphere.

Table 2. Analytical chamber dust concentrations of a moderately nonfree-flowing powder[a] dispersed by the Upjohn dust generator

Sampling Time Intervals (min)	Concentration, $\bar{X}$±S.D.[b,c] (mg/l)	Deviation (%)
2	1.98±0.36	18
6	2.45±0.08	3
10	2.46±0.26	11
14	2.63±0.36	14
18	2.37±0.30	13
22	2.64±0.61	23
26	2.55±0.52	20
30	2.35±0.45	19
45	2.44±0.22	9
58	2.43±0.15	6
Average	2.48±0.33[d]	13.6

Footnotes:

[a]= dust generated from a mixture of 2 parts diatomaceous earth and 1 part talcum powder

[b]= each entry represents the mean of 4 values obtained in 4 separate experiments

[c]= samples were taken at the exhaust side of the chamber

[d]= average dust concentrations at equilibrium (only samples taken at 6 to 58 minutes were considered)

PARTICLE SIZE DISTRIBUTION

The effectiveness of the puffing action in dispersing and deagglomerating the powder was studied by analysing the particle size distribution of a homogeneous powder (air-milled to 3μ optical diameter) in the dust atmosphere. An Andersen® 1 ACFM ambient particle sizing sampler was used for taking the chamber dust atmosphere at 1, 2, 3, and 4 hour time points of a four-hour run. The chamber atmosphere was drawn into the sampler at the rate of 28.3 l/min for 15 or 30 seconds. Thereafter, the weight of dust particles retained on each of the eight stages was determined gravimetrically and the percentages by weight for each size category were calculated. The results on the analyses of several experimental atmospheres for an acute LC_{50} toxicity study are presented in Table 3. It can be seen that the mass median aerodynamic diameter (MMAD) of approximately 3μ for the dust particles in the atmosphere agreed well with the optical mean length diameter. The geometric standard deviation of approximately 2 indicated that the particle size distribution was fairly homogenous. The MMAD appeared to be independent of the concentration of the dust in the chamber atmosphere under the present experimental conditions.

CONCLUSIONS

The aforementioned new dust generator is compact and effective in metering and aerosolizing powdery materials which have flow properties ranging from moderately free-flowing to moderately non-free-flowing. The rate of dust dissemination can be regulated by regulating the pressure and airflow of the reservoir, and the speed of the rotating disk. The stability of dust output was found to be acceptable for several hours as long as there was adequate supply of powder in the reservoir.

The pressurized "puffing" action in discharging each finite quantity of powder is effective in dispersing and deagglomerating both moderately free-flowing and moderately non-free-flowing powders.

This new dust generator can be operated for several hours with little or no attention.

Table 3. The nominal and analytical concentrations, and particle size distribution of a powdery product[a] in the chamber atmosphere of a 4-hour inhalation toxicity study.

Quantity of compound dispersed (g/4 hr)	Calculated rate of compound dispersion (mg/min)	Total chamber airflow (l/min)	Nominal conc. (mg/l)	Analytic[b] concentration (mg/l)	Mean mass medium aerodynamic diameter (μ)	Geometric standard deviation
11.8	49.2	50	1.0	0.5±0.4[c]	2.98±0.23[c]	1.81±0.24[c]
14.0	58.5	50	1.2	0.5±0.6	3.11±0.32	2.24±0.15
28.0	116.8	50	2.3	0.4±0.1	3.25±0.33	1.82±0.13
43.0	179.3	50	3.6	1.0±0.1	3.25±0.19	1.90±0.14
50.8	211.7	50	4.2	1.5±0.8	3.26±0.18	1.85±0.42

Footnotes:

[a] a powdery product which has been air-milled to have mean optical diameter of 3 micrometers

[b] represents the concentration of particles which were fine enough to remain suspended in the air during the sampling period

[c] number of samples = 4

REFERENCES

Carr, R. L. (1965a) Classifying flow properties of solids. Chemical Engineering, Albany, NY, 72, 69-72.

Carr, R. L. (1965b) Evaluating flow properties of solids. Chemical Engineering, Albany, NY, 72, 163-168.

Dill, R.S. (1938) A test method for air filters. Trans. Am. Soc. Heat. Vent. Eng. 44, 379-386.

Leong, B.K.J. (1979) A powder metering device. United States Patent, No. 4, 177, 941.

Leong, B.K.J., Powell, D.J., Pochyla, G.L., and Lummis, M.G. (1981) An active dispersion inhalation exposure chamber. (this symposium volume)

Marple, V.A., Liu, V.Y.H. and Rubons, K.L. (1978) A dust generator for laboratory use. Amer. Ind. Hyg. Assoc. J. 39, 26-32.

Silver, S.D. (1946) Constant flow gassing chambers: Principles influencing design and operation. J. Lab. Clin. Med. 31, 1153-1161.

Silverman, L. and Billings, C.E. (1956) Method of generating solid aerosols. J. Air Poll. Control Assoc. 6, 1-8.

Wright, B.M. (1949) British Provisional Patent, No. 33262.

Wright, B.M. (1950) A new dust-feed mechanism. J. Sci. Inst. 27, 12-15.

A Large Flow Rate Fluidized Bed Aerosol Generator

JUGAL K. AGARWAL, and PETER A. NELSON
TSI Incorporated
P.O. Box 43394
St. Paul, Minnesota 55164

ABSTRACT

A new dust generator has been developed for chronic and sub-chronic exposures. It utilizes a fluidized bed of 100 μm bronze beads for deagglomeration of particles. A very stable output over long periods of time is characteristic of the fluidized bed.

A detailed description of the generator is discussed. The ouput stability of the generator is shown.

INTRODUCTION

An acceptable method of generating particles is a significant area of concern for inhalation toxicologists. Often times when particles are generated in air from a bulk form powder they are not generated as discreet particles. This can bias respirable levels of exposure due to generated particles not being of its unitary size.

Another area of concern is the stability of the mass concentration output. Some generators have highly fluctuating particle concentration densities. These fluctuations cause excursions in mass concentration which are usually undesirable for exposure studies.

Any aerosol generator for animal exposure studies must meet the following two criteria:

a. It must deagglomerate the powder to its unitary size.

b. The output of the generator should be reasonably constant.

It has been shown that a well designed fluidized bed aerosol generator meets these requirements (Willeke et al, 1974; Marple et al, 1978). However, most fluidized bed aerosol generators are small generators designed for instrument calibration. When one tries to design a large flow rate aerosol generator based on the same principle, the following two additional problems occur (Moreno and Blann, 1976):

1. In a large fluidized bed, there is a tendency for the air to flow unevenly through certain portions of the bed.

2. The powder to be dispersed must be evenly distributed to each part of the fluidized bed.

In this paper a fluidized bed (TSI Model 9310) having a flow rate of 450 liters per minute is described. The problem of uneven flow and that of distributing the powder in the fluidized bed is solved by unique design.

DESCRIPTION

The fluidized bed aerosol generator is schematically shown in Figure 1. It consists of a 4.5 inch diameter, 8 inch long powder reservoir and a 10 inch diameter, 10 inch long fluidized bed chamber.

The powder to be dispersed is stored in the powder reservoir. A powder dispenser driven by a variable speed motor drops the powder into a horizontal channel through a powder feed orifice. The powder is then transported to the fluidized bed chamber via a spring rotated by a constant speed motor. The bottom of the fluidizied bed chamber is made of a microporous stainless steel screen. The chamber holds a 1" thick bed of 100 μm diameter bronze beads. In this fluidized bed chamber, the powder to be aerosolized is mixed with the bronze beads by a 4 blade mixer driven by another constant speed motor.

Compressed air is introduced at the bottom of the fluidized bed which strips the powder from the bronze beads. The powder ladden air (aerosol) comes out at the top of the fluidized bed chamber.

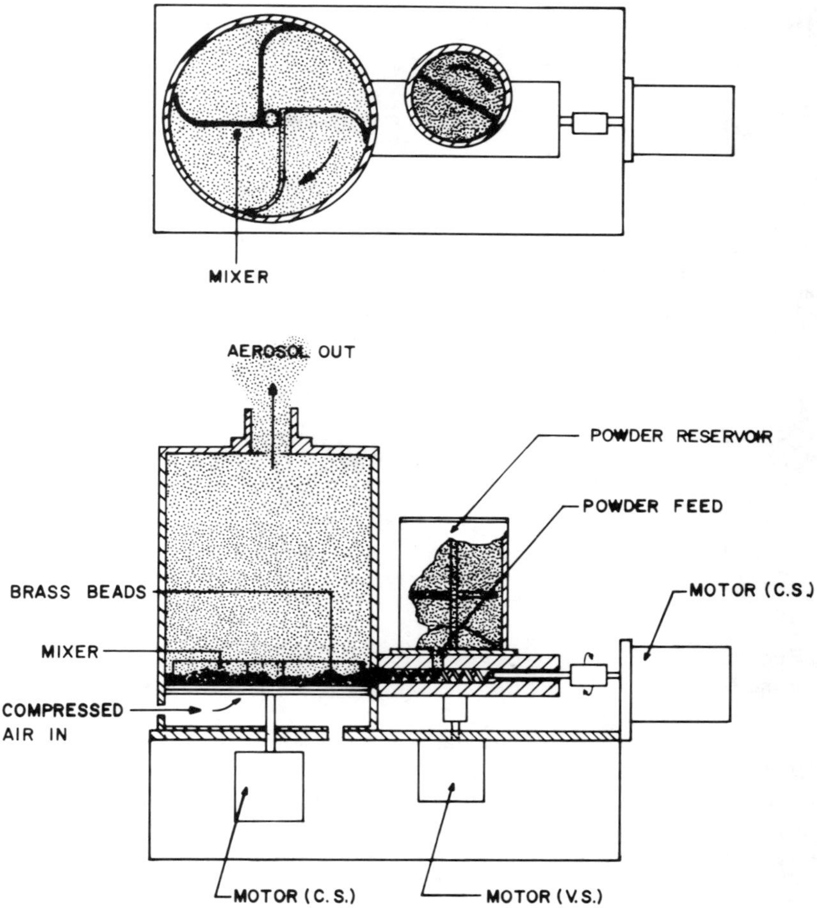

Figure 1. Schematic of Fluidized Bed Aerosol Generator

The problem of nonuniform flow through the fluidized bed is solved by partially masking off the microporous stainless steel screen (Figure 2). The compressed air is introduced into the fluidized bed in the form of high velocity circumferential air jets through the unmasked portion. The ratio of unmasked vs. masked area must be carefully selected for proper operation.

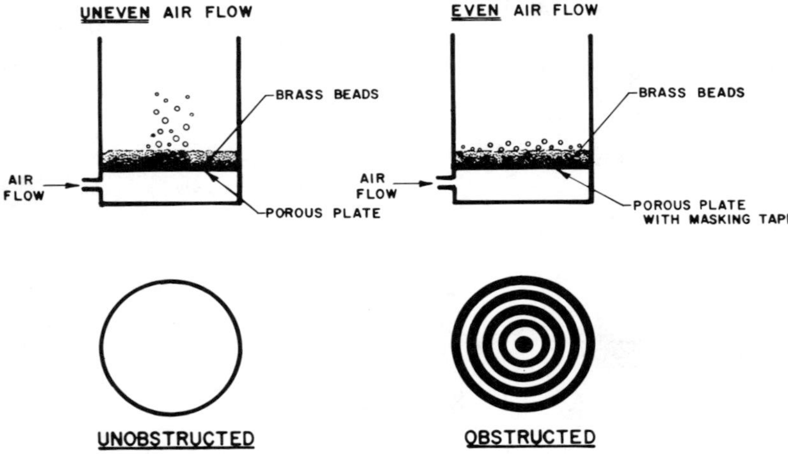

Figure 2. Evenflow is created by masking off the porous plate

The problem of distributing the powder throughout the fluidized bed is solved by use of the rotating mixer. Even though the powder is fed to the bed at a single point, the mixer keeps the powder and the beads well mixed, thereby distributing the powder throughout the bed.

PERFORMANCE

The generator has been used to disperse several powders, one of which is silica powder. Figure 3 shows the electron microscope photograph of silica particles. The silica aerosol was generated by Model 9310 and the sample was collected on a glass slide by an electrostatic aerosol sampler (TSI Model 3100). The principle and operation of the electrostatic sampler has been described by Liu et. al. From Figure 3, it is clear that the fluidized bed aerosol generator completely deagglomerates the silica particles.

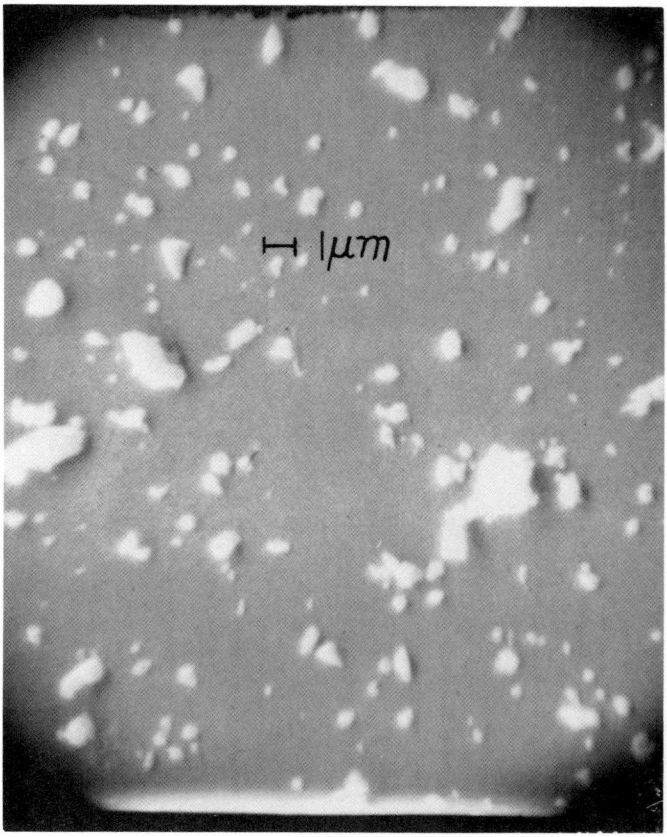

Figure 3 Photo of Silica Particles

Figure 4 shows 10 mass concentration measurement taken every 6 seconds. The measurements were taken by an Automatic Piezobalance (TSI Model 5000) which is described by Sem and Quant. Figure 5 shows the mass concentration measurements taken over a 6 hour period. The Automatic Piezobalance has a sampling period for 1 minute and a down time for 2 minutes during which its sensor is cleaned and dried. Thus, each data point shown in Figure 5 is a 10 minute average taken over 30 minute periods. These measurements show the stability of output concentration on a short term as well as long term basis.

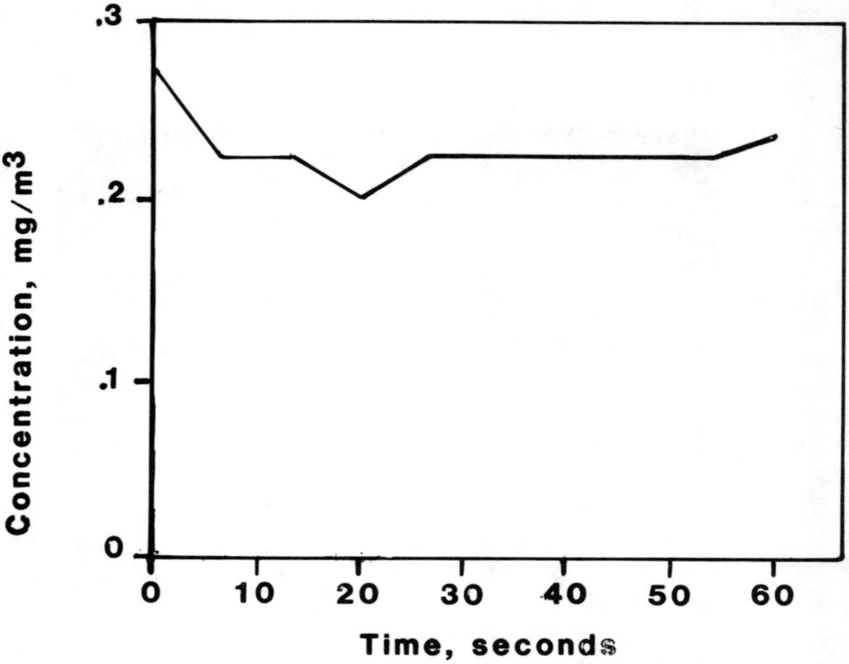

Figure 4. Concentration Change Over 1 Minute Period

We have continuously operated the prototype of this generator for more than six months, without any mechanical failures or wear. Since all one needs to do is to fill the powder chamber when it is empty, it is extremely easy to use. Another feature of this generator is that the output of the generator can be fed into a system under pressure.

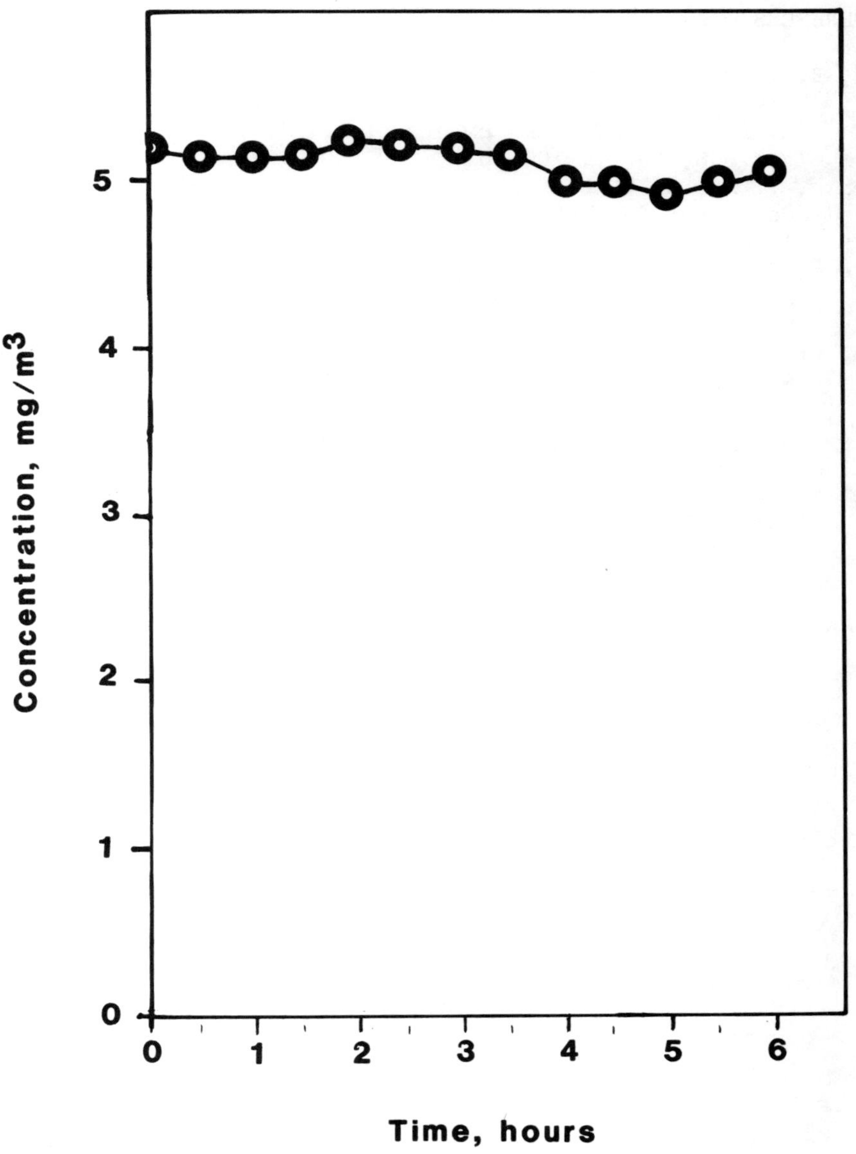

Figure 5 Concentration Change Over 6 Hour Period

REFERENCES

Liu, B. Y. H., K. T. Whitby and H. H. S. Yu. (1967) Electrostatic Aerosol Sampler for Light and Electron Microscopy. The Review of Scientific Instruments, Vol. 38, No. 1, 100-102.

Marple, V. A., B. Y. H. Liu and K. L. Rubow. (1978) A Dust Generator for Laboratory Use. American Ind. Hyg. Assoc. J. 39, 26.

Moreno, F. and D. Blann. (1976) Large Flow Rate Redispersion Aerosol Generator in Fine Particles (B.Y.H. Liu, ed.), Academic Press, Inc.

Sem, G. J. and F. R. Quant. An Automatic Piezobalance Respirable Aerosol Mass Monitor for Unattended Real Time Measurement. To be presented at the International Symposium on Aerosols in Mining and Industrial Work Environment, Minneapolis, Nov. 1981.

Willeke, K., C. S. K. Lo and K. T. Whitby. (1974) Particulate Dispersion by Means of a Fluidized Bed. J. Aerosol Science 5, 449.

An Instrument for Real Time Aerodynamic Particle Size Analysis Using Laser Velocimetry

JUGAL K. AGARWAL, RICHARD J. REMIARZ, and PETER A. NELSON
TSI Incorporated
P.O. Box 43394
St. Paul, Minnesota 55164

ABSTRACT

A new commercially available technique for measurement of aerodynamic particle diameter in real time is described. The technique utilizes a two spot laser velocimeter which measures the velocity of particles as they leave an accelerating nozzle. The particle velocity is inversely proportional to aerodynamic diameter.

The accelerating nozzle and signal processing are described in detail. Calibration methods are discussed and typical calibration data shown. The measurement results with monodisperse aerosol indicate extremely good accuracy in contrast to commonly used optical particle counters.

INTRODUCTION

When studying inspirable particle behavior the most commonly accepted parameter for characterization of a particle is its aerodynamic diameter - "the diameter of a unit density sphere with the same settling velocity as the particle in question". Historically, this characterization has been done with impaction or cyclonic separation followed by a counting or weighing procedure. This approach is tedious and time consuming and has instigated development of real time instrumentation for aerodynamic characterization.

Original work done by Olin, Sem and Christenson[1] and Chuan[2] on utilizing piezoelectric crystals for sensing mass enabled other researchers to utilize this sensing technique with aerodynamic size fractionating devices. The primary drawback of this approach is the frequent and time consuming maintenance required by the piezoelectric crystals since there have not been provisions for automatic crystal cleaning.

The most common approach for sizing particles in the 0.5 to 10.0 μm range has been optical particle counters. The problem common to these instruments is that they sense an "equivalent light scattering diameter". Liu et.al. have demonstrated the dependence of the instruments to refractive index and, in the case of irregular particles the dependence of particle shape. Van Buijtenen and Oeseberg have shown the light scattering diameter measured by an optical counter can vary from the aerodynamic diameter by a factor of 1.2 to 2.4 and from geometric diameter by a factor of 1.3 to 3.2. As reported by Gebhart, laser based optical particle counters are useful for sizing particles smaller than the wavelength of the monochromatic illumination source. But for particles greater than the wavelength of the monochromatic source, the response curve is subject to oscillations. Some white light instruments also demonstrate oscillations in their response curves.

In recent years, researchers have developed other techniques to measure aerodynamic diameter of aerosol particles in real time. In all cases, the particles were first made to acquire a velocity which was related to their aerodynamic diameter. The velocity of the particle is then measured by using a laser velocimeter. Dr. William Yanta was perhaps the first researcher to work in this area. He measured the particle velocity after a normal shock in a Mach 3 nozzle with a laser Doppler velocimeter and showed that the measured particle velocity correlates with the particle size. A device described by Dahneke utilizes a jet to accelerate the particles. Chaby and Bright describe a chamber in which particles settle and their settling velocity is measured using a laser Doppler velocimeter. Kirsch and Mazumder subjected particles to acoustic excitation and measured the particle relaxation time, and hence, aerodynamic diameter, with a differential laser Doppler velocimeter.

Another technique was reported by Wilson and Liu when they used an accelerating nozzle and measured the particle velocity as a function of aerodynamic diameter at the exit of the nozzle. This work was resumed by Agarwal and Fingerson (1978) in a device which simultaneously measured the aerodynamic diameter and equivalent light scattering diameter of a particle. This device was further modified to measure the size distribution of a polydisperse aerosol and was reported by Agarwal and Fingerson (1979).

The commercial version of the instrument developed by Agarwal and Fingerson is being reported here. The fundamental difference in the commercial technique from that reported earlier is the use of a two spot laser velocimeter in comparison to a laser Doppler velocimeter.

DESCRIPTION

The aerodynamic particle size analyzer measures the velocity of the particles at the exit of an accelerating nozzle. Since the particles will lag behind the air according to their aerodynamic size, the measured particle velocity will be inversely related to the aerodynamic diameter of the particle. The instrument is pictured in Figure 1. It consists of three primary modules (i) the sensor, (ii) the signal processor and multi-channel accumulator and (iii) a microcomputer for data analysis and display. A description of these three modules is given below.

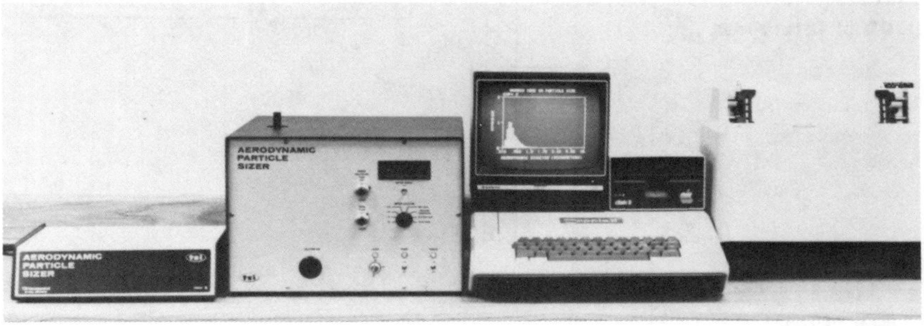

Figure 1. Photo of aerodynamic particle sizer

(i) Sensor Module
The sensor module consists of an accelerating orifice and a laser velocimeter. The accelerating orifice of the instrument is schematically shown in Figure 2. It consists of a 1.0 mm diameter outer orifice and 0.8 mm diameter inner nozzle. About 20 percent of the sample aerosol goes through the inner nozzle. The remaining 80 percent of the sampled aerosol passes through a filter and a flowmeter and is reintroduced to the system as sheath air. The primary function of the sheath air is to confine the aerosol particles to the central region of the jet where the air velocity is uniform.

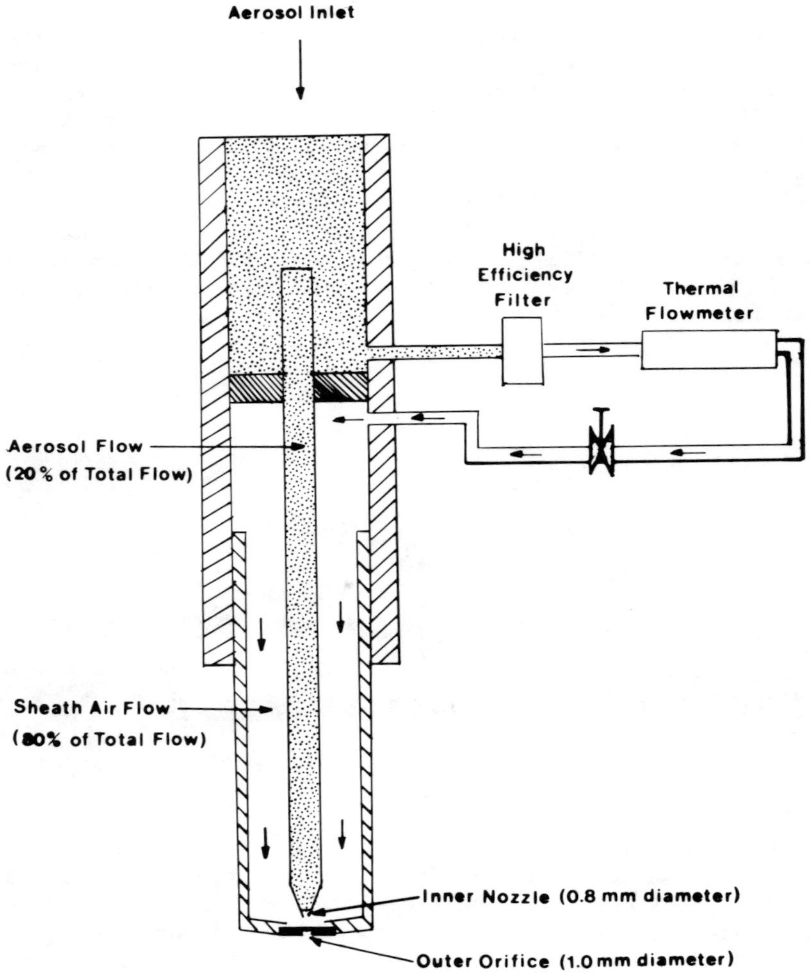

Figure 2. Diagram of accelerating nozzle

In the instrument, a nozzle exit velocity of approximately 150 m/sec is maintained by keeping the sensing chamber at a pressure of 125 cm of water below the ambient inlet pressure. The total flow through the outer orifice is approximately 83 cm^3/ sec. The true aerosol flow is about 20% or 16.6 cm^3/sec (1.00 L/min).

For proper operation of the instrument, it is important that both the air velocity through the orifice and the aerosol flow rate through the inner nozzle are maintained at their respective values at which the instrument was calibrated. The instrument has provision so that these two operating parameters can be monitored and manually adjusted to their set values. The monitoring devices are highly sensitive thermal type mass flow meters.

The velocity of the individual particles exiting from the outer orifice are then measured by a two spot laser velocimeter. The laser beam is split into two beams and then focused to form two parallel rectangular spots in front of the accelerating nozzle. The main beams are then stopped. The light scattered by the particles exiting from the accelerating orifice is collected (in near forward direction) and focused onto a photo-detector. A particle passing through the two beams will produce two electrical pulses. The time interval, τ, between the two pulses is proportional to the particle velocity.

The optical arrangement of the two spot laser velocimeter is schematically shown in Figure 3. It uses a 2 mW He-Ne laser as the light source. The laser beam is first expanded (about 3 times) with a combination of a negative and positive lens. The beam is then split into two beams. A combination of a positive lens and a positive cylindrical lens is used to focus the beams into two parallel narrow rectangular spots.

Figure 4 shows the photo-detector outputs of an aerodynamic particle size analyzer. Figure 4(a) corresponds to a 0.797 μm Dow Polystyrene Latex (PSL) particle and Figure 4 (b) corresponds to a 1.09 μm PSL particle. It may be noted that τ (time taken by the particle to travel the distance between the two slots) is about 876 ns for the 0.79μm particle and is about 940 ns for the 1.09μm

The time, τ , is measured with better than 4ns accuracy.

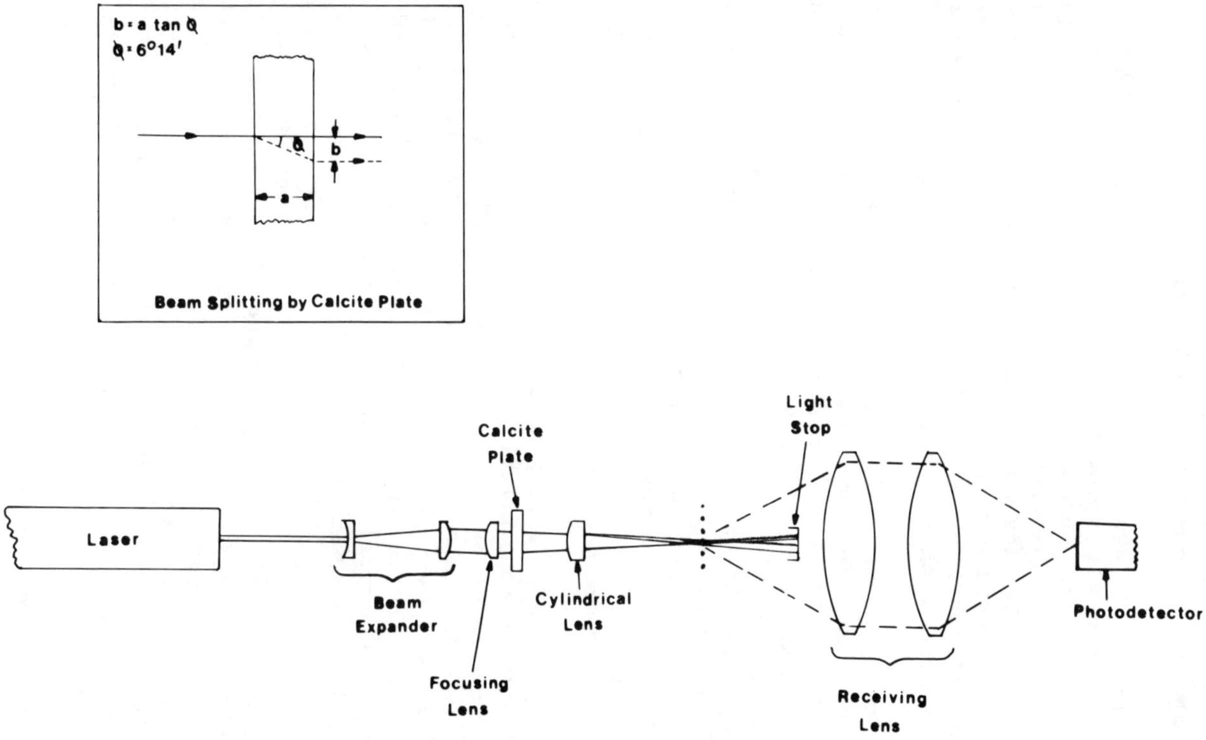

Figure 3. Schematic of Optical Arrangement

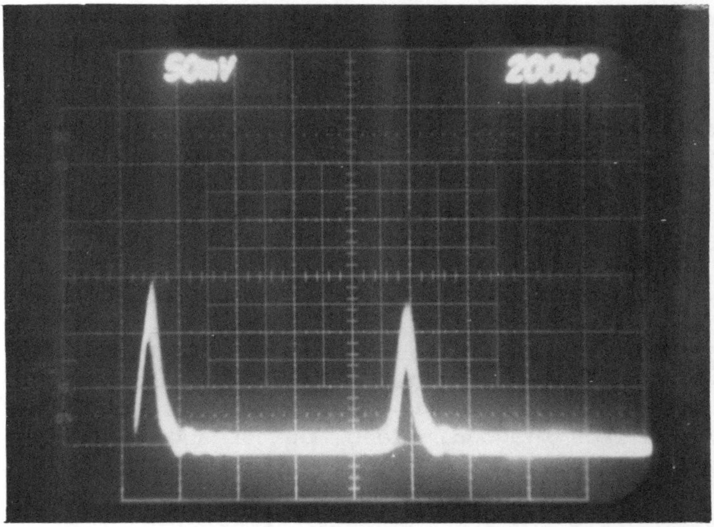

Figure (a)

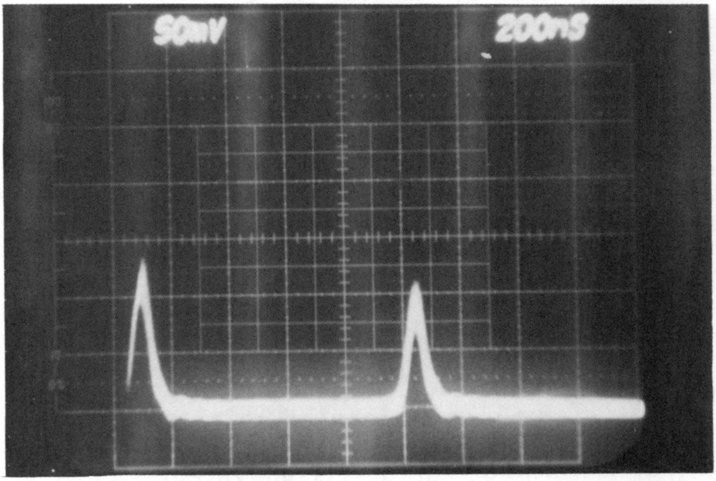

Figure (b)

Figure 4. Response of Photo-detector Figure (a) is for 0.797 PSL. Figure (b) is for 1.091 PSL

(ii) Signal Processing

The output of the photodetector is two pulses separated by the time, τ , which ranges from 0.8 to 3 ηs. It is this time that is a measure of particle size. The time interval between the two pulses is measured by a high speed digital ECL clock. The time measured by the clock is passed on to a Multi channel accumulator (MCA) and the clock is reset to measure the next particle. The MCA increments an accumulator corresponding to the time interval of the particle measured. The MCA has a total of 1024 accumulators each capable of counting to greater than 10 million. The MCA is also interfaced to a microcomputer which performs the time interval to particle size conversion after the sample is complete.

(iii) Microcomputer for Data Analysis and Display

This version of the instrument includes an Apple II PLUS (with 48K memory) microcomputer, Disk II Drive and Controller (microcomputer system manufactured by Apple Computer, Incorporated, Cupertino, California 95014), Sanyo 9-inch Diagonal Video Monitor and an IDS-445 Impact Printer.

After a programmable sample period, the computer reads each register of the multi-channel accumulator, translates the various channel numbers to particle sizes (using a stored calibration curve) and displays the measured size distribution in the form of a histogram. The printer provides a hard copy of the particle size distribution.

CALIBRATION

Calibration of the instrument is carried out with two types of monodisperse aerosols. Dioctyl phthalate (DOP) particles in the size range of 1.4 to 15 μm are generated using a Vibrating Orifice Monodisperse Aerosol Generator TSI Model 3050 (Berglund and Liu). Monodisperse aerosol in the size range from 0.5 to 3.44 μm is generated by atomizing a dilute suspension of PSL uniform spheres.

The system to generate PSL aerosol is schematically shown in Figure 5. The first step of this method is to prepare a very dilute suspension of PSL particles by mixing the original suspension in distilled water. This suspension is atomized in an atomizer (TSI Model 9302). The resulting aerosol is passed through a diffusion drier (TSI Model 3062). The diffusion dryer consists of two coaxial cylinders; the outer one of plastic and the inner one of wire mesh. The space between the two cylinders is filled with silica gel.

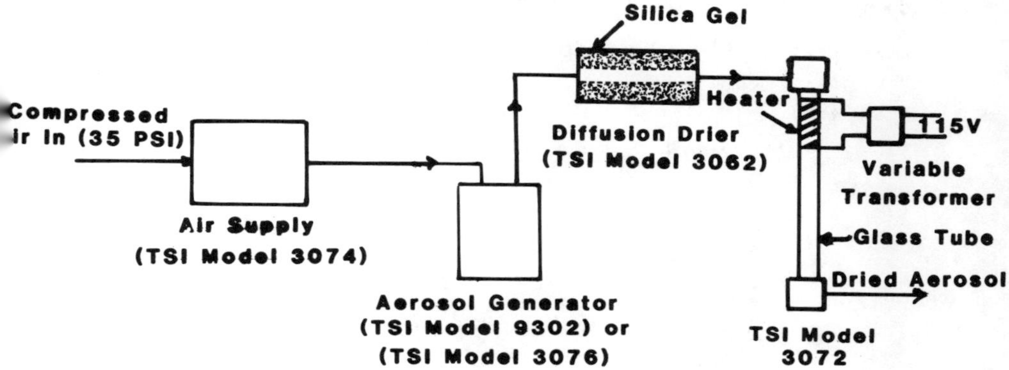

Figure 5. Generation System for PSL aerosol

As the aerosol passes down the axis of the unobstructed inner cylinder, moisture diffuses to the silica gel. The aerosol then passes through a heated glass tube (TSI Model 3072) to ensure complete drying of the PSL particles.

The calibration procedure of the instrument consists of generating a monodisperse aerosol of specific size, sampling the aerosol by the instrument, and noting the channel number containing maximum counts. Then a monodisperse aerosol of another size is generated and the procedure is repeated. The instrument has a calibration curve similar to the one shown in Figure 6. This is derived from the typical data points shown in Table 1.

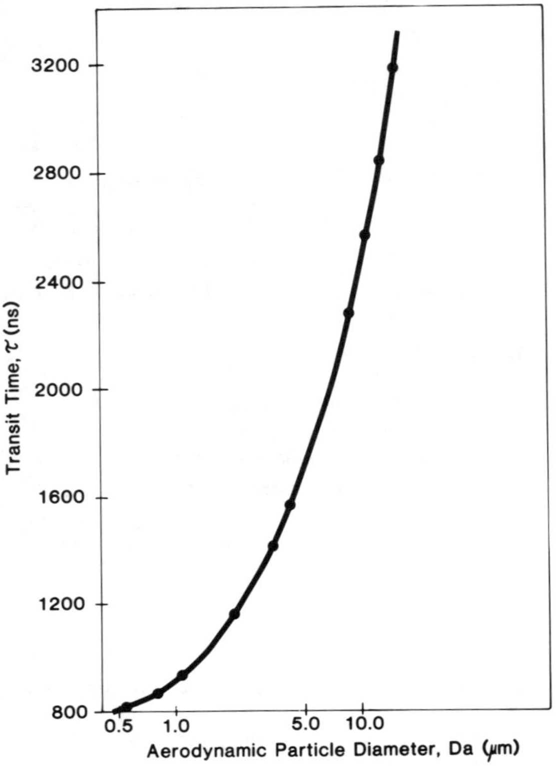

Figure 6. Calibration Curve

Geometric Diameter Dp,μm	Particle Density ρ,g/cc	Aerodynamic Diameter (14) Da,μm	Transit Time T, ns
.546	1.027	0.55431	820
.797	1.05	0.81852	874
1.091	1.05	1.1198	940
2.02	1.027	2.0481	1160
3.526	0.9861	3.5008	1408
4.44	0.9861	4.4084	1562
8.891	0.9861	8.8284	2288
11.202	0.9861	11.123	2572
12.99	0.9861	12.898	2842
16.32	0.9861	16.205	3192

TABLE 1 Calibration points for accelerating nozzle

DISCUSSION

For characterizing aerodynamic size of particles, the new instrument described here is preferable and superior to other commercial techniques. This technique measures aerodynamic diameter irrespective of refractive index, shape, or laser power. It is also not subject to the ambiguity of an oscillating response curve typical of those instruments dependent on classical Mie scattering theory. Shape and density only affect the this instruments measurement as they would the particles' aerodynamic behavior.

The superior size resolution of the instrument is demonstrated by its ability to characterize the monodispersity of aerosols. Ideally, if an aerosol is truly monodisperse, and the instrument has infinite resolving power, the instrument should classify all the particles into a single channel ($\sigma_g = 1$). In practice, however, a monodisperse aerosol is invariably classified into more than one channel. In the APS, 99% of the monodisperse PSL aerosol generated by an atomizer was sampled into 11 channels. The cumulative percentages of the size channels is shown in Figure 7. The measured standard deviation of the aerosol was 1.015 while the standard deviation specified by the manufacturer of the PSL was 1.0067.

Typically, optical particle counters rarely indicate σ_g less than 1.1 due to the non-uniformity of the light intensity in the viewing volume.

One non-trivial matter are the oscillations of the response curve associated with other instrument designs. If signals as shown in Figure 4 were processed utilizing pulse height analysis, the larger particle would be interpreted as being smaller, even though it is actually 35% greater in size. The aerodynamic particle sizer avoids problems due to pulse height since the measurement parameter is the transit time, not pulse height.

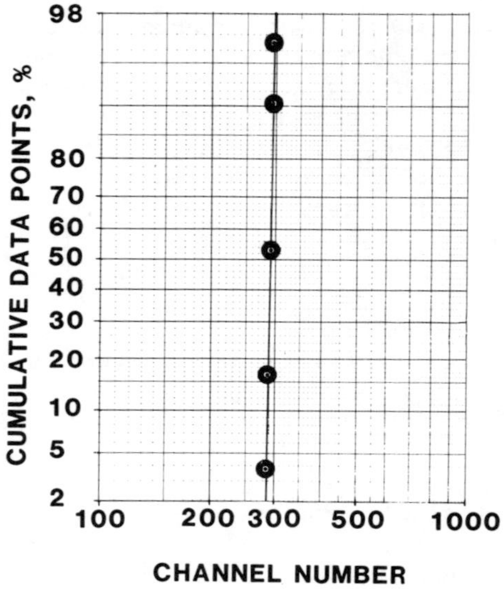

Figure 7. Cumulative distribution of data points showing σ g of 1.015 for PSL aerosol of 1.0067 σg.

FURTHER DEVELOPMENTS

Significant further activity is planned for the Aerodynamic Particle Sizer. It is the opinion of the authors that a superior technique is at hand, however, the performance of the instrument on several aerosols of varying properties needs to be addressed. Also, through further development, the authors feel this technique can be extended to larger and smaller particle sizes.

There continues to be a need for the comparison of this technique to other techniques associated with aerodynamic particle size.

REFERENCES

Agarwal, J. K. and Fingerson, L. M. (1978) Evaluation of Various Particles for Their Suitability as Seeds in Laser Velocimetry. In: Proceedings of the Third International Workshop on Laser Velocimetry, held at Purdue University.

Agarwal, J. K. and Fingerson, L. M. (1979) Real Time Aerodynamic Particle Size Measurement with a Laser Velocimeter. TSI Quarterly, Vol. V, Issue 1.

Berglund, R. N. and Liu, B. Y. H. (1973) Generation of Monodisperse Aerosol Standards. Environmental Science & Technology, Vol. 7, pp. 147-153.

Chabby, I. and Bright, D. S. (1977) Measurement of the Size Distribution of Liquid and Solid Aerosols by Laser Doppler Shift Spectroscopy. J. Colloid Interface Sci. 63, 304-309.

Chuan, R. L. (1970) An Instrument For the Direct Measurement of Particulate Mass. Aerosol Science, Vol. 1, pp. 111-114.

Dahneke, B. and Flachsbart, H. (1972) An Aerosol Beam Spectrometer. J. Aerosol Sci., 3, 345-349.

Gebhart, J., Heyden, J., Roth, C., and Stahlhofen, W. (1976) Optical Size Spectrometry Below and Above the Wavelength of Light - A Comparison. In: Fine Particles: Aerosol Generation, Measurement, Sampling, and Analysis. Academic Press, New York (B.Y.H. Liu, ed.)

Kirsch, K. J. and Mazumdar, M. K. (1975) Aerosol Size Spectrum Analysis Using Relaxation Time Measurement. Appl. Phys. Letters, 26, 193-195.

Liu, B. Y. H., Berglund, R. N. and Agarwal, J. K. (1974) Experimental Studies of Optical Particle Counters. Atmospheric Environment, Vol. 8, pp. 717-732.

Olin, J. G., Sem, G. J. and Christenson, D. L. (1971) Piezoelectric-electrostatic Aerosol Mass Concentration Monitor. American Industrial Hygiene Association Journal, Vol. 32, April.

Raabe, O. G. (1976) Aerosol Aerodynamic Size Conventions for Inertial Sampler Calibration. J. Air Pollution Control Association 26, 856-860.

Van Buijtenen, C. J. P. and Oeseburg, F. (1974) Comparison of "Light Scattering Diameter" Based on Forward Scattering Measurements and Aerodynamic Diameter of Aerosol Particles. Atmospheric Environment, Vol. 8, pp. 885-896.

Willeke, K. and Liu, B. Y. H. (1976) Single Particle Optical Counter: Principle and Application. In: Fine Particles, Academic Press Inc. (B.Y.H.Liu, ed.).

Wilson, J. C. and Liu, B. Y. H. (1979) Aerodynamic Particle Size Measurement by Laser - Doppler Velocimetry. Submitted to J. Aerosol Science.
Yanta, W. J. (1973) Measurements of Aerosol Size Distribution with a Laser Doppler Velocimeter. Presented at AIAA 6th Fluid and Plasma Dynamics Meeting, Palm Springs, CA.

Dust Explosion Hazards in the Pharmaceutical Industry

RICHARD P. POSKA
Pharmacy Research
The Upjohn Company
Kalamazoo, MI 49001

ABSTRACT

This review explores the concepts of fluidized bed processing, the explosion potential associated with this processing and the methods of minimizing this explosion hazard. The film presented illustrates the methods of limiting explosions. This work of Dr. Bartknecht, of the CIBA-GEIGY Corporation, has led to many structural improvements in the fluid-bed systems now marketed and has led to a better understanding of the dust explosion hazard in the pharmaceutical industry.

INTRODUCTION

Fluidization of powders can be defined as the process of allowing air to flow upward through a bed of powder at a velocity greater than the settling velocity of the particles and less than the velocity required for pneumatic conveying of the powders. Under these conditions, the powder becomes partially suspended in the air stream and behaves similar to fluids, hence the name fluidized.

Since each particle is completely surrounded by the drying air when fluidized, a very efficient heat transfer is realized and even allows for the drying of heat sensitive materials without the need of large temperature differentials. The 2-6 fold advantage in thermal efficiency over traditional oven/tray drying results in less handling and faster drying times.

This fluidization also lends itself to allow for the efficient granulation of powders when a binding liquid is sprayed onto the suspended particles. The resultant agglomerates are almost immediately dried which makes the traditional two stage granulating/drying procedure a one step operation. The following is a diagram of a typical Fluid-bed dryer-granulator.

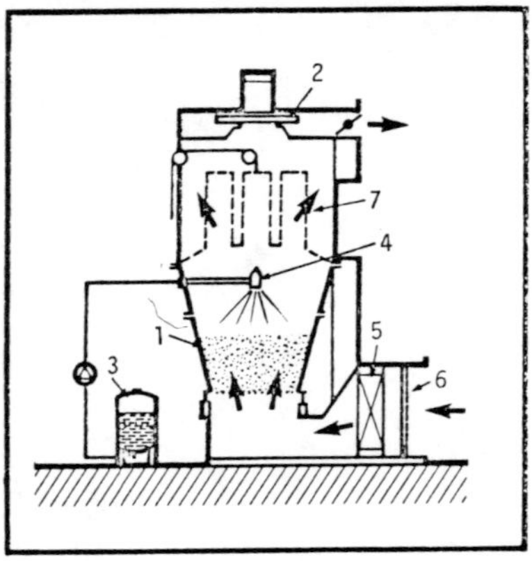

Fig. 1 Fluid-bed granulator. 1 Container, 2 suction fan, 3 spraying liquid, 4 nozzle, 5 heat exchanger, 6 inlet, and 7 exhaust filters

(Courtesy of Aeromatic Inc.)

EXPLOSION HAZARDS

The above advantages have contributed greatly to the increased popularity of fluid-bed systems in the pharmaceutical industry over recent years. However, a major disadvantage of these systems is the explosion potential which has been realized by a few unfortunate firms.

For any fire or explosion to occur, the concurrent existence of three basic components within the same space is essential and comprise the fire triangle. These three primary components are fuel, oxygen and ignition source. If any one of these components is lacking, a fire cannot start. However, once started, a fire can become self-sustained as long as an adequate supply of fuel and oxygen is provided.

The fuel portion of the triangle is readily apparent when granulating with a commonly used flammable solvent such as alcohol. However, less obvious fuel sources such as dust can explode in the absence of a solvent. Combined, the dust and solvent form hydrid mixtures which can explode with greater force than the solvent alone.

Although it is very difficult to identify the actual ignition source of these explosions, the energy of ignition required for many dusts (without solvents) can be generated by a small static spark. It is interesting to note in the following table that a commonly used powder in pharmaceutical processing, corn starch, requires less severe conditions to ignite than coal dust.

TABLE I

DUST-EXPLOSION CHARACTERISTICS OF VARIOUS POWDERS

Type of powder	Ignition temperature of dust cloud, deg C	Minimum spark energy required to ignite dust cloud, millijoules	Minimum explosive concentration, oz per cu ft	Maximum explosion pressure, psi	Rates of pressure rise, lb/sq in./sec: Average	Maximum	Limiting oxygen percentage to prevent ignition of dust cloud by electric sparks
Zirconium	[a]	15	0.040	50	1450	5000	[b]
Magnesium	520	20	0.020	72	4400	4750	[b]
Aluminum	645	20	0.035	89	2150	5700	3
Titanium	480	..	0.045	52	750	1650	[b]
Rosin	390	10	0.015	56	1250	3000	14
Phenolic resin	500	10	0.025	61	1350	3150	14
Polyethylene	450	80	0.025	83	400	1250	15
Allyl alcohol resin	500	20	0.035	68	1750	3550	..
Cellulose propionate	460	60	0.025	66	1350	2350	..
p-Oxybenzaldehyde	430	15	0.020	58	2150	3150	..
Hard rubber; crude	350	50	0.025	57	850	3350	15
Coal	610	40	0.035	46	350	800	16
Sulphur	190	15	0.035	41	700	1950	11
Phenothiazine	540	..	0.015	43	600	1450	16
Cornstarch, modified	470	40	0.045	72	1050	2150	..
Soap	430	60	0.045	60	660	1300	..
Aluminum stearate	400	15	0.015	62	750	2100	..

[a] When zirconium powder was dispersed into air at room temperature it ignited under some conditions, apparently through static electric discharge between particles in dust cloud.

[b] Oxygen-reduction tests were made in air-CO_2 mixtures. Dust clouds of zirconium, magnesium, titanium, and certain magnesium-aluminum alloys ignited in pure CO_2.

...Robin Beach, "Industrial Fires and Explosions from Electrostatic Origin," Mechanical Engineering, April, 1953.

During an explosion, the pressure increases rapidly to a maximum amount and then drops slowly. The speed at which the pressure increases (dP/dt) indicates how violently the explosion takes place.

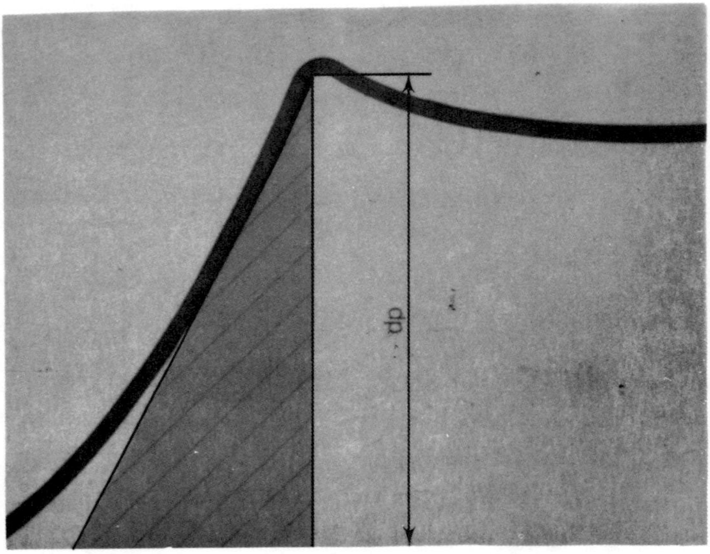

(Courtesy of Aeromatic, Inc.)

Fig. 2 Pressure Increases Upon an Explosion

Vessel volume is known to contribute to explosion intensity. This can be explained using the "cubic law" which relates vessel volume (v) and rate of pressure rise (dP/dt) to an anticipated violence of explosion (K).

$$K = \frac{(dP)max}{(dt)max} \cdot V^{1/3}$$

The following figure illustrates this using volumes of 20 cubic meter, 1 cubic meter and .001 cubic meter.

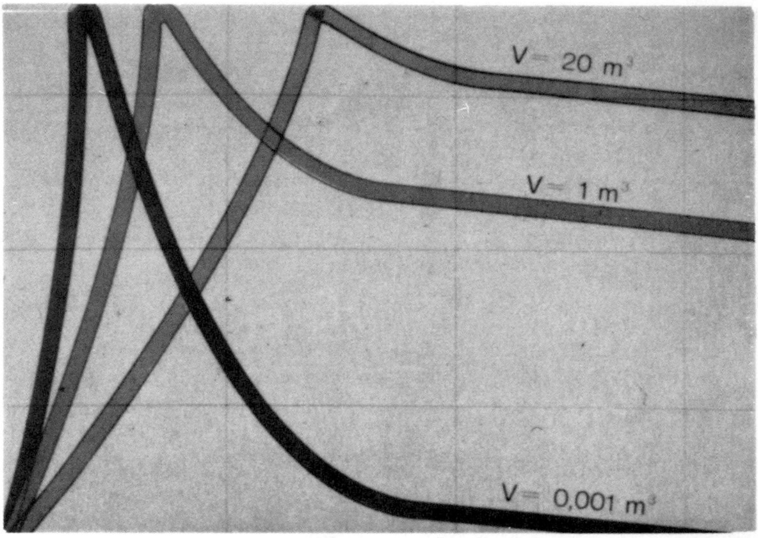

(Courtesy of Aeromatic, Inc.)

Fig. 3 Volume Effects on Explosion Intensity
(with the same quantity of combustible material)

Powder particle size also effects explosion intensity. Generally, the finer the dust the higher the explosion pressure will be. An example of the effects of methyl cellulose particle size and explosion pressure is shown below.

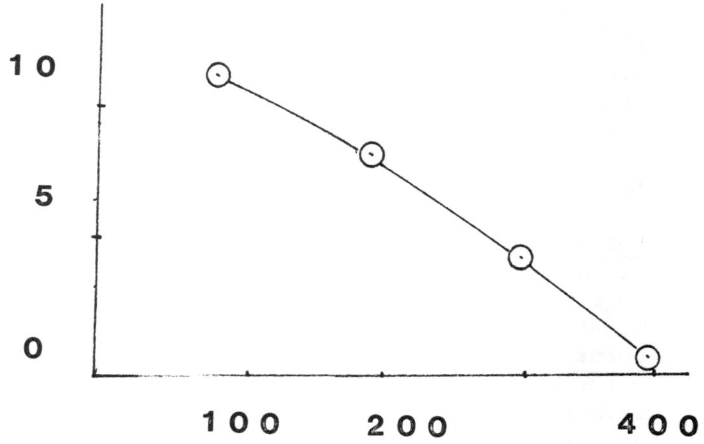

Fig. 4 Particle Size Effects on Explosion Intensity

SAFETY MEASURES

Explosion proof electric will minimize the chance of ignition by electrical spark. However, it will not prevent static sparks which also can ignite an explosion.

Probably the most common and most important safety measure taken to prevent static is the grounding of equipment. Even though grounding is not absolute, it will help minimize the chance of ignition from a static charge.

Other safety measures are available to lessen the hazard after an explosion has occurred. These methods will not prevent explosions but only lessen the hazards. They include:

1. Isolation by buildings
2. Separation by walls
3. Pressure relief
4. Suppression
5. Environment dilution

Isolation--The most uneconomical method of protecting a plant from a hazardous operation is by construction of a separate facility to isolate the process subject to an explosion. This measure offers no protection for operator safety unless the operation is fully automated and there is no need for personnel in the building.

Separation--Walls can be constructed within a given building to separate the operation from the rest of the building. These walls must be constructed to withstand the magnitude of blast predicted for the given operation. As in isolation, this method offers no protection for the operator unless the operation is fully automated. It offers less plant protection since the operation is actually located within a given facility.

Relief--By far the most economical and practical method of decreasing explosion hazards is by pressure relief. However, for relief to be effective, the equipment that might be subjected to an explosion must be properly constructed. This means reinforced construction to withstand a minimum of 2 bar pressure, and explosion relief plates that will blow out into a reinforced duct at less than the 2 bar construction. Most manufacturers of fluid bed systems offer these safety features on their new models. However, one manufacturer recommends larger than normal vent areas thereby claiming an exemption to the need for reinforcement. This relief plate is usually located on top of or on the side of the fluid bed system as is illustrated in the drawings below. It is essential that safety considerations be given to the area at the end of the relief duct. This area must have controlled limited access since this is where the flame will exit in the event of an explosion. A fenced-in area of adequate size would be appropriate if no natural means of control, such as a pond, are available.

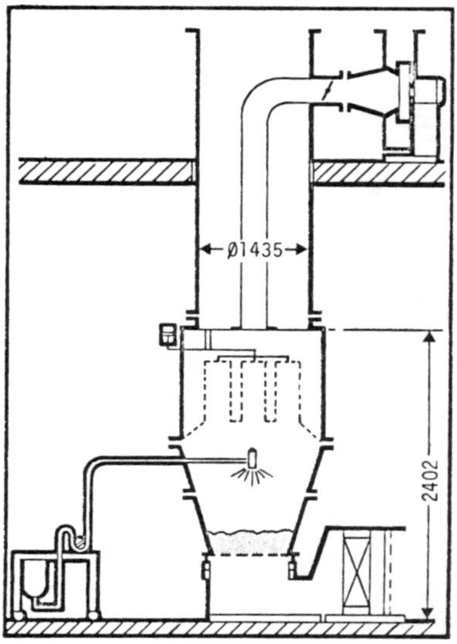

Modular fluid bed plant with vertical explosion relief channel venting through roof

Fig. 5

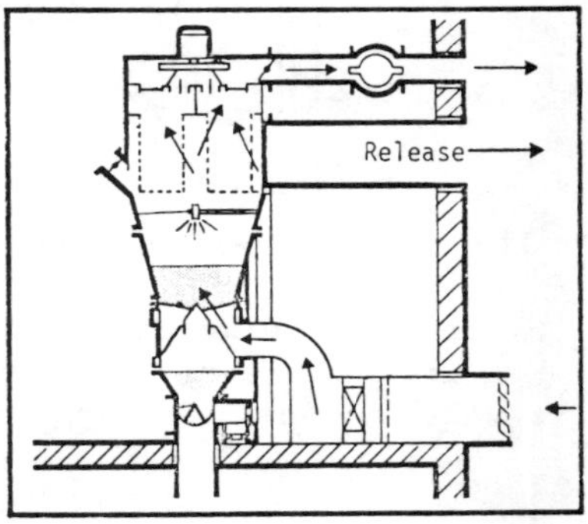

Modular fluid bed plant with horizontal explosion relief channel

Fig. 6

(Courtesy of Aeromatic, Inc.)

For either relief method, the relief duct should withstand 2 bar pressure and be of larger diameter than the relief plates so that the plate will not lodge in the duct and obstruct the venting of the explosion pressures. The duct should reach outdoor atmosphere (through wall or ceiling) within 15 feet. Ideally the duct should be straight or without any bends greater than 22°. Some companies recommend 1 square foot of venting for every 10 cubic foot of volume.

Suppression--Explosion suppression can also be considered in supplementing pressure relief to minimize hazards of explosions. These systems require specialized maintenance and are expensive.

The suppression system is comprised of pressure sensors located within the dryer housing. These sensors pick up the increase in pressure at the inception of an explosion, trigger the release of an extinguishing medium inside a pressure container, and blows it through a ball jet into the housing. The following diagram shows this schematically.

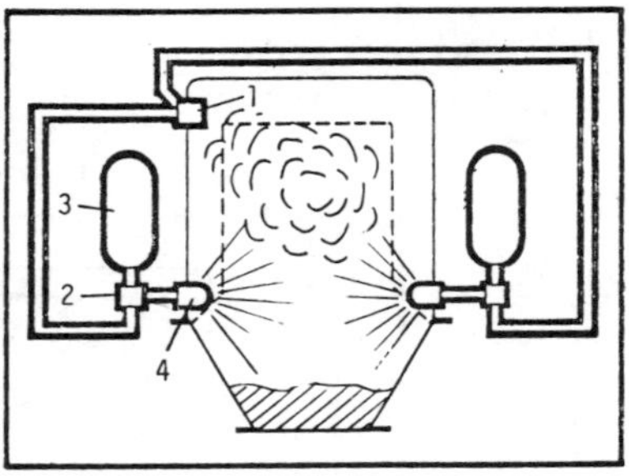

Schematic diagram of explosion suppression.
1 Pressure sensor, 2 percussion cap triggered valve, 3 ammonium phosphate, 4 ball nozzle

Fig. 7

(Courtesy of Aeromatic, Inc.)

Generally this extinguishing medium is ammonium phosphate, although halon and water have been tried. Due to the lag time between pressure detecting and extinguishing medium release, this sytem will not prevent but will only minimize explosion pressures and the spreading of flames. Since there is a lag time involved, it is not recommended as an alternative to pressure relief venting. Also, since an increase in container volume will increase the time required for an explosion to reach its maximum pressure, the suppression systems work best with production size equipment.

Environment Dilution--By reducing the amount of oxygen by fluidizing with inert gases instead of air, the formation of explosive mixtures can be prevented. With typical operation of fluidized systems, the air for fluidization and drying is exhausted after one pass through the machine. The cost of using an inert gas instead of air would make this substitution cost prohibitive. Some manufacturers, however, offer a closed system at extra cost which recirculates the gas used for fluidization and drying, thereby minimizing the amount of inert gas needed. This closed system could also offer an advantage in solvent granulation by recovering the solvent vapors normally vented to the outdoors.

STRUCTURAL REINFORCEMENT

As mentioned earlier, for a pressure relief system to work successfully, the construction of the fluid bed dryer must be reinforced to render it explosion proof. This means that the unit, exclusive of the relief ports should withstand a minimum of 2 bar pressure. This includes the observation ports and access door which in earlier models were inadequately reinforced. Other features include sieve bases that are firmly connected to the dryer, thereby preventing dislocation with an increase in pressure. This is needed due to the forces of explosion as shown by the diagram below.

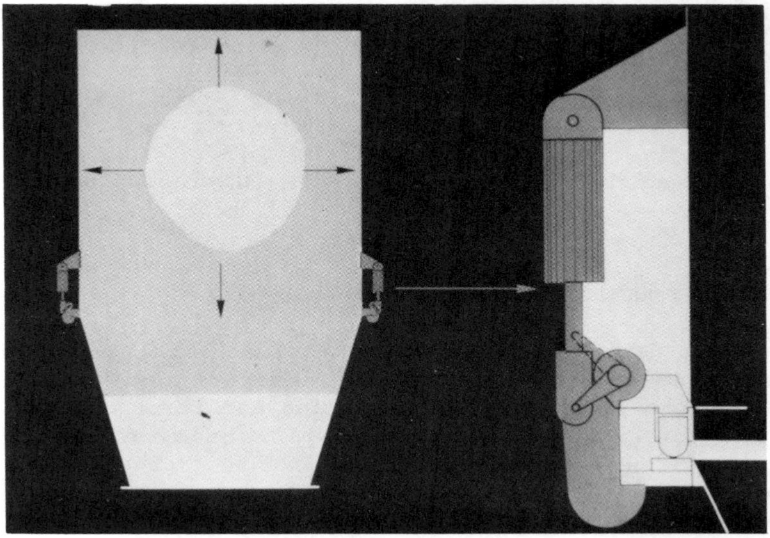

Fig. 8 Explosion Forces   Fig. 9 Hydraulic Clamp

(Courtesy of Aeromatic, Inc.)

Either hydraulic clamps as illustrated above, manual clamps or hydraulic supports (illustrated below) have been used to prevent the dislodging of the sieve base upon an explosion.

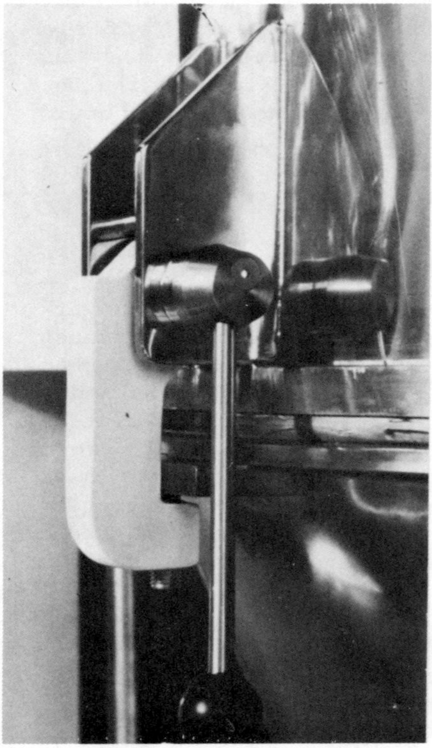

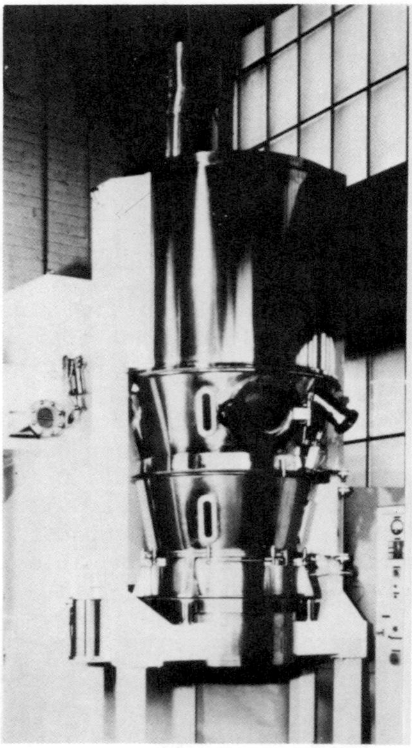

Fig. 10 Manual Clamp

Fig. 11 Hydraulic Supports

(Courtesy of Aeromatic, Inc.)

EXHAUST AIR DUCT PROTECTION

There is a danger of a secondary explosion in exhaust air ducts longer than 6 m. These secondary explosions, which may be due to preliminary condensation and turbulences, can be stronger than the primary explosion from the main apparatus. These exhaust air ducts can be protected by the installation of a membrane detector for pressure which will actuate the closing of a safety valve, which is incorporated into some company's models.

MISCELLANEOUS SAFETY

Additional precautions can be taken to increase operator safety when working with fluid bed systems. Antistatic shoes are highly recommended as is flame retardent clothing.

This clothing would offer some protection to an operator that might be caught in the flame path in the unfortunate case of an inadequately relieved explosion. If flame retardent clothing is not practical for one reason or another, all cotton clothes (including underwear) should be worn instead of the synthetic fibers such as polyester. In the presence of flames, cotton will simply burn with little or no melting but the synthetic fibers will actually melt onto the skin, compounding the resultant burn.

The turbulent dusts found in a fluid bed dryer can explode with similar, if not greater violence than non-turbulent gases, causing severe structural damage and a life threatening potential. The following are a few case histories supplied by the Aeromatic Corp.

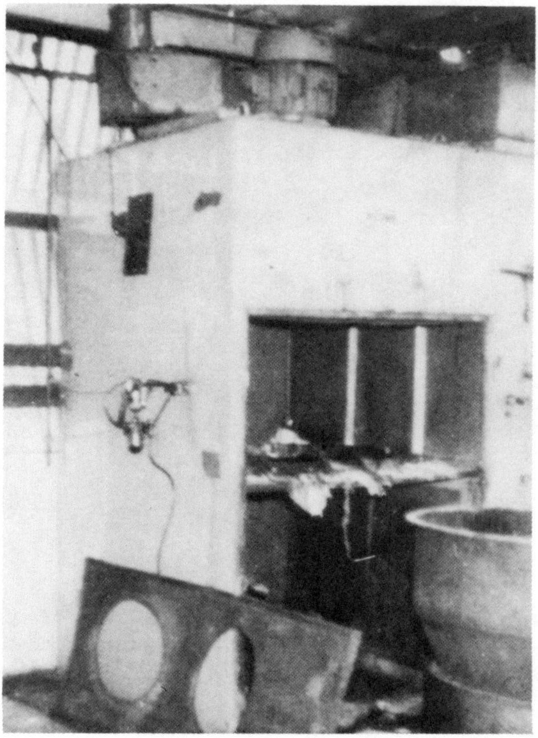

Fig. 12 This apparatus was not equipped with explosion flaps and the explosion took place during the drying of a pharmaceutical product moistened with solvent. The operation door was blown off by the force of the explosion. Nobody was injured but a great deal of damage was done resulting in an inconvenient interruption in production.

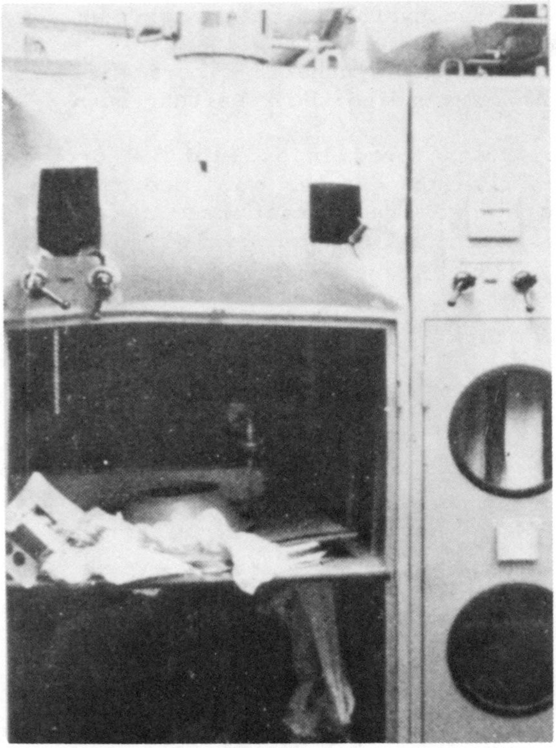

Fig. 13

This photograph shows an early installation of three units supplied to an American customer fitted side by side without, however, explosion relief flaps.

The explosion occurred in one of the outer machines during the drying of pharmaceutical product containing ethanol forming a hybrid mixture with the dust of the material. As with other explosions the source of ignition could not be traced.

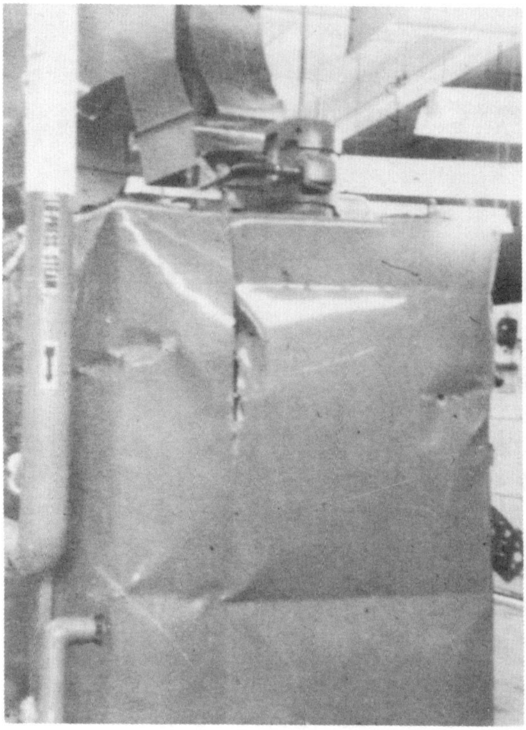

Fig. 14

This picture shows the impact caused by a dust explosion. The whole outside wall of the apparatus as well as the outlet air duct are completely blown out. It was indeed fortunate that none of the operators were standing in the vicinity of the apparatus.

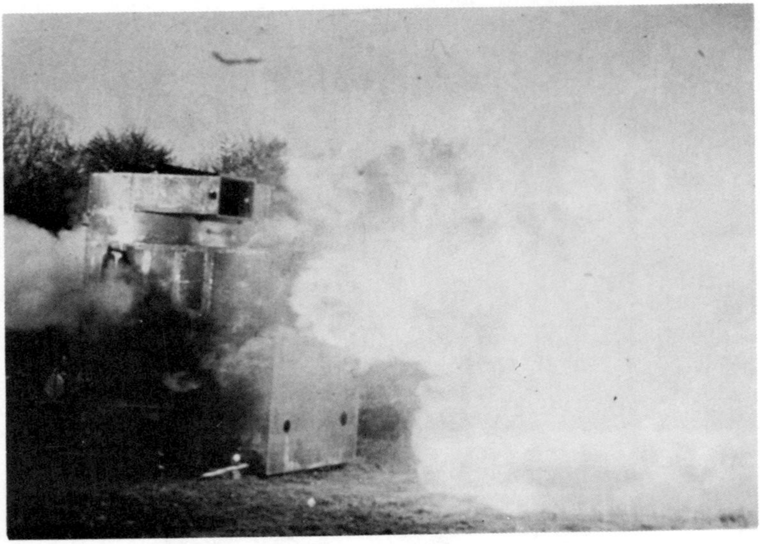

Fig. 15

The safety department of CIBA-GEIGY arranged a large number of explosion tests with various models of fluid bed dryers. During these experiments also, safety devices were tested and data for the design of these elements were accumulated. This picture shows how important it is to lead the explosion duct directly to the outside.

ACKNOWLEDGMENTS

The technical advice and assistance of Jesse F. Glasscock and Chester Sperry, and the generous supply of information from both the CIBA-GEIGY Corporation and Aeromatic, Inc. are deeply appreciated.

BIBLIOGRAPHY

Baier, W. H. (1980) The Theory and Practice of Fluid Bed Drying. The Fitzpatrick Co., May.

Bartknecht, W. (1975) Explosion Protection Measures on Fluidized Bed Spray Granulators and Fluidized Bed Dryers. CIBA-GEIGY Ltd., 4 August.

Kulling, W. (1976) Measures and Installations for Making Fluid Bed Dryers and Fluid Bed Spray Granulators Safe Against Dust and Solvent Explosions. Aeromatic AG, March.

Simon, E. (1978) Containment of Hazards in Fluid-Bed Technology. Manufacturing Chemist and Aerosol News, January.

INHALATION TOXICOLOGY

Toxicological Evaluation of Airborne Chemical Irritants and Allergens Using Respiratory Reflex Reactions

YVES ALARIE
Department of Industrial Environmental Health Sciences
Graduate School of Public Health
University of Pittsburgh
Pittsburgh, PA 15261

ABSTRACT

Numerous sensory endings are located at the surface of the respiratory tract, from the nose to the alveolar level. They are easily stimulated by a variety of chemicals and their stimulation is followed by a variety of reflex responses. By measuring the intensity of these responses, the potency of the chemicals can be evaluated. It appears that two general models may be of use in inhalation toxicology. The first model with chemicals capable of stimulating nerve endings in the nasal mucosa can be used to predict levels of sensory irritation in humans, i.e. burning, stinging sensation of the eyes, nose and throat. This model seems useful to predict acceptable levels of exposure for humans. The second model with chemicals capable of stimulating pulmonary nerve endings can be used to evaluate airborne chemicals which in general produce pulmonary edema or congestion. The ratio of the potency of each chemical for sensory irritation vs. pulmonary irritation may be useful to indicate the hazard associated with accidental and industrial exposures. The second model can also be used to evaluate allergic reactions to inhaled foreign proteins or haptens.

INTRODUCTION

Afferent endings located in the nasal mucosa belong to the trigeminal nerve and are cholinergic in nature (Cauna et. al. 1969). The innervation of the lung is more complex, with afferent endings of various types located around the conducting airways as well as at the alveolar level (Nagaishi, 1972, Richardson 1979). When inhaled chemicals impinge on the surface of the respiratory tract these nerve endings are stimulated and a variety of reflex responses are initiated (Alarie 1973, Widdicombe, 1974). The purpose of this presentation is to explore how animal models can be used to evaluate the potency of airborne chemicals as sensory irritants (i.e.: trigeminal stimulation) or pulmonary irritants (i.e.: stimulation of any afferent nerve endings in the lung regardless of their nature or location) by measuring characteristic reflex responses occuring from stimulation of sensory receptors. This paper also explores the possibility of predicting safe levels of exposure for humans on the basis of the response observed in these animal models.

Part I: Sensory irritation

Basis of the animal model

In 1870, Kratschmer described the action of a variety of chemicals on the nasal mucosa and demonstrated that inhibition of respiration occured reflexively from stimulation of the trigeminal nerve endings. This was further confirmed by Magne et. al. (1925a, b) and other researchers (see Alarie, 1973, for review). If respiration is recorded by a barometric body plethysmographic method, the pattern observed during exposure to a sensory irritant displays a characteristic pause during expiration as shown in figure 1.

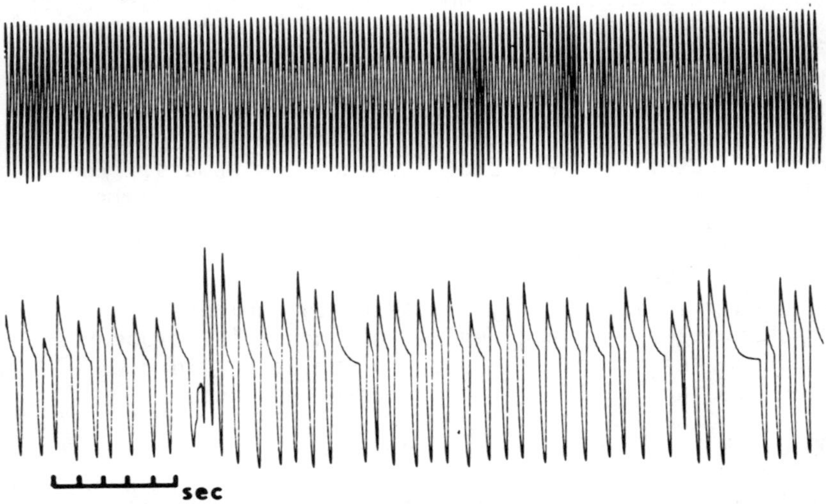

Figure 1. Characteristic decrease in respiratory rate in mice during exposure to sensory irritants (bottom trace) in comparison to control conditions (top trace).

The higher the concentration of irritant, the longer the pause and the larger the decrease in respiratory rate. Thus concentration-response relationships can be obtained by plotting the percentage decrease in respiratory rate vs. the logarithm of the exposure concentration (Alarie, 1966). From this relationship, the RD50, the concentration necessary to evoke a 50% decrease in respiratory rate, is obtained. The potency of a variety of chemicals can be compared on the basis of RD50 values, provided that concentration-response curves are reasonably parallel. A series of curves obtained for a wide variety of chemicals is presented in figure 2.

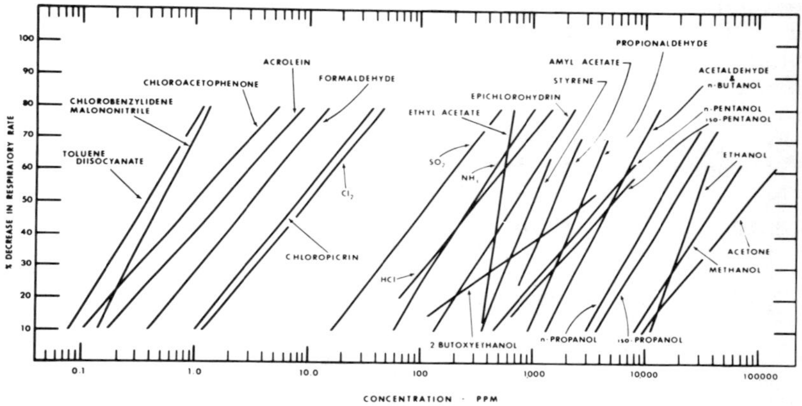

Figure 2. Concentration-response relationships obtained in Swiss-Webster mice with exposure to a variety of sensory irritants.

These curves are reasonably parallel with two exceptions: those for ethyl acetate and 2 butoxyethanol.

Qualitative Predictions

In order to use this model for qualitative prediction of sensory irritation in man, a wide variety of chemicals were tested in both mice and humans at approximately the same concentration. Additionally, reports from the literature of human responses were used for comparison with results in mice (Alarie, 1966, Alarie, 1973, Kane et. al. 1979). The characteristic decrease in respiratory rate occurred in mice during exposure to chemicals reported by humans to be sensory irritants. No such decrease was observed for chemicals lacking sensory irritation properties. Thus a perfect correlation existed and the model appears appropriate for use in testing new chemicals as well as complex mixtures of chemicals (Kane and Alarie, 1978, Alarie et. al. 1980).

Quantitative Predictions

In order to use this model for quantitative prediction of sensory irritation in humans and to predict acceptable levels of exposure in industrial situations, various approaches have been suggested, all based on the RD50 value found in mice (Alarie, 1973, Barrow et. al. 1977, Kane et. al. 1979, Alarie et. al. 1980). Recently, it has been proposed that 0.03 RD50 found in male Swiss-Webster mice can be used to predict acceptable levels of exposure for industrial situations, i.e. a time-weighted average threshold limit value (TLV-TWA). The relationship found between 0.03 RD50 values for 26 chemicals and the 1980 TLV-TWA for them is presented in figure 3. It can be seen that by using this model a good prediction of possible TLV-TWA can be made for airborne chemicals. Obviously, other toxicological studies must be undertaken to establish a TLV-TWA for each chemical but 0.03 RD50 certainly indicates that such a level is likely to be the maximum acceptable in industrial situations.

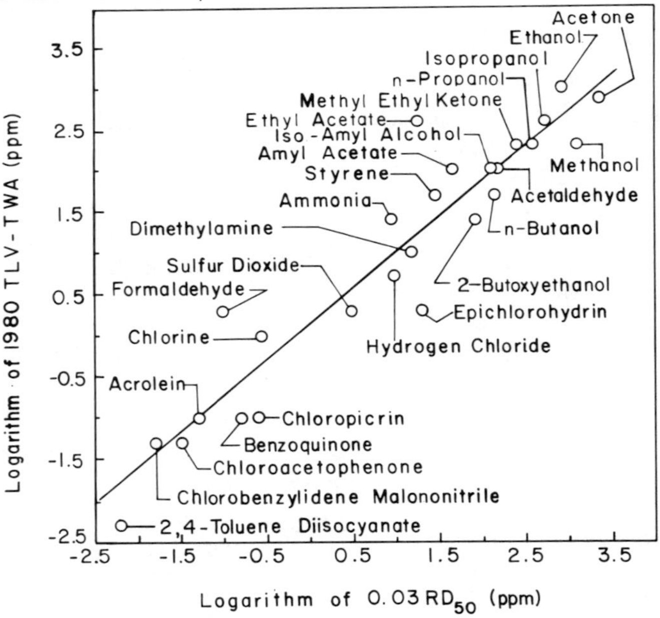

Figure 3. Relationship between log 0.03 RD50 obtained in mice and the 1980 TLV-TWA value for 26 chemicals. Regression equation: Y = 0.126 + 0.865X, standard deviation of Y about the regression line = 0.507, r^2 = 89.4%, r^2 adjusted for 24 degrees of freedom = 88.9%

Part II: Pulmonary Irritation

Basis of the model

Magne et. al. (1925a, b) pointed out that the chemicals capable of stimulating the nasal trigeminal nerve endings were also capable of stimulating nerve endings in the lung and that the reflex response was characterized by a rapid shallow breathing pattern as shown in figure 4.

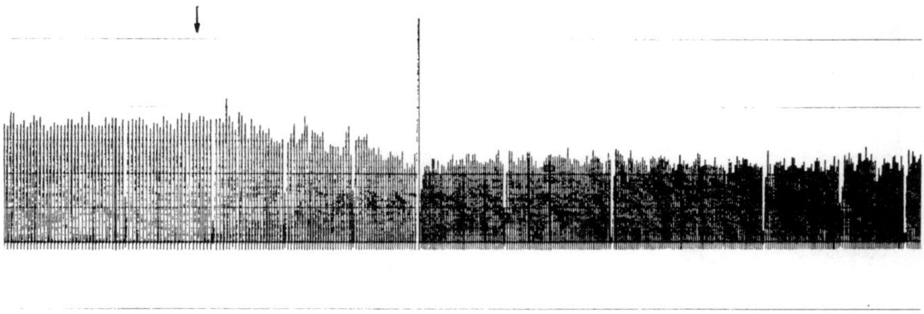

Figure 4. Rapid shallow breathing in rabbit during inhalation via tracheal cannula, of an aerosol of FPL 52757. Inspiratory volume amplitude measured by integrator automatic reset to baseline after each inspiration. Aerosol exposure starts at arrow.

However, if the chemical is a potent sensory irritant, the trigeminal reflex will predominate and the pulmonary reflex can be observed only when the chemical is inhaled via a tracheal cannula, thus by-passing the nose. If, on the other hand, the chemical is not retained by the nose or has little potency as a sensory irritant it can be studied in intact animals. The increase in respiratory rate occurs in several animal species and has been observed with a variety of chemicals (Alarie, 1973). Table I shows the chemicals and animals studied. Of interest is the fact that this rapid shallow breathing also occurs in man, as shown in Table I. Equally important is the fact that in sensitized animals challenged with antigens via inhalation the rapid shallow breathing is also observed. A variety of animals respond in this manner as shown in Table II and the pattern is similar to the one obtained with inhalation of histamine,(see Table I)

Table I. Studies demonstrating a rapid shallow breathing pattern during inhalation of airborne chemicals*

Chemicals and Animals	References
Guinea-pigs	
acrolein	Davis et. al., 1967
cigarette smoke	Davis et. al., 1967
formaldehyde	Davis et. al., 1967
nitrogen dioxide	Murphy et. al., 1964
ozone	Murphy et. al., 1964
sulfur dioxide	Davis et. al., 1967
histamine	Bennet and Lockett, 1964
histamine	Amdur, 1966
histamine	Douglas et. al., 1972
histamine	Noelpp and Noelpp Eschenhagen, 1952
Cats	
sulfur dioxide	Widdicombe, 1954a
sulfur dioxide	Widdicombe, 1954b
sulfur dioxide	Grunstein et. al., 1977
phosgene	Whitteridge, 1948
ammonia	Banister et. al., 1950
o-chlorobenzylidene malononitrile	Brimblecombe et. al., 1972
trichloroethylene	Grunstein et. al., 1977
Monkeys	
histamine	Michoud et. al., 1978
sulfuric acid mist	Alarie et. al., 1973
nitrogen dioxide	Coate and Busey, 1972
Rabbits	
ammonia	Sellick and Widdicombe, 1969
ammonia	Allen, 1929
benzene	Allen, 1929

Table I. (continued)

Chemicals and Animals	References
Rabbits (continued)	
bromacetone	Magne et. al., 1925b
chlorine	Magne et. al., 1925b
chloroform	Magne et. al., 1925b
ether	Mills et. al., 1970
ozone	Scheel et. al., 1959
ozone	Alpert and Lewis, 1971
toluene	Allen, 1929
histamine	Mills et. al., 1970
Dogs	
ozone	Lee et. al., 1977
ozone	Lee et. al., 1979
ozone	Lee et. al., 1980
phosgene	Rossing, 1964
phosgene	Laqueur and Magnus, 1921
chloropicrin	Magne et. al., 1925b
chlorine	Magne et. al., 1925b
histamine	Bleecker et. al., 1976
histamine	Lee et. al., 1979
prostaglandin	Lee et. al., 1979
Humans	
sulfuric acid mist	Amdur et. al., 1952
ozone	Griswold, et. al.
ozone	DeLucia and Adams, 1977
ozone	Folinsbee et. al., 1975
carbachol	Dautrebande, 1962

*Note: In most instances inhalation of these chemicals occured via tracheal cannulation, see text for details.

Table II. Studies demonstrating a rapid shallow breathing pattern in immediate and delayed type reactions upon challenge of sensitized animals by aerosolized antigens

Antigens and Animals	References
Dogs	
keyhole limpet haemocyanin	Schatz et. al., 1977
ascaris suum	Cotton et. al., 1977
ascaris suum	Booth et. al., 1970
ragweed pollen	Patterson, 1960
ovalbumin	Noelpp and Noelpp-Eschenhagen, (1952)
Monkeys	
ascaris suum	Patterson et. al., 1976
ascaris suum	Patterson et. al., 1977
ascaris suum	Patterson and Talbot, 1969
ascaris suum	Michoud et. al., 1978
ascaris suum	Pare et. al., 1976
Calves	
pasteurella haemolytica	Wilkie et. al., 1980
micropolyspora faeni	Wilkie, 1976
Goats	
ovalbumin	Noelpp and Noelpp-Eschenagen, (1952)
Guinea-pigs	
killed tubercle bacilli	Miyamoto and Kabe, 1971
purified protein derivative	Miyamoto et. al., 1971
ovalbumin	Karol et. al., 1978
p-azobenzearsonate-ovalbumin	Karol et. al., 1978
p-tolylureido ovalbumin	Karol et. al., 1978
hexyl isocyanate-ovalbumin	Karol et. al., 1979
p-tolylisocyanate-bacterial amylase	Karol et. al., 1980

Table II (continued)

Antigens and Animals	References
Guinea-pigs (continued)	
purified protein derivative	Karol et. al., 1981
ovalbumin	Noelpp and Noelpp-Eschenhagen, 1952
Humans	
not given	Dautrebande, 1962
not given	Miyamoto et. al., 1968
not given	Noelpp and Noelpp-Eschenhagen, 1952
Rats*	
ovalbumin	Piechuta et. al., 1979
DNP-ovalbumin	Carswell and Oliver, 1978a
DNP-ovalbumin	Carswell and Oliver, 1978b

* In this species a decrease in respiratory rate was observed see text for details.

Thus, this response can be used to evaluate the pulmonary response in sensitized animals (Karol, et. al. 1978). However, as pointed out by Noelpp and Noelpp-Eschenhagen (1952) this rapid shallow breathing, which they observed in dogs, goats, horses, guinea pigs and man will change to a slow breathing pattern during severe asthmatic attacks. The same phenomena were reported in guinea pigs by Karol et. al. 1978 and was also observed with histamine. However, at high concentrations, histamine decreases the respiratory rate without first increasing it (Amdur 1966, Douglas et. al. 1972). This must be taken into account in toxicological evaluation (Karol, et. al. 1978). Similarly, with very high concentrations of chemicals listed in Table I we may expect a decrease in respiratory rate following the initial increase. Nevertheless, the evidence accumulated indicates that the rapid shallow breathing pattern is a characteristic of pulmonary irritation by a variety of chemicals which if inhaled for a period of time typically induce pulmonary edema or congestion.

Quantitative predictions

It is impossible at this time to make quantitative

predictions of pulmonary damage in man from an increase in respiratory rate in animals. Unfortunately we do not have good concentration-response relationships for the chemicals listed in Table I with the exception of ozone and nitrogen dioxide presented by Murphy et. al. (1964). From the data presented by Murphy et. al. (1964) a concentration-response relationship was obtained by plotting the percentage increase in respiratory rate vs. the logarithm of the exposure concentration (Alarie, 1973). From the concentration-response relationships the concentration necessary to increase respiratory rate by 50% (RI 50) was found to be approximately 0.8 ppm for ozone and 8 ppm for NO_2. This factor of 10 is in line with the potency of these two gases as edemagenic agents and also their respective TLV-TWAs. As a guide, 0.1 RI50 obtained in guinea-pigs may be suggested as a "safe" level of exposure in man but this is only a "best guess" at this time. It is, however, of interest to note that ozone concentrations effective in increasing respiratory rate in humans (see Table I) are within the range found to be effective in guinea-pigs.

Some disadvantages of this model

A major disadvantage of this model for toxicological evaluation of pulmonary irritation with airborne chemicals is that the majority are also sensory irritants and therefore tracheal cannulation must be employed. The model can be used in long-term studies with pulmonary irritants, or with sensory irritants at concentration below which sensory irritation occurs, to see if this rapid breathing will develop due to cumulative pulmonary damage (Alarie et. al. 1973, Coate and Busy, 1972). The model can also be used in intact animals with aerosolized antigens or with hapten-protein conjugates since they are devoid of sensory irritation properties.

Possible animal model for toxicological investigation of pulmonary irritation

The first attempts to develop concentration-response relationships measuring the reflex increase in respiratory rate for airborne chemicals which have sensory irritating properties were with rabbits fitted with a tracheal cannula and under anesthesia. Dogs and monkeys were ruled out because they were too expensive for a screening test. Guinea pigs were ruled out because although their response under anesthesia was marked, it was difficult to maintain a stable and reproducible degree of anesthesia in all animals. This inconsistancy may in turn influence the degree of response. Using rabbits, reproducible results were obtained and a concentration-response curve for FPL-52757 was determined (Melnick 1974). From the concentration response relationship the concentration necessary to evoke a 50% increase in respiratory rate (RI50) was found to be 132 mg/m^3. This chemical, a chromone, was initially found to be a pulmonary irritant during a toxicological study in monkeys. In some animals the gavage tube accidentally entered the trachea and the chemical, delivered to the lung, induced pulmonary edema followed by death. Surprisingly, this chemical is a pulmonary irritant when given via intratracheal injection or when inhaled as an aerosol but has no pulmonary effect when given orally or intravenously, even at high doses (Melnick 1974). However in an attempt to reproduce these results in a second series of rabbits, some rabbits were totally unresponsive while in others the anticipated level of response was observed. The RI50 for the second series was 87 mg/m^3 excluding the non-reactors. This phenomenon was also reported to us by Fisons Pharmaceutical, England, using the same procedure and the same chemical. It was therefore decided to proceed with another animal species. Barrow et. al. (1977) had reported a moderate (16-18%) increase in respiratory rate in mice breathing 17 ppm chlorine via tracheal cannulation. This concentration is almost twice the RD50. Several chemicals shown in figure 1 were also tested in a similar manner using the RD50 or about twice the RD50 yielding for the majority of chemicals no decrease in respiratory rate or sometimes a brief increase in respiratory rate. It was therefore decided to use mice fitted with a tracheal cannula and higher concentrations of some of the sensory irritants listed in figure 1 as well as FPL-52757 to determine if this species could be used for toxicological evaluation of pulmonary irritation.

Part III: Pulmonary irritation in mice

Procedure

Male Swiss-Webster mice from Hilltop Laboratories were anesthetized with pentobarbital, (40-50 mg/kg.) given intramuscularly. Following a skin incision in the neck, the trachea was cut and a thin polytetrafluoroethylene tube was inserted. Skin sutures were made to hold firm the cannula and the area was infiltrated with local anesthetic. While recovering from anesthesia each mouse was inserted in a body plethysmograph attached to a glass exposure chamber. The exposure system has been described by Barrow et. al., 1977 for exposure of normal mice to airborne chemicals. This system permits exposure of a group of four mice while monitoring their tidal volume and respiratory rate. Average respiratory rate of the group was continuously monitored prior to, during and following exposure. As the mice were recovering from anesthesia their respiratory rate returned to the pre-anesthesia level, approximately 250 breaths/minute. Exposure to each chemical was initiated 10 to 15 minutes after this level was achieved. For each chemical listed in Table III a 10 minute control period was observed,

Table III. Concentration necessary to induce a 50% decrease in respiratory rate in normal mice (RD50) or in mice breathing via a tracheal cannula (RD50TC) during a 10 minute exposure to airborne irritants. Concentration necessary to produce 50% mortality in normal mice (LC50) and in mice breathing via a tracheal cannula (LC50TC) following a 10 minute exposure to airborne irritants within a 3-hour observation period

RD50 ø (ppm) and 95% C.L.	RD50TC (ppm) and 95% C.L.	RD50TC/ RD50	LC50 (ppm) and 95% C.L.	LC50TC (ppm) and 95% C.L.
Acrolein				
1.68 (1.2-2.2)	142 (86-352)	84.5	687 (548-861)	416 (313-553)
Ammonia				
303 (159-644)	1603 (1,226-2,287)	5.3	4115 (3,244-5,218)	12,578 (6,112-25,925)
Chlorine				
9 (6.6-14.1)	12.4 (8.9-31.4)	1.4	302 (266-344)	131 (99-174)
Hydrogen chloride				
309 (241-410)	540 (399-788)	1.7	10,138 (7,893-13,022)	1,095 (866-1,385)
Formaldehyde				
3.7 (1.5-6.7)	114 (82-179)	30.8	2,162 (1,687-2,770)	2,422 (1,691-3,467)
Nitrogen dioxide				
349 (297-460)	344 (276-495)	0.99	204 (148-281)	305 (217-429)

Table III. (continued)

RD50 ø (ppm) and 95% C.L.	RD50TC (ppm) and 95% C.L.	RD50TC/ RD50	LC50 (ppm) and 95% C.L.	LC50TC (ppm) and 95% C.L.
Sulfur dioxide				
117 (107-128)	380 (233-636)	3.2	1380 (1,108-1,718)	1,628 (989-2,680)
FPL-52757*				
50.6 (26-79)	179 (125-310)	3.5	--	--
o-chlorobenzylidene Malononitrile*				
4.0 (2.7-6.1)	177**	44.3	--	--

ø From concentration-response relationships shown in figure 2, except for nitrogen dioxide and FPL 52757, this report.

* Values for these chemicals are in mg/m^3.

** Extrapolated RD50TC value, see text.

followed by a 10 minute period of exposure and a 30 minute recovery period. The percent change in respiratory rate was calculated from the level observed at the end of the 10 minutes of exposure in comparison with the pre-exposure level. In order to obtain concentration-response relationships exposure of several groups of animals were made at different concentrations of each chemical. The pulmonary irritation effects of thermal decomposition products of a variety of polymers, as listed in Table IV were also investigated. The thermal decomposition products were generated by placing various amounts of each sample in a furnace which was heated, at the rate of 20°C/minute (Alarie and Anderson, 1979). When 0.2% weight loss was recorded from the sample, exposure to the thermal decomposition products was initiated and continued for 10 minutes, followed by a 30-minute recovery period. Concentration-response relationships were obtained by placing different amounts of samples in the furnace. For comparison, LC50 values were also determined for the chemicals listed in Table III. These were obtained by exposing groups of four animals, in the same exposure chamber described above, for 10 minutes and recording mortality which occured during the following 3 hour period.

Table IV. Concentration necessary to induce a 50% decrease in respiratory rate in normal mice (RD50) or in mice breathing via a tracheal cannula (RD50TC) during a 10 minute exposure to thermal decomposition products of various polymers

Polymers	RD50*ø and 95% C.L.	RD50TC* and 95% C.L.	RD50TC/ RD50
GM-21: Flexible polyurethane foam	3.7 (2.9-5.4)	810 (696-999)	218.9
Douglas Fir	34 (24-53)	1,736 (1,370-2,300)	51.1
Polytetrafluoroethylene	17.4 (12-27)	660 (550-790)	37.9
Polyvinylchloride, 46% homopolymer with filler and plasticizer (PVC-A)	15.9 (13-20)	437	27.5
Cellulose Insulation, with flame retardant	12.6 (9.0-18.0)	1,400 (1,080-1,980)	111.1
Wool Fibers (undyed)	360 (252-557)	940 (730-1,390)	2.6

* Concentration is given as milligram of sample loaded in the furnace to produce sufficient thermal decomposition products to evoke a 50% decrease in respiratory rate.

ø From Alarie and Anderson, 1979.

RESULTS

When mice were exposed to the chemicals listed in Tables III and IV a decrease in respiratory rate was observed instead of the expected increase in respiratory rate as would be predicted from the results obtained on a variety of animal species. The decrease in respiratory rate was shown to be concentration dependent and a concentration-response relationship was observed, as shown for formaldehyde, in figure 5.

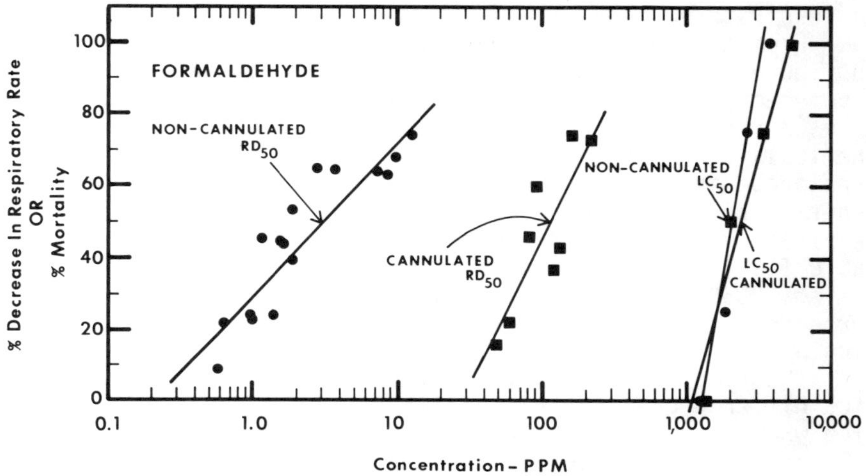

Figure 5. Concentration-response relationships obtained with formaldehyde in normal mice and mice breathing via tracheal cannulation.

The breathing pattern responsible for this decrease in respiratory rate is shown in figure 6. It can be seen that this

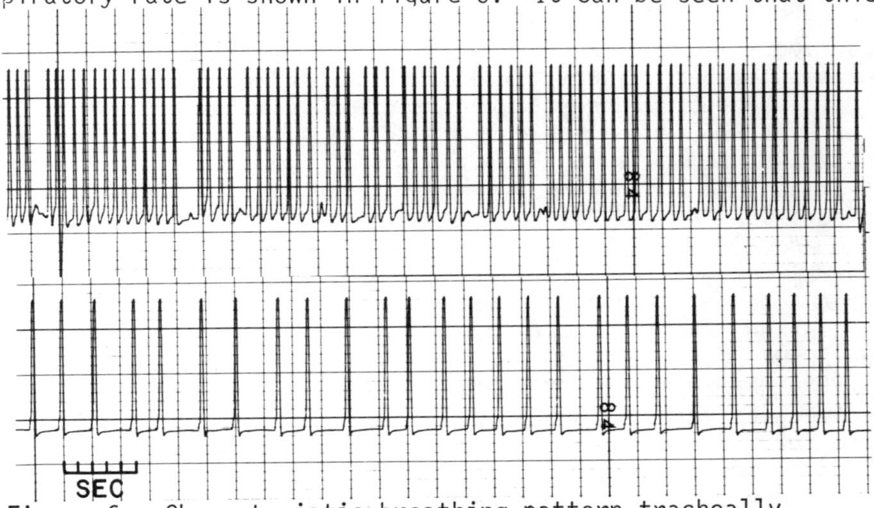

Figure 6. Characteristic breathing pattern tracheally cannulated mice during exposure to irritants at moderate (top trace) and high (lower trace) concentrations.

pattern is completely different from the one observed during exposure of normal mice to the same irritants, as shown in figure 1. The decrease in respiratory rate is due to a pause between each breath and this pause increased with the concentration of the irritant, resulting in a net decrease in respiratory rate.

From the concentration-response relationship presented in figure 5, a RD50TC, the concentration necessary to evoke a 50% decrease in respiratory rate in tracheally cannulated mice can be calculated. Values of RD50TC for a variety of chemicals are given in Table III. For one chemical, o-chlorobenzylidene malononitrile, it was impossible to generate an aerosol concentration high enough to depress the respiratory rate by more than 35-40% and the RD50TC given in Table III is an extrapolated value. Also given in Table III are the RD50 values for each chemical and the LC50 values for each chemical in normal as well as tracheally cannulated mice.

The time-response relationship obtained in cannulated mice differed greatly from those observed in non-cannulated mice where response results from sensory irritation. With sulfur dioxide and formaldehyde, a fade in the response occurred at the RD50 during the 10 minutes of exposure (Alarie et. al. 1973, Kane et. al. 1977). At RD50TC for these chemicals there was a slow recovery following exposure. For acrolein recovery occurred immediately following exposure at RD50 (Kane et. al. 1977). However, at RD50TC there was no recovery following exposure. For chlorine and hydrogen chloride (Barrow et. al. 1977) and nitrogen dioxide there is a slow recovery following exposure at RD50. No recovery was observed following exposure to these chemicals at RD50TC. For o-chlorobenzylidene malononitrile (Alarie, et. al. 1973) and for FPL- 52757 the recovery is immediate following exposure at RD50 and a rapid recovery was also observed for these two chemicals at RD50TC.

The same approach was taken for exposure to thermal decomposition products of various polymers. The values for RD50 and RD50TC are presented in Table IV. The least potent thermal decomposition products for production of pulmonary irritation were those released from Douglas fir and Cellulose insulation. Again, the recovery patterns from exposure at the RD50TC concentration were markedly different from those of RD50 exposures (Barrow et. al. 1978). In addition, recovery patterns at RD50TC differed greatly among polymers with the slowest recovery being observed with polyvinylchloride and the fastest with Douglas fir.

The results of LC50 determinations given in Table III indicate that in most cases the toxicity of these chemicals was similar in normal mice and mice undergoing exposure via tracheal cannulation. The most notable exceptions were hydrogen chloride where a factor of ten difference was found between the two conditions, and ammonia where a factor of three difference was found. Thus the nose of the animals seems to be a more effective scrubber for these two gases than for the others. These gases are the most water soluble of the group.

DISCUSSION

Since the RD50 in mice is a concentration which will produce intolerable sensory irritation in humans (Kane et. al. 1979), the ratios RD50TC/RD50 presented in Table III and IV are useful guides to indicate the acute hazard of accidental exposure to these chemicals. The lower the ratio the less warning an individual has of exposure to a chemical capable of inducing pulmonary irritation. It would seem that the ratios, (taking nitrogen dioxide as 1.0) are in general agreement with what is known about the pulmonary toxicity of these chemicals with the possible exception of acrolein which appears to be too high. Nevertheless, this approach seems to be a good starting point to investigate new chemicals. The same methodology was used to study unknown complex mixtures of thermal decomposition products, from polymers. The lowest ratio observed was obtained with wool and the next highest with polyvinylchloride. The results for polyvinylchloride are not surprising since a large amount of hydrogen chloride is released from this polymer. The agent responsible for pulmonary irritation with wool has not been identified.

It is interesting to speculate on the difference in the reflex reaction observed in cannulated mice as opposed to other species listed in Table I. In the other species, the variety of stimuli known to elicit a rapid shallow breathing are often associated with apneic periods prior to the increase in respiratory rate (Widdicombe 1974, Alarie 1973). It may be that in mice the stimulation of these receptors induces a decrease in respiratory rate which is not followed by the increase as observed in other species. Also responding in a totally opposite manner than the species noted in Table II is the rat during inhalation challenge by various antigens. In this species a decrease in respiratory rate was noted, having the same pattern (Carswell and Oliver, 1978a, b, Pietchuta et. al. 1979) observed in mice with pulmonary irritants as shown in figure 6. It could also be possible that mice and rats follow a similar pattern as seen in guinea-pigs, i.e. an increase in respiratory rate followed by a decrease in respiratory rate (Karol et. al. 1978) but that the increase in respiratory rate is much smaller and therefore missed. Barrow et. al. (1977) had reported a small increase with chlorine but we have not consistently observed this with chlorine or with the other irritants tested.

In using this animal model some caution is indicated since the pattern of respiratory depression obtained with pulmonary irritants can also be observed in other circumstances. With general anesthetics and the chemical asphyxiants carbon monoxide and hydrogen cyanide, after a brief stimulation of respiratory rate, depression will occur with a breathing pattern similar to the one observed with pulmonary irritants (Alarie and Anderson, 1979). However, in these instances, escape movements of the animals from the plethysmograph are completely absent due to general depression (Alarie and Anderson, 1979) and this can be used to differentiate the two conditions. From the recovery patterns observed following exposure of normal vs. tracheally cannulated mice it appears that the reaction for pulmonary irritation is not solely due to stimulation of pulmonary receptors. At the beginning of exposure these pulmonary irritants may stimulate lung receptors directly. With the high concentrations used it is probable that interstial edema may be induced within the 10 minute of exposure. This and other pathological changes, which are known to evoke the same reflex actions (Widdicombe, 1974, Alarie, 1973) may then prevent recovery to occur rapidly.

SUMMARY AND CONCLUSIONS

Two methods have been presented to evaluate effects of airborne chemicals on the respiratory tract. The first method relies upon measurement of the reflex decrease in respiratory rate which occurs with stimulation of trigeminal nerve endings in the nasal mucosa. This model can be used to predict sensory irritation of the eyes, nose and throat in man and to predict the maximum acceptable level in industrial situations. The second method relies upon measurement of the reflex decrease in respiratory rate which occurs with stimulation of pulmonary nervous structures in mice inhaling chemicals via a tracheal cannula. This method can be used to indicate pulmonary irritation. Both methods are simple, yield concentration-response relationships from which comparison of potency can be made and can be used to rapidly evaluate new chemicals or mixtures of chemicals.

ACKNOWLEDGEMENT

Supported under National Bureau of Standards grant No. NB79NADA0009. Dr. L.E. Kane, Dr. R.C. Anderson, Mrs. M.F. Stock and Mrs. R. Dombroske participated in the development of the pulmonary irritation model. Figures 1 and 3 reprinted with permission from CRC Press and A. Wheaton Co.

REFERENCES

Alarie, Y. (1966). Irritating properties of airborne materials to the upper respiratory tract. Arch. Environ. Health 13: 433-449.

Alarie, Y. (1973). Sensory irritation by airborne chemicals. CRC Crit. Rev. Toxicol. 2: 299-363.

Alarie, Y. and Anderson, R.C. (1979). Toxicologic and acute lethal hazard evaluation of thermal decomposition products of synthetic and natural polymers. Toxicol. Appl. Pharmacol. 51: 341-362.

Alarie, Y., Kane, L. and Barrow, C. (1980). Sensory irritation: the use of an animal model to establish acceptable exposure to airborne chemical irritants. In Toxicology: Principles and Practice, Vol. 1, A.L. Reeves, Ed. John Wiley and Sons, Inc. N.Y.

Alarie, Y., Wakisaka, I. and Oka, S. (1973). Sensory irritation by sulfur dioxide and chlorobenzylidene malononitrile. Environ. Physiol. Biochem. 3: 53-64.

Alarie, Y., Busey, W.M., Krumm, A.A. and Ulrich, C.E. (1973). Long-term continuous exposure to sulfuric acid mist in cynomolgus monkeys and guinea-pigs. Arch. Environ. Health, 27: 16-24.

Allen, W.F. (1929). Effect on respiration, blood pressure and carotid pulse of various inhaled and insufflated vapors when stimulating one cranial nerve and various combinations of cranial nerves, II, vagus and vagotomy experiments. Am. J. Physiol. 87: 558-565.

Alpert, S.M. and Lewis, T.R. (1971). Unilateral pulmonary function study of ozone toxicity in rabbits. Arch. Environ. Health 23: 451-458.

Amdur, M.O. (1966). The respiratory response of guinea-pigs to histamine aerosol. Arch. Environ. Health 13: 29-37.

Amdur, M.O., Silverman, L. and Drinker, P. (1952). Inhalation of sulfuric acid mist by human subjects. Arch. Ind. Hyg. Occ. Med. 6: 305-313.

Banister, J., Fegler, G. and Hebb, C. (1950). Initial responses to intratracheal inhalation of phosgene and ammonia. Q.J. Exp. Physiol. 35: 233-250.

Barrow, C.S., Alarie, Y. and Stock, M.F. (1978). Sensory irritation and incapacitation evoked by thermal decomposition products of polymers and comparisons with known sensory irritants. Arch. Environ. Health 33: 79-88.

Barrow, C., Alarie, Y., Warrick, J. and Stock, M. (1977). Comparison of the sensory irritation response in mice to chlorine and hydrogen chloride. Arch. Environ. Health 32: 68-76.

Bennett, A. and Lockett, M.F. (1964). Method for recording respiratory changes induced in guinea-pigs by aerosols of histamine or of specific antigen, and for assessing drugs which antagonise bronchoconstriction. J. Pharm. Pharmacol. 16: 241-249.

Bleecker, E.R., Cotton, D.J., Fischer, S.P., Graf, P.D., Gold, W.M. and Nadel, J.A. (1976). The mechanism of rapid shallow breathing after inhaling histamine aerosol in exercising dogs. Amer. Rev. Resp. Disease 114: 909-916.

Booth, B.H., Patterson, R. and Talbot, C.H. (1970). Immediate-type hypersensitivity in dogs: cutaneous, anaphylactic and respiratory responses to ascaris. Lab. Clin. Med. 76: 181-189.

Brimblecombe, R.W., Green, D.M. and Muir, A.W. (1972). Pharmacology of o-chlorobenzylidene malononitrile (CS). Br. J. Pharmacol. 44: 561-576.

Carswell, F. and Oliver, J. (1978). The respiratory response in sensitized rats to aerosol challenge. Immunology, 34: 465-470.

Carswell, F. and Oliver, J. (1978). Site of respiratory reaction in allergic rats challenged via the airways. Int. Archs. Allergy Appl. Immun. 57: 358-363.

Cauna, N., Hinderer, K.H. and Wentges, R.T. (1969). Sensory receptor organs of the human nasal respiratory mucosa. Amer. J. Anat. 124: 187-209.

Coate, W.B. and Busey, W.M. (1972). Chronic exposure of cynomolgus monkeys to nitrogen dioxide singly and in binary combination with certain airborne pollutants. Hazleton Laboratories, Inc. Report to Coordinating Research Council Project CAPM - 6 - 68.

Cotton, D.J., Bleecker, E.R., Fischer, S.P., Graf, P.D., Gold, W.M. and Nadel, J.A. (1977). Rapid, shallow breathing after Ascaris suum antigen inhalation: role of vagus nerve. J. Appl. Physiol.: Respirat. Environ. Exercise Physiol. 42: 101-106.

Dautrebande, L. (1962). Microaerosols, pp. 108-112, Academic Press, N.Y.

Davis, T.R.A., Battista, S.P. and Kensler, C.J. (1967). Mechanism of respiratory effects during exposure of guinea-pigs to irritants. Arch. Environ. Health 15: 412-419.

DeLucia, A.J. and Adams, W.C. (1977). Effects of O_3 inhalation during exercise on pulmonary function and blood biochemistry. J. Appl. Physiol. 43: 75-81.

Douglas, J.S., Dennis, M.W., Ridgway, P. and Bouhuys, A. (1972). Airway dilation and constriction in spontaneously breathing guinea-pigs. J. Pharmacol. Expt. Therap. 180: 98-109.

Folinsbee, L.J., Silverman, F. and Shepard, R.J. (1975). Exercise responses following ozone exposure. J. Appl. Physiol. 38: 996-1001.

Griswold, S.S., Chambers, L.A. and Motley, H.L. (1957). Report of a case of exposure to high ozone concentrations for two hours. A.M.A. Arch. Indust. Health 15: 108-110.

Grunstein, M.M., Hazucha, M., Sorti, J. and Milic-Emili (1977). Effect of SO_2 on control of breathing in anesthetized cats. J. Appl. Physiol. 43: 844-851.

Kane, L.E. and Alarie, Y. (1977). Sensory irritation to formaldehyde and acrolein during single and repeated exposures in mice. Amer. Ind. Hyg. Assoc. J. 38: 509-522.

Kane, L. and Alarie, Y. (1978). Sensory irritation of some select experimental photochemical oxidants. Arch. Environ. Health 33: 244-250.

Kane, L., Barrow, C.S. and Alarie, Y. (1979). A short-term test to predict acceptable levels of exposure to airborne sensory irritants. Am. Ind. Hyg. Assoc. J. 40: 207-229.

Karol, M.H., Hauth, B.A. and Alarie, Y. (1979). Pulmonary hypersensitivity to hexyl isocyanate-ovalbumin aerosol in guinea-pigs. Toxicol. Appl. Pharmacol. 51: 73-80.

Karol, M.H., Dixon, C., Brady, M. and Alarie, Y. (1980). Immunologic sensitization and pulmonary hypersensitivity by repeated inhalation of aromatic isocyanates. Toxicol. Appl. Pharmacol. 53: 260-270.

Karol, M.H., Ioset, H.H., Riley, E.J. and Alarie, Y.C. (1978). Hapten-specific respiratory hypersensitivity in guinea-pigs. Amer. Ind. Hyg. Assoc. J. 39: 546-556.

Karol, M.H., Underhill, D.W., Stadler, J. and Alarie, Y. (1981). Monitoring delayed respiratory hypersensitivity in guinea-pigs. The Toxicologist, in press.

Kratschmer, F. (1870). Uber reflexe von der Nasenchleimbaut auf ahtmung und Kreislauf. Akad. Wiss. Lit. Abh. Math.-Naturwiss. Kl. (Mainz), 62: 147-170.

Laqueur, E. and Magnus, R. (1921). Uber Kampfgas-vergiftugen III. Experimentelle Pathologie des Phosgenvergiftung. Z. Gesamte Exp. Med. 13: 31-179.

Lee, L.Y., Bleecker, E.R. and Nadel, J.A. (1977). Mechanism of rapid shallow breathing after ozone exposure in conscious dogs. J. Appl. Physiol.: Respirat. Environ. Exercise Physiol. 46: 1108-1114.

Lee, L.Y., Djokic, T.D., Dumont, C., Graf, P.D. and Nadel, J.A. (1980). Mechanism of ozone-induced tachypneic response to hypoxia and hypercapnia in conscious dogs. J. Appl. Physiol.: Respirat. Environ. Exercise Physiol. 48: 163-168.

Lee, L.Y., Dumont, C., Djokic, T.D., Menzel, T.E. and Nadel, J.A. (1979). Mechanism of rapid shallow breathing after ozone exposure in conscious dogs. J. Appl. Physiol.: Respirat. Environ. Exercise Physiol. 46: 1108-1114.

Magné, H., Mayer, A. and Plantefol, L. (1925a). Recherches sur les action reflexes produites par l'irritation des voies respiratoires. Ann. Physiol. 1: 394-427.

Magné, H., Mayer, A. and Plantefol, L. (1925b). La mort par inhibition et l'irritation des premieres voies respiratoires. Ann. Physiol. 1, 428-443.

Melnick, F.B. (1974). A model for pulmonary irritation using FPL-52757. Master degree essay. Graduate School of Public Health, University of Pittsburgh.

Michoud, M.C., Paré, P.D., Boucher, R. and Hogg, J.C. (1978). Airway response to histamine and metacholine in ascaris suum-allergic rhesus monkeys. J. Appl. Physiol.: Respirat. Environ. Exercise Physiol. 45: 846-851.

Mills, J.E., Sellick, H. and Widdicombe, J.G. (1970). Epithelial receptors in the lungs, in Breathing: Hering-Breur Centenary Symposium, Porter, R. Ed., Churchill, London 1970, 77-99.

Miyamoto, T. and Kabe, J. (1971). The lungs as the site of delayed-type hypersensitivity reactions in guinea-pigs. J. Allergy 47: 181-185.

Miyamoto, T., Kabe, J., Noda, M., Kobayashi, N. and Miura, K. (1971). Physiologic and pathologic respiratory changes in delayed type hypersensitivity reaction in guinea-pigs. Amer. Rev. Resp. Disease 103: 509-515.

Miyamoto, T., Reynolds, L.B., Patterson, R., Cugell, D.W. and Kettel, L.J. (1968). Respiratory changes in passively sensitized dogs and monkeys as models of allergic asthma. Am. Rev. Resp. Disease 97: 76-88.

Murphy, S.D., Ulrich, C.E., Frankowitz, S.H. and Xintaras, C. (1964). Altered function in animals inhaling low concentrations of ozone and nitrogen dioxide. Am. Ind. Hyg. Assoc. J. 25: 246-252.

Nagaishi, C. (1972). Functional anatomy and histology of the lung. University Park Press, Baltimore, MD.

Noelpp, B. and Noelpp-Eschenhagen, I. (1952). Das experimentelle Asthma bronchiale des Meerschweinchens IV. Mitteilung Zum Modellcharakter des experimentellen Meerschweinchenasthmas. Intern. Arch. Allergy Immun. 3: 207-217.

Paré, P.D., Michoud, M.C. and Hogg, J.C. (1976). Lung mechanics following antigen challenge of ascaris suum-sensitive rhesus monkeys. J. Appl. Physiol. 41: 668-676.

Patterson, R. (1960). Investigations of spontaneous hypersensitivity of the dog. J. Allergy 31: 351-363.

Patterson, R. and Kelley, J.F. (1974). Animal models of the asthmatic state. Annu. Rev. Med. 25: 53-68.

Patterson, R. and Talbot, C.H. (1969). Respiratory responses in subhuman primates with immediate type hypersensitivity. J. Lab. Clin. Med. 73: 924-933.

Patterson, R., Harris, K.E. and Susko, I.M. (1977). Sequential immunologic stimuli to the respiratory tract. Amer. Rev. Resp. Disease 115: 929-936.

Patterson, R., Harris, K.E., Suszko, M. and Roberts, M. (1976). Reagin-mediated asthma in rhesus monkeys and relation to bronchial cell histamine release and airway reactivity to carbocholine. J. Clin. Invest. 57: 586-593.

Pietchuta, H., Smith, M.E., Share, N.N. and Holme, G. (1979). The respiratory response of sensitized rats to challenge with antigen aerosols. Immunology 38: 385-392.

Richardson, J.B. (1979). Nerve supply to the lungs. Amer. Rev. Resp. Disease 119: 785-802.

Rossing, R.G. (1964). Physiologic effects of chronic exposure to phosgene. J. Appl. Physiol. 207: 265-272.

Schatz, M., Patterson, R., Sommers, H.M., Harris, K.E., Suszko, I.M. and Roberts, M. (1977). Immediate-type hypersensitivity to heyhole limpet haemocyanin in the dog. Immunology 32: 95-101.

Scheel, L.D., Dobrogorski, O.J., Mountain, J.T., Svirbely, J.L. and Stokinger (1959). Physiologic, biochemical immunologic and pathologic changes following ozone exposure. J. Appl. Physiol. 14: 67-80.

Sellick, H. and Widdicombe, J.G. (1969). The activity of lung irritant receptors during pneumothorax, hyperpnea and pulmonary vascular congestion. J. Physiol. 203: 359-381.

Whitteridge, D. (1948). The action of phosgene on the stretch receptors of the lung. J. Physiol. 107: 107-114.

Whitteridge, D. and Bulbring, E. (1944). Changes in activity of pulmonary receptors in anesthesia and their influence on respiratory behavior. J. Pharmacol. Exp. Therap. 81: 340-359.

Widdicombe, J.G. (1954a). Respiratory reflexes from the trachea and bronchi of the cat. J. Physiol. 123: 55-70.

Widdicombe, J.G. (1954b). Receptors in the trachea and bronchi of the cat. J. Physiol. 123: 71-104.

Widdicombe, J.G. (1974). Reflex control of breathing. In: Respiratory Physiology, Vol. 2, J.G. Widdicombe Ed. University Park Press, Baltimore MD.

Widdicombe, J.G. (1977). Defensive mechanisms of the respiratory system. In: International Review of Physiology, Respiratory Physiology II, Volume 14 J.G. Widdicombe Ed. University Park Press, Baltimore, MD.

Wilkie, B.N. (1976). Experimental hypersensitivity pneumonitis. Humoral and cell-mediated immune response of cattle to micropolyspora faeni and clinical response to aerosol challenge. Int. Archs. Allergy Appl. Immun. 50: 359-373.

Wilkie, B.N., Markham, R.J.F. and Shewen, P.E. (1980). Responses of calves to lung challenge exposure with pasteurella haemolytica after parenteral or pulmonary immunization. Am. J. Vet. Res. 41: 1773-1778.

Immunologic Response of the Respiratory System to Industrial Chemicals

MERYL H. KAROL
Department of Industrial Environmental Health Sciences
Graduate School of Public Health
University of Pittsburgh
Pittsburgh, Pennsylvania

ABSTRACT

Inhalation of gases, vapors or dusts may induce immunologic hypersensitivity reactions within the respiratory tract. In order to assess the sensitizing potencies of various industrial materials, an animal model for pulmonary hypersensitivity has been developed. In the model, guinea pigs are sensitized by exposures designed to simulate those experienced in the industrial situation; i.e., exposure via inhalation and dermal contact. Using the industrial chemical, toluene diisocyanate, (TDI) a dose-response relationship has been detected between exposure concentration of TDI and development of immunologic response. Extension of the animal model to ascertain a "no-response" concentration should enable the setting of Threshold Limit Values for industrial workers to protect against industrial sensitization.

INTRODUCTION

Exposure of workers to certain organic as well as inorganic chemicals in the workplace may result in the development of pulmonary hypersensitivity. Examples of such allergenic chemicals are presented in Table I. The hypersensitivity response is thought to be immunologic in nature since prior exposure to the chemical is required, and very small amounts are subsequently sufficient to trigger a response. Onset of respiratory reactions may occur either within minutes of re-exposure, or may be delayed and occur hours following exposure.

Table I. Respiratory Hypersensitivity from Industrial Chemicals

Industrial Compound	Symptoms	Reference
Amprolium hydrochloride	Asthma	Greene and Freedman, 1976
Beryllium	Rhinitis, cough, dyspnea, cyanosis	Hardy and Tabershaw, 1946
Cement dust	Asthma	Kobayashi, 1974
Chloramine	Asthma	Bourne _et al_., 1979
Diphenylmethane diisocyanate (MDI)		Zeiss _et al_., 1980; Konzen _et al_., 1966
Enflurane	Asthma	Schwettmann and Casterline, 1976
Ethylenediamine	Asthma	Lam and Chan-Yeung, 1980
Formalin	Asthma	Hendrick and Lane, 1975
Naphthylene diisocyanate	Asthma	Harries _et al_., 1979
Nickel sulfate	Asthma	McConnell _et al_., 1973
Persulfate salts	Asthma, dermatitis	Pepys _et al_., 1976 Baur _et al_., 1979
Phenylglycine acid chloride	Asthma	Kammermeyer and Mathews, 1973
Phenylmercuric proprionate	Asthma, urticaria	Koszewski and Hubbard, 1956; Mathews, 1968; Morris, 1960
Phthalic anhydride	Asthma, rhinitis	Kern, 1939; Maccia _et al_., 1976

Table I. (cont'd.)

Industrial Compound	Symptoms	Reference
Platinum salts	Asthma, dermatitis	Freedman and Krupey, 1968; Cleare *et al*., 1976
Sodium bichromate	Asthma	Kobayashi, 1974
Spiramycin	Asthma, dermatitis	Davies and Pepys, 1975
Tannic acid	Asthma, urticaria, rhinitis	Johnston *et al*., 1951
Tetracycline	Asthma	Menon and Das, 1977
Toluene diisocyanate (TDI)	Asthma, urticaria	Avery *et al*., 1969; Pepys *et al*., 1972; Karol *et al*., 1979b
Trimellitic anhydride	Asthma	Zeiss *et al*., 1977

Due to the severe, sometimes life-threatening nature of pulmonary hypersensitivity reactions, it is essential to understand the process of sensitization to industrial chemicals. For many years, effort has been directed toward development of an animal model for inhalation sensitization where exposure to foreign materials occurs via the respiratory tract. Using this route, several investigators have been successful in achieving pulmonary hypersensitivity (see Table II). Using inhalation exposure, sensitization has been achieved with natural products, such as dander, molds and spores (Ratner *et al*., 1927), as well as by inhalation of purified proteins (Schatz *et al*., 1977). Inhalation sensitization has been achieved in several animal species including guinea pigs (Ratner, 1939; Swineford, 1968), calves (Wilkie, 1976), and rabbits (Salvaggio *et al*., 1975). By contrast, sensitization to low molecular weight chemicals via inhalation exposure, has been achieved only very recently in this laboratory (Karol *et al*., 1980) by repeated inhalation of p-tolyl isocyanate and toluene diisocyanate vapors. Respiratory sensitivity was apparent 2 weeks following exposure. The ability to experimentally produce sensitivity as a result of inhalation of chemicals is the first step toward understanding industrial respiratory sensitivity and preventing future sensitization of industrial workers.

Table II. Experimental Induction of Pulmonary Hypersensitivity Using Aerosol Exposure

Antigen	Animal Species	Reference
Ragweed extract	Dog	Patterson and Kelly, 1974; Patterson et al., 1963
Ascaris	Dog	Booth et al., 1970
Keyhold limpet haemocyanin	Dog	Schatz et al., 1977
Ascaris	Monkey	Weiszer et al., 1968
Micropolyspora faeni, Bovine serum albumin	Rabbit	Salvaggio et al., 1975
Benzylpenicilloyl bovine gamma globulin	Horse	Lazary et al., 1974
Micropolyspora faeni	Cow	Wilkie, 1976
Horse dander	Guinea pig	Ratner et al., 1927; Ratner, 1939; Herxheimer and West, 1955
Egg white	Guinea pig	Swineford, 1968
Diastase	Guinea pig	Kobayashi, 1974
Bacterial amylase	Guinea pig	Yagura et al., 1970; Yamamura et al., 1974
Picryl-bacterial amylase	Guinea pig	Yamamura et al., 1974
Bacillus subtilus subtilopeptidase A	Guinea pig	Markham and Wilkie, 1976
Ovalbumin, Bovine serum albumin	Guinea pig	Matsumura, 1970

Table II. (cont'd.)

Antigen	Animal Species	Reference
Ovalbumin, p-Azobenzenearsonate ovalbumin, p-tolyl isocyanate ovalbumin	Guinea pig	Karol *et al*., 1978
Hexyl isocyanate ovalbumin	Guinea pig	Karol *et al*., 1979a
p-Tolyl isocyanate, Toluene diisocyanate	Guinea pig	Karol *et al*., 1980

To safeguard workers, it is essential to know the concentration of chemical and the exposure conditions which induce sensitivity. Such information can be obtained using an animal model for inhalation sensitization. The following report describes use of the guinea pig animal model (Karol *et al*., 1978, 1979a, 1980) to investigate sensitization of the respiratory tract to an industrial chemical, toluene diisocyanate.

MATERIALS AND METHODS

Female, English smooth-haired guinea pigs (Hilltop Lab Animals) were used for sensitization. Animals were exposed to toluene diisocyanate (TDI, 80/20 mixture of 2,4/2,6 isomers) using a "head-only" exposure system as described previously (Karol *et al*., 1980). Animals were placed in body plethysmographs with heads extending through a latex collar into a 10 liter plexiglass inhalation chamber. Chamber concentrations of TDI were generated by bubbling metered quantities of dried air through a glass impinger containing TDI. Concentrations in the inhalation chamber were determined by sampling from the chamber during animal exposure and analyzing samples using the method of Marcali (Marcali, 1957). For sensitization, animals were exposed to TDI vapor for 3 hours a day on 5 consecutive days.

To test for the presence of pulmonary sensitivity, guinea pigs were challenged with low concentrations of TDI (below 0.02 ppm) while restrained in body plethysmographs. Sensitivity was assessed by measuring respiratory rates and tidal volumes of animals during bronchial provocation challenge and comparing the values during challenge with those immediately preceeding challenge when ambient air was drawn through the chamber. Respiratory rate increases during inhalation challenge with specific antigen is known to occur in numerous species of animals including rabbits, calves, dogs, monkeys, sheep, guinea pigs and man (Patterson and Kelly, 1974; also reviewed by Karol et al., 1980). In studies reported here, a respiratory rate increase of 47% or greater was considered significant. This value is equivalent to the mean + 3 SD respiratory rate found in control non-sensitized guinea pigs when challenged with antigen by inhalation.

Skin Sensitization

Animals were sensitized to TDI by application of 25 ul onto each of 2 shaved, depilated sites on the dorsal area of guinea pigs. Fourteen days later animals were bled for serologic study.

Antibody Evaluation

Blood was drawn from the nail bed of guinea pigs. Sera were evaluated for cytotrophic antibodies using the passive cutaneous anaphylaxis assay (PCA). In the assay, 0.1 ml of serial dilutions of sera, in saline, were injected into backs of normal guinea pigs. After a six hour latent period, antibodies were detected by intravenous injection of a TDI-guinea pig serum albumin (TDI-GSA) conjugate together with Evans blue dye. Preparation of the conjugate antigen has been detailed elsewhere (Karol et al., 1978). Antibody titers were defined as the highest serum dilution which yielded a blue reaction site of at least 5 mm D.

RESULTS

Groups of guinea pigs were exposed to known amounts of TDI vapor on each of five consecutive days. During exposure, respiratory rates of animals were measured. Typically respiratory rates fell by 50% to 80% during exposure to 0.25, 0.50, and 1.00 ppm TDI. This response was due to the sensory irritating properties of TDI on the nasal mucosa as shown to occur in mice (Sangha and Alarie, 1979) and guinea pigs (Karol et al., 1980).

Blood was obtained from animals 21 days following the first day of exposure and evaluated for cytotrophic antibodies. As seen in Table III, antibody titers were highest in those animals which had the greatest exposures to TDI.

Exposure to 1.00 ppm TDI resulted in antibody production in all animals with titers ranging from 8 to 256 (Table III). By contrast, exposure of animals to 0.25 ppm TDI resulted in minimal antibody production. At that concentration antibodies were detected in only 5 of the 16 TDI-exposed guinea pigs and titers never exceeded 2-4. These results indicate a dose-response relationship between exposure concentration of TDI and stimulation of the immune system to produce TDI-specific cytotrophic antibodies.

Table III. Antibody Production in Guinea Pigs to TDI Vapor

TDI Concentration	Total ppm-hours[1]	No. Animals Tested	PCA Antibody Titer
0.25 ppm	3.75	16	0,0,0,0,0,0,0,0,0 0,0,2,2,2,4,4
0.50 ppm	7.50	8	0,0,0,2,8,8,8,64
1.00 ppm	10.0	14	8,32,32,32,32,64, 64,64,64,64,64 128,128,256

[1] Calculated from: exposure concentration in ppm x hours of exposure.

Pulmonary sensitivity

Cytotrophic antibodies attach to cells along the respiratory tract. Subsequent contact of cell-bound antibody with inhaled antigen causes release of mediators, vasodilatation and contraction of smooth muscle (Patterson et al., 1978). The production of specific cytotrophic antibodies in animals exposed to toluene diisocyanote thus implies the possibility of pulmonary sensitivity in these animals. Accordingly, guinea pigs were evaluated for pulmonary sensitivity by bronchial provocation challenge using TDI-GSA conjugate. Results in Table IV indicate that a percentage of the animals possessing antibodies to TDI (Table III) responded with pulmonary sensitivity reactions. The number of animals responding increased with the TDI exposure. These pulmonary hypersensitivity reactions were specific for TDI since none of the animals responded when challenged with aerosols of non-conjugated GSA.

Table IV. Pulmonary Sensitivity in Guinea Pigs Repeatedly Exposed to TDI Vapor

TDI Concentration	No. Animals	#Animals Responding[1]/Total
0.25 ppm	16	0/16
0.50 ppm	8	2/8
1.00 ppm	14	8/14

[1] Pulmonary sensitivity was evaluated by bronchial provocation challenge using TDI-GSA aerosol. A respiratory rate increase of 47% from pre-challenge levels was considered a significant response.

Effect of route of exposure

Sensitization of animals to toluene diisocyanate has been accomplished by repeatedly exposing animals to vapors of TDI as described above. It has also been possible to sensitize animals to TDI exclusively by dermal contact (Karol et al., 1981). Animals exposed to TDI by the latter route develop TDI-specific contact sensitivity and produce TDI-specific antibodies. Additionally, as in the situation with inhalation exposure, a proportion of animals sensitized by dermal contact demonstrate TDI-specific respiratory hypersensitivity when challenged with TDI or TDI-GSA antigen. One can compare the immunogenic potency of TDI when administered to animals by the two routes of exposure; i.e., inhalation and dermal. Results of such a comparison are presented in Table V.

Calculation of the total amount of TDI received during inhalation sensitization was made as follows assuming complete retention of TDI vapor for each breath: chamber conc. TDI (ug/l) x min. exposure x respir. rate x tidal vol. (in ml) x 10^{-3} (l/ml). Values for the respiratory rate and tidal volume of animals were obtained by body plethysmography during exposure. It is apparent that inhalation exposure to TDI is *much* more potent than dermal exposure for inducing an immunologic response. A dose of 60 mg TDI onto the skin was required to achieve an antibody response comparable to that obtained following inhalation of 42 ug TDI. Whether the immunogenic potency of TDI when administered by inhalation results from the route of administration, the vapor state of the chemical, or a combination of both factors remains to be investigated.

Table V. Immunogenicity of TDI: Comparison of Inhalation and Dermal Routes of Exposure

TDI Dose (ug)	Route of Exposure	PCA Antibody Titers
42	inhalation	8,32,32,32,64,64,64,64,64,65,128 128,264
600	dermal	0,0,0,0,0
6000	dermal	0,0,2,4,4,16
60,000	dermal	32,32,32,32,32,64,64,64

DISCUSSION

Many chemicals have been recognized as causing industrial hypersensitivity reactions. In order to protect workers from becoming sensitized to these materials, it is essential to determine if the sensitization process is controlled by a dose-response relationship. The existence of such a relationship can only be ascertained by employing an animal model for industrial sensitization where exposure route and concentration can be carefully controlled. Use of the animal model described here to obtain dose-response relationships between exposure concentration and development of hypersensitivity will allow evaluation of the sensitizing potency of individual chemicals and permit comparison of the relative potencies of several industrial chemicals. This data should enable threshold limit values to be set for the *first time* which will likely prevent immunologic sensitization of workers by small organic molecules capable of acting as haptens.

ACKNOWLEDGMENTS

This work was supported by funds from grant R01-ES01532 from the National Institute of Environmental Health Sciences and grant R01-OH00865 from the National Institute for Occupational Safety and Health.

REFERENCES

Avery, S. B., Stetson, D. M., Pan, P. M. and Mathews, K. P. (1969). Immunological investigation of individuals with toluene diisocyanate asthma. Clin. exp. Immunol. 4, 585-596.

Baur, X., Fruhmann, G. and v. Liebe, V. (1979). Persulfat-Asthma und Persulfat-Dermatitis bei zwei Industriearbeitern. Respiration 38, 144-150.

Booth, B. H., Patterson, R. and Talbot, C. H. (1970). Immediate-type hypersensitivity in dogs: cutaneous, anaphylactic and respiratory responses to Ascaris. J. Lab. Clin. Med. 76, 181-189.

Bourne, M. S., Flindt, M. L. H. and Walker, J. M. (1979). Asthma due to industrial use of chloramine. Brit. Med. J. 2, 10-12.

Cleare, M. J., Hughes, E. G., Jacoby, B. and Pepys, J. (1976). Immediate (type I) allergic responses to platinum compounds. Clin. Allergy 6, 183-195.

Davies, R. J. and Pepys, J. (1975). Asthma due to inhaled chemical agents - the macrolide antibiotic spiramycin. Clin. Allergy 5, 99-107.

Freedman, S. D. and Krupey, J. (1968). Respiratory allergy caused by platinum salts. J. Allergy Clin. Immunol. 42, 233-238.

Greene, S. A. and Freedman, S. (1976). Asthma due to inhaled chemical agents - amprolium hydrochloride. Clin. Allergy 6, 105-108.

Hardy, H. L. and Tabershaw, I. R. (1946). Delayed chemical pneumonitis occurring in workers exposed to beryllium compounds. J. Indust. Hyg. Toxicol. 28, 197-211.

Harries, M. G., Burge, P. S., Samson, M., Newman-Taylor, A. J. and Pepys, J. (1979). Isocyanate asthma. Respiratory symptoms due to 1,5-naphthylene di-isocyanate. Thorax 34, 762-766.

Hendrick, O. J. and Lane, D. J. (1975). Formalin asthma in hospital staff. Brit. Med. J. 1, 607-608.

Herxheimer, H. and West, T. (1955). Sensitization of guinea pigs by inhalation. J. Physiol. 127, 564-571.

Johnston, T. G., Cazort, A. G., Marvin, H. N., Pringle, R. B. and Sheldon, J. M. (1951). Bronchial asthma, urticaria and allergic rhinitis from tannic acid. J. Allergy. 22, 494-499.

Kammermeyer, J. K. and Mathews, K. P. (1973). Hypersensitivity to phenylglycine acid chloride. J. Allergy Clin. Immunol. 52, 73-84.

Karol, M. H., Dixon, C., Brady, M. and Alarie, Y. (1980). Immunologic sensitization and pulmonary hypersensitivity by repeated inhalation of aromatic isocyanates. Toxicol. Appl. Pharmacol. 53, 260-270.

Karol, M. H., Hauth, B. A., Riley, E. J. and Magreni, C. M. (1981). Dermal contact with toluene diisocyanate (TDI) produces respiratory tract hypersensitivity in guinea pigs. Toxicol. Appl. Pharmacol. (in press).

Karol, M. H., Ioset, H. H., Riley, E. J., and Alarie, Y. (1978). Hapten-specific respiratory hypersensitivity in guinea pigs. Amer. Ind. Hyg. Assoc. J. 39, 546-556.

Karol, M. H., Hauth, B. A. and Alarie, Y. (1979a). Pulmonary hypersensitivity to hexyl isocyanate-ovalbumin aerosol in guinea pigs. Toxicol. Appl. Pharmacol. 51, 73-80.

Karol, M. H., Sandberg, T., Riley, E. J. and Alarie, Y. (1979b). Longitudinal study of tolyl-reactive IgE antibodies in workers hypersensitive to TDI. J. Occup. Med. 21, 354-358.

Kern, R. A. (1939). Asthma and allergic rhinitis due to sensitization to phthalic anhydride; report of a case. J. Allergy 10, 164-165.

Kobayashi, S. (1974). Occupational asthma due to inhalation of pharmacological dusts and other chemical agents with some reference to other occupational asthmas in Japan. In Allergology, Proceedings of the VIII International Congress of Allergology (Y. Yamamura, O. L. Frick, Y. Horiuichi, S. Kishimoto, T. Miyamota, P. Naranjo and A. deWeck, eds.), p. 124. American Elsevier Publishing Co., New York.

Konzen, R. B., Croft, B. F., Schell, L. D., Gorski, C. H. (1966). Human response to low concentrations of p,p-diphenylmethane diisocyanate (MDI). Am. Ind. Hyg. Assoc. J. 27, 121-127.

Koszewski, B. J. and Hubbard, T. F. (1956). Immunological agranulocytosis due to mercurial diuretics. Am. J. Med. 20, 958-963.

Lam, S. and Chan-Yeung, M. (1980). Ethylenediamine-induced asthma. Am. Rev. Resp. Dis. 121, 151-155.

Lazary, S., Gerber, H., Friedrich, W., Schatzman, U., Straub, R., Rivera, E., and deWeck, A. L. (1974). Hypersensitivity in the horse with special reference to reaction in the lung. In Allergology, Proceedings of the VIII International Congress of Allergology (Y. Yamamura, O. L. Frick, Y. Horiuchi, S. Kishimoto, T. Miyamoto, P. Naranjo and A. deWeck, eds.), p. 501-508 American Elsevier Publishing Co., New York.

Maccia, C. A., Bernstein, I. L., Emmett, E. A. and Brooks, S. M. (1976). In vitro demonstration of specific IgE in phthalic anhyride hypersensitivity. Am. Rev. Resp. Dis. 113, 701-704.

Marcali, K. (1957). Microdetermination of toluene diisocyanates in atmosphere. Anal. Chem. 29, 552-558.

Markham, R. J. F. and Wilkie, B. N. (1976). Influence of detergent on aerosol allergic sensitization with enzymes of Bacillus subtilis. Int. Archs. Allergy appl. Immun. 51, 529-543.

Mathews, K. P. (1968). Immediate-type hypersensitivity to phenyl mercuric compounds. Am. J. Med. 44, 310-318.

Matsumura, Y. (1970). The effects of ozone, nitrogen dioxide, and sulfur dioxide on the experimentally induced allergic respiratory disorder in guinea pigs. I. The effect on sensitization with albumin through the airway. Am. Rev. Resp. Dis. 102, 430-437.

McConnell, L. H., Fink, J. N., Schleuter, D. P. and Schmidt, M. D. (1973). Asthma caused by nickel sensitivity. Ann. Intern. Med. 78, 888-890.

Menon, M. P. S. and Das, A. K. (1977). Tetracycline asthma - a case report. Clin. Allergy 7, 285-290.

Moore, V. L., Hensley, G. T. and Fink, J. N. (1975). An animal model of hypersensitivity pneumonitis in the rabbit. J. Clin. Invest. 56, 937-944.

Morris, G. E. (1960). Dermatosis from phenyl-mercuric salts. Arch. Environ. Health 1, 53-55.

Patterson, R. and Kelly, J. F. (1974). Animal models of the asthmatic state. Annu. Rev. Med. 25, 53-68.

Patterson, R., Pruzansky, J. J., and Chang, W. W. Y. (1963). Spontaneous canine hypersensitivity to ragweed. Characterization of the serum factor transferring skin, bronchial, and anaphylactic sensitivity. J. Immunol. 90, 36-41.

Patterson, R., Suszko, I. M. and Harris, K. E. (1978). The in vivo transfer of antigen induced airway reactions by bronchial lumen mast cells. J. Clin. Invest. 62, 519-524.

Pepys, J. Hutchcroft, B. J. and Breslin, A. B. X. (1976). Asthma due to inhaled chemical agents - persulfate salts and henna in hairdressers. Clin. Allergy 6, 399-404.

Pepys, J., Pickering, C. A. C., Breslin, A. B. X. and Terry, D. J. (1972). Asthma due to inhaled chemical agents - tolylene diisocyanate. Clin. Allergy 2, 225-236.

Porter, C. V., Higgins, R. L., and Scheel, L. D. (1975). A retrospective study of clinical, physiologic and immunologic changes in workers exposed to toluene diisocyanate. Am. Ind. Hyg. Assoc. J. 36, 159-168.

Ratner, B. (1939). Experimental asthma. Am. J. Dis. Child. 58, 699-733.

Ratner, B., Jackson, H. C., and Gruehl, H. L. (1927). Respiratory anaphylaxis. Sensitization, shock, bronchial asthma and death induced in the guinea pig by the nasal inhalation of dry horse dander. Am. J. Dis. Child. 34, 23-52.

Salvaggio, J., Phanuphak, P., Stanford, R., Bice, D., and Claman, H. (1975). Experimental production of granulomatous pneumonitis. Comparison of immunological and morphological sequelae with particulate and soluble antigens administered via the respiratory route. J. Allergy Clin. Immunol. 56, 364-380.

Sangha, S. K. and Alarie, Y. (1979). Sensory irritation by toluene diisocyanate in single and repeated exposures. Toxicol. Appl. Pharmacol. 50, 533-547.

Schatz, M., Patterson, R., Sommers, H. M., Harris, K. E., Suszko, I. M. and Roberts, M. (1977). Immediate-type hypersensitivity to keyhold limpet haemocyanin in the dog. Immunol. 32, 95-101.

Schwettman, R. S. and Casterline, C. L. (1976). Delayed asthmatic response following occupational exposure to enflurane. Anesthesiol. 44, 166-169.

Swineford, O. Jr. (1968). Active sensitization of guinea pigs by inhalation of aerosols of antigen. Ann. Allergy 26, 28-32.

Weiszer, I., Patterson, R. and Pruzansky, J. J. (1968). Ascaris hypersensitivity in the rhesus monkey. I. A model for the study of immediate type hypersensitivity in the primate. J. Allergy. 41, 14-36.

Wilkie, B. N. (1976). Experimental hypersensitivity pneumonitis. Int. Archs. Allergy appl. Immun. 50, 359-373.

Yagura, T., Miyagawa, T. and Yamamura, Y. (1971). Experimental allergic asthma in guinea pigs. In: New Concepts in Allergy and Clinical Immunology, Proc. VII International Congress Allergol., Florence, 1970 (U. Serafini, A. W. Frankland, C. Masala and J. M. Jamar, eds.) p. 266-274 Excerpta Medica, Amsterdam.

Yamamura, Y., Yagura, T. and Miyake, T. (1974). Experimental allergic asthma in guinea pigs. In: Allergology, Proceedings of the VIII International Congress of Allergology (Y. Yamamura, O. L. Frick, Y. Horiuchi, S. Kishi moto, T. Miyamoto, P. Naranjo, and A. deWeck, eds.) p. 509-515 American Elsevier Publishing Co., New York.

Zeiss, C. R., Kanellakes, T. M., Bellone, J. D., Levitz, D., Pruzansky, J. J. and Patterson, R. (1980). Immunoglobulin E-mediated asthma and hypersensitivity pneumonitis with precipitating anti-hapten antibodies due to diphenylmethane diisocyanate (MDI) exposure. J. Allergy Clin. Immunol. 65, 346-352.

Zeiss, C. R., Patterson, R., Pruzansky, J. J., Miller, M. M., Rosenberg, M. and Levitz, D. (1977). Trimellitic anhydride-induced airway syndromes: Clinical and immunologic studies. J. Allergy Clin. Immunol. 60, 96-103.

Aerosol Administration for Specific Pharmacologic Activity on the Tracheobronchial Tree

MARTIN A. WASSERMAN, ROBERT L. GRIFFIN, and PETER E. MALO
Department of Hypersensitivity Diseases Research
The Upjohn Company
Kalamazoo, Michigan 49008

ABSTRACT

In order to investigate the pharmacologic effects of test substances on the respiratory system, the oral, parenteral, or aerosol routes of administration are conveniently accessible. However, both the oral and parenteral routes are fraught with problems and concerns including: extraneous, perhaps undesirable effects on other systems, binding to tissues or blood-borne products, and absorption-distribution kinetics. Thus, aerosolization of drugs would be the most direct, accurate, and judicious method for detecting and evaluating bronchopulmonary activities.

In dogs and guinea pigs, one can examine many different potential bronchoconstrictors and bronchodilators, especially those of the sympathetic, prostaglandin, and anticholinergic classes. Laboratory animals can be anesthetized or conscious and can be normal or hyperreactive to specific antigens, thus permitting aerosol provocation to be either pharmacologic or immunologic. With these various options, one can analyze mechanistically how and where bronchoconstriction occurs in the tracheobronchial tree and, therapeutically, which drugs may be useful as aerosols in predictive models of acute, reversible airways disorders, e.g., bronchial asthma.

INTRODUCTION

Even though pharmacotherapeutic agents are most rapidly absorbed intravenously (I.V.) or most conveniently and economically administered orally, that method most applicable to direct accessability to the respiratory system is aerosolization/nebulization (Davies, 1975). Side effects on other systems, absorption-distribution kinetics and binding to blood-borne products represent only a few reasons for selecting the more specific aerosol route of administration, rather than oral or I.V., when investigating the local bronchopulmonary actions of experimental drugs and/or treating airway and lung disorders clinically. Inhalation is usually the preferred route (Brain and Valberg, 1979):

-to relieve bronchospasm, edema, allergy, inflammation, infection, and congestion which may be present in pulmonary disorders, e.g., asthma or emphysema.

-for provocational testing, e.g., methacholine, in asthmatics.

-to decrease mucosal viscosity and hasten its clearance.

-to humidify the airways.

-to achieve relatively high local (topical) therapeutic levels without unwanted systemic effects.

-to permit convenient and rapid access for systemic actions, if so desired.

-for drugs with difficult access to the lung parenchymal surfaces.

Those physical characteristics of aerosols which may determine efficacy include: penetration into the various branches of the tracheobronchial tree, deposition of suspended particles on the target surface, retention of particles to initiate physiologic or biochemical events, and appropriate clearance (Brain and Valberg, 1979).

Those particular classes of aerosolized agents which have been proven efficacious in the pharmacotherapy of bronchial asthma are: β-adrenergic sympathomimetics, anticholinergics, prostaglandin E's, corticosteroids, α-adrenergic antagonists, and mast cell stabilizers, while those agents with potential efficacy include: antihistamines, mucolytics, e.g., mucous rheology regulators, vasoactive peptides, local anesthetics, xanthines, and minor tranquilizers/anxiolytics.

Our research in the intact animal has focused on an understanding of the mechanisms underlying bronchoconstriction and the vast array of agents which can reverse this cardinal feature of bronchial asthma. In this paper, several animal models are described which have enabled us to perform successful pulmonary pharmacologic experiments with aerosol drugs. Examples of each model will highlight our results with these experimental investigations.

MATERIALS AND METHODS

Anesthetized Dogs: Beagle dogs of either sex (8-11 kg) were anesthetized with sodium pentobarbital (30 mg/kg) given I.V. Supplemental doses were administered as required to maintain a light level of anesthesia throughout the experiment. Test agents were administered intrabronchially as aerosols. All animals were permitted to breathe room air spontaneously.

Pulmonary mechanics, i.e., pulmonary resistance (R_L) and dynamic lung compliance (C_{DYN}) were estimated by the technique of Diamond (1972). This method for the anesthetized dog is a modification of the procedure introduced by Amdur and Mead (1958) for the unanesthetized guinea pig and has been described at length previously (Wasserman and Griffin, 1979; Wasserman et al., 1980a,b). Briefly, airflow rate ($\dot{V}$), tidal volume (V_T) and transpulmonary pressure (P_{TP}) were monitored simultaneously by established pharmacologic techniques (Figure 1). When there is no airflow and the airways are open, the

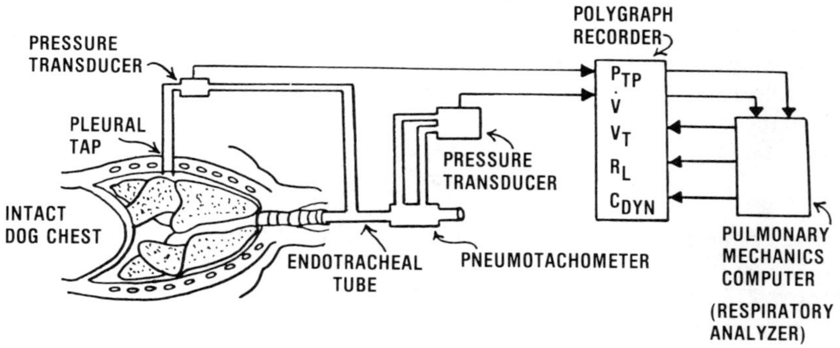

Figure 1 - Schematic depicting the anesthetized canine model used to detect pulmonary mechanical changes following aerosolized bronchoconstrictors and bronchodilators. Transpulmonary pressure (P_{TP}), airflow rate ($\dot{V}$), tidal volume (V_T), pulmonary resistance (R_L), and dynamic lung compliance (C_{DYN}) are monitored continuously on a breath-to-breath basis.

pressure at the mouth equals the pressure in the alveoli. Output signals representing P_{TP}, $\dot{V}$. and V_T were amplified and fed on-line into an analog Pulmonary Mechanics Computer (Buxco Electronics, Inc.). This device provided a continuous breath-by-breath analysis of the mechanical properties of the airways and lungs (Giles et al., 1971). The computer performed the necessary calculations at precisely the exact instant for measuring R_L and C_{DYN}; the output was displayed on a direct-writing Grass Model 7B polygraph. Between five and ten consecutive breaths were analyzed at the height of the response after treatment. The frequency of breathing (f) could be counted manually as the number of breaths/min.

After this initial preparation of the dogs and calibration of the equipment, a standard provocation was assessed. Either a bolus I.V. injection of $PGF_{2\alpha}$ (3 μg/kg) or an aerosol of acetylcholine (0.01%) produced a transient, yet reproducible, bronchoconstriction, which could be attenuated by known or test bronchodilators.

Aerosols were generated by a Mark VII Bird® Respirator with an in-line micronebulizer. This device was completely integrated with the bellows action of the animal's chest wall so as to minimize inspiratory effort and shift the work of breathing from animal to respirator. The flowrate, sensitivity and pressure settings on the respirator were adjusted to keep constant the volume of drug nebulized per breath. No attempt was made to estimate exactly how much drug was actually inhaled, but rather by knowing the concentration of each drug used and the average volume nebulized per breath (0.007 ml), the total amount of drug delivered over a uniform number of breaths could be approximated. The on-line, automatic, mainstream micronebulizer propelled particles in the range of 0.5-4.0 micrometer (μm) (mass median aerodynamic diameter).

Differences in bronchodilator activites were analyzed statistically by the "t" test for nonpaired data according to Snedecor (1956). A "p" value of 0.05 or less was selected as the level of significance.

Conscious dogs: The irritant liability of inhaled substances, e.g., PGE_2, was tested in a group of conscious beagle dogs by modifying the cat model of Gardiner et al. (1978). Dogs were trained to remain comfortably restrained in a modified sling for periods as long as 30-60 min (Figure 2). A plexiglas® head dome (4L.), adapted with a miniature crystal microphone and air intake/exhaust ports, was secured over the dog's head by interlocking brackets. Lining the circumference of the head dome was a rubber gasket to insure a hermetic seal. Variations in neck size were compensated by using an inflatable cuff positioned between the stanchion and dog's neck. The microphone/amplification system was developed by a medical electronics specialist (The Upjohn Company) and used to monitor sounds within the head dome,

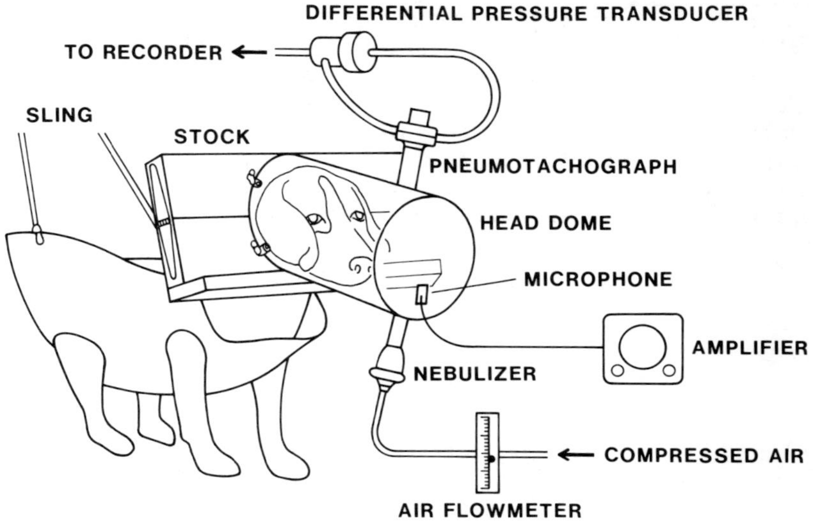

Figure 2 - Animal head dome model for detecting and evaluating the irritation and discomfort of inhaled substances, in conscious dogs. (Reprinted with permission of The Williams and Wilkins Co.; Wasserman et al., J. Pharmacol. Exp. Ther. 214: 68-73, 1980).

i.e., coughing, choking, or vocalizing. A modified DeVilbiss Model #45 nebulizer generated all aerosols and was affixed to the inhalation port. This nebulizer produced particles of suitable and effective size (0.3-2.0 μm) to reach the deeper recesses of the respiratory system. A constant 4L/min airflow was delivered through this nebulizer; at this flow, the volume of drug aerosolized was calculated to be 0.066 ml/min. Expired gas escaped through a heated mesh-screen pneumotachograph affixed to the exhaust port. Breathing patterns were displayed on and recorded from an oscilloscope (Electronics for Medicine DR-8) via a differential pressure transducer (Statham PM5 ± 0.15-350) connected to the pneumotachograph (Figure 2).

All dogs were given a one min. exposure to each of two control environments, i.e., compressed air and sterile distilled water, in order to acclimatize them to the system.

Then, they were exposed to aerosols of PGE_2 (0.2% or 1.0% for 3 min). Coughing, aggravated irregular airflow patterns, and general discomfort were taken as the subjective/objective indicators of relative aerosol-induced irritation.

Guinea Pigs: Asthma-like bronchoconstriction was induced in normal, male guinea pigs of the Hartley strain (250-500 g) by exposing them to an aerosol of a 0.25% aqueous solution of histamine diphosphate. This method is similar to the "microshock" technique of Herxheimer (1952). An inverted glass battery jar (9L.), into which a DeVilbiss #40 glass nebulizer was properly adapted, served as the aerosol chamber (Figure 3). The amount of aerosol produced was calculated to be 0.5 ml/60 sec. when generated under an air pressure of 5 psig. Before any animal was placed into the chamber,

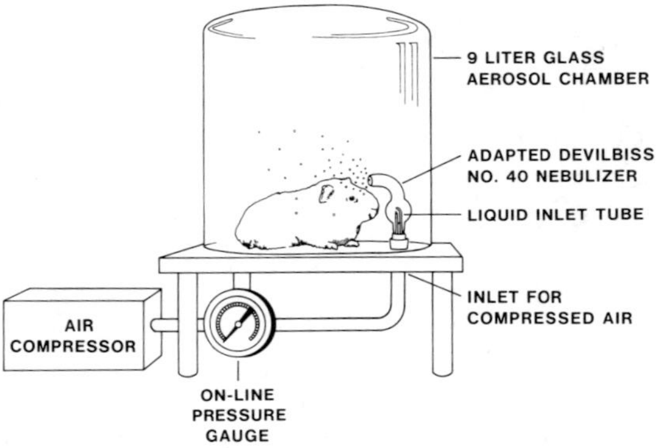

Figure 3 - *In vivo* conscious guinea pig system for evaluating the aerosol effects of potential bronchoconstrictors and bronchodilators.

histamine was aerosolized for 20 sec. in order to completely fill the system. The onset of near-fatal asphyxial collapse was found to be a consistent and reproducible endpoint and was taken to represent bronchoconstriction. The pre-asphyxial time was recorded for each guinea pig. Animals were removed quickly from the chamber after collapse and resuscitated as necessary. Recovery was usually complete within minutes. Once control responses to histamine were complete, groups of animals were subjected to aerosols of bronchodilators or vehicle alone for one min and, then, challenged with histamine one min later. The degree of protection from bronchospasm was assessed from the increased time to asphyxia; 420 sec was selected arbitrarily as the time of complete protection.

Another group of guinea pigs was used to evaluate immunologically-induced respiratory distress. A modification of the Herxheimer (1952) method was used for sensitization. Briefly, animals were injected i.m. (biceps femoris) with 0.7 ml of a 5% ovalbumin (OA) suspension prepared in isotonic saline Seven days later, this procedure was repeated. Fourteen days following this second injection, animals were exposed to an OA aerosol (0.5%) in the same type of chamber as described above. The anaphylactic syndrome following antigen-antibody interaction is characterized by deep abdominal breathing. The onset of this severe dyspnea within 420 sec was selected as the experimental endpoint. Those sensitized guinea pigs which did not exhibit anaphylaxis within 420 sec were omitted from further study. Test drugs were aerosolized and evaluated as before.

RESULTS AND DISCUSSION

Anesthetized Dogs: A brief exposure to the cholinergic agonist, acetylcholine (ACh) (1.0%; 3 tidal breaths), produces an immediate bronchospasm in anesthetized dogs, which is readily reversible when preceded by an inhalation of the anticholinergic, methscopolamine bromide (0.01%; 20 tidal breaths) (Figure 4). Since ACh has been implicated as a

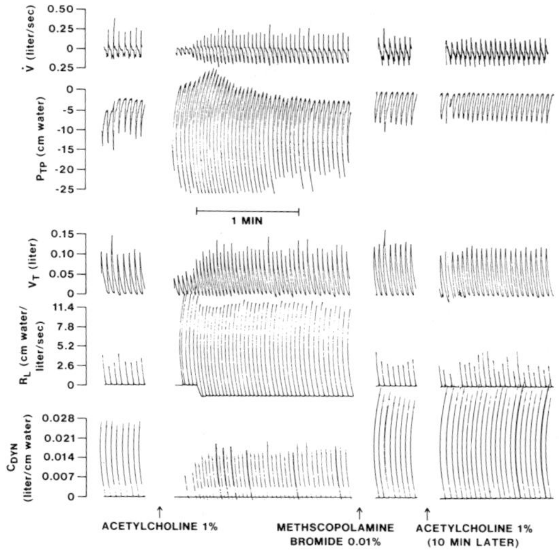

Figure 4 - Bronchopulmonary responses to aerosolized acetylcholine before and after an aerosol exposure to methscopolamine bromide in the anesthetized dog. (Reprinted with permission of The Williams and Wilkins Co.; Wasserman and Griffin, J. Pharmacol. Exp. Ther. 211: 159-166, 1979).

potentially important mediator of the asthmatic bronchospasm (Eppinger and Hess, 1915; Yu et al., 1972; Gold, 1973), it may follow logically that anticholinergics, e.g., methscopolamine bromide, would add to the physician's armamentarium against this disease (Solomon et al., 1955: Wasserman and Griffin, 1979).

When beagle dogs were exposed to aerosols of potential prostaglandin bronchodilators, i.e., PGI_2, PGE_1, or PGE_2, the potent bronchoconstrictor effects of I.V. $PGF_{2\alpha}$ were inhibited in a concentration-dependent fashion (Figures 5 and 6).

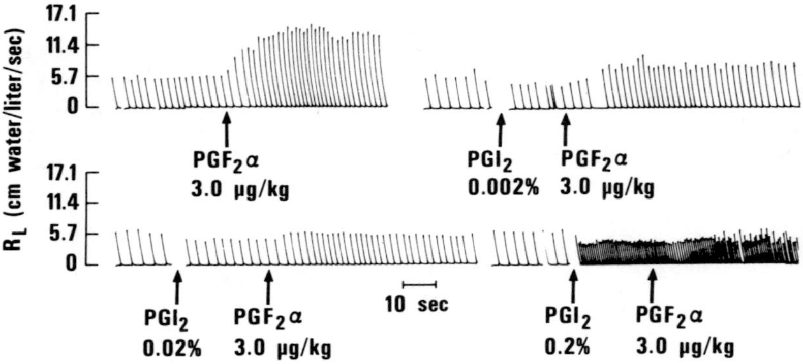

Figure 5 - Concentration-dependent inhibitory effects of aerosolized PGI_2 on the increase in pulmonary resistance (R_L) induced by I.V. $PGF_{2\alpha}$ in the anesthetized dog.

Successful bronchodilation by PGI_2 aerosols (0.002-0.2%) is displayed clearly in Figure 5. Although this inhibition could be comparably demonstrated when PGI_2 is given I.V., systemic cardiovascular side effects are less intense via the more direct aerosol route (Table 1). PGI_2 (0.3-30 g/kg, I.V.) results in vasodepression, i.e., a decrease in mean systemic arterial blood pressure (MAP), and tachycardia, i.e., an increase in heart rate (HR), but when administered via the aerosol route, PGI_2 remains a highly effective bronchodilator, but without the unnecessary effects on the cardiovascular system (Table 1; Wasserman et al., 1980b).

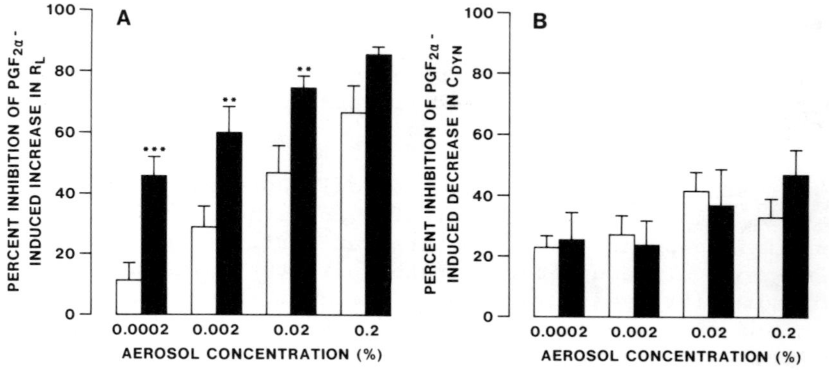

Figure 6 - Comparative inhibitory effects of aerosolized PGE_1 (□) and PGE_2 (■) against (A) the increase in pulmonary resistance (R_L) and (B) the decrease in dynamic lung compliance (C_{DYN}) induced by I.V. $PGF_{2\alpha}$ in anesthetized dogs. Each bar represents the mean ± SE percentage inhibition from four animals. $^{**}P<0.01$; $^{***}P<0.001$, comparing PGE_1 to PGE_2. (Reprinted with permission of The Williams and Wilkins Co.; Wasserman et al., J. Pharmacol. Exp. Ther. 214: 68-73, 1980).

Table 1. Comparison of the Bronchopulmonary and Cardiovascular Actions of Prostacyclin Administered by Intravenous (I.V.) Injection and by Aerosol to Anesthetized Dogs

Route	Dose	R_L (%Inhibition)	C_{DYN} (%Inhibition)	ΔMAP (mm Hg)	ΔHR (Beats/Min)
I.V.	(ug/kg)				
	0.3	26.8 ± 4.3	8.4 ± 5.6	-21 ± 4	17 ± 5
	1.0	47.8 ± 4.4	27.5 ± 7.6	-37 ± 5	22 ± 5
	3.0	58.1 ± 6.2	24.2 ± 4.5	-45 ± 5	18 ± 5
	10.0	78.0 ± 5.8	49.3 ± 7.0	-47 ± 4	19 ± 7
	30.0	86.3 ± 5.9	66.7 ± 3.3	-55 ± 5	16 ± 7
Aerosol	(%)				
	0.002	32.2 ± 13.1	18.4 ± 8.1	-3 ± 4	0
	0.02	70.0 ± 9.6	38.4 ± 13.8	-2 ± 1	7 ± 4
	0.2	84.1 ± 5.0	59.7 ± 10.2	-21 ± 14	-15 ± 11

Both PGE_1 and PGE_2 aerosols significantly inhibited $PGF_{2\alpha}$-induced changes in R_L and C_{DYN} (Figure 6; Wasserman et al., 1980a). However, observe that both test drugs affect R_L more than C_{DYN}, thus implying a greater preference for central airways, since variations in R_L may be reflected in alterations of these larger conducting airways, where the greatest resistance to airflow is detected (Colebatch et al., 1966).

Conscious Dogs: Although it would appear that PGE aerosols might be useful clinically in asthma, their use has been limited because of an unfortunate irritant property upon inhalation. This upper respiratory irritation is manifest in pharyngeal/laryngeal discomfort, wheezing, coughing, headache, and retrosternal soreness (Cuthbert, 1971; Herxheimer and Roetscher, 1971; Kawakami et al., 1973). Our conscious dog model demonstrates an apparent concentration-related irritant action of inhaled PGE's (Wasserman et al., 1980a). A representative example shows that when PGE_2 (0.2%) is aerosolized for 3 min, no overt subjective or objective breathing changes occur; however, when the concentration is raised to 1.0%, the animals become aggressive, restless, hold their breath, cough, and exhibit irregular airflow rate patterns (Figure 7). Thus, these intolerable irritant effects may be achieved at some critical concentration, below which effective bronchodilation and absence of irritation may be attainable.

Guinea Pigs: When exposed to the noxious vapors of histamine alone (0.25%) in our aerosol chamber, normal guinea pigs undergo the signs of respiratory distress (bronchoconstriction) in the following sequence: coughing, dyspnea, and then, asphyxial collapse (Figure 8). Animals pretreated with a vehicle aerosol afforded little protection vs. histamine, whereas various concentrations of PGE_1, PGE_2, or β-adrenergic agonists, isoproterenol and isoetharine, were highly effective in prolonging the onset of asphyxia (Figure 8). In this study, PGE aerosols were shown to be more effective than the sympathomimetics as potential bronchodilators vs. a pharmacologic provocation in normal guinea pigs (Wasserman et al., 1980a).

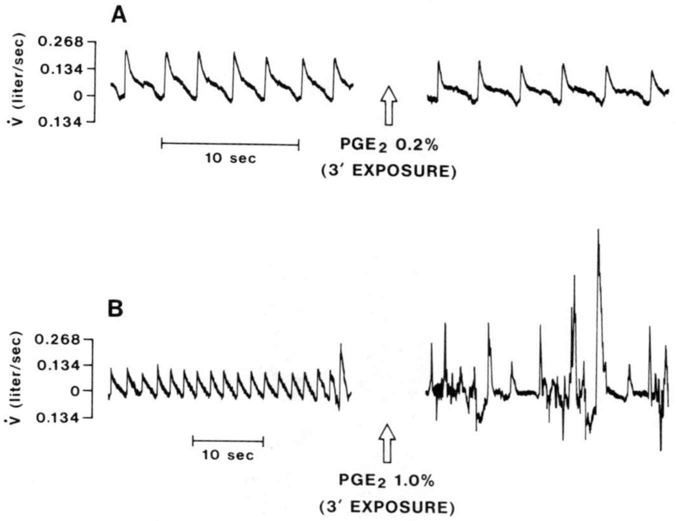

Figure 7* - Representative tracings from the head dome model in the conscious dog illustrating (A) an unchanged pattern of breathing following exposure to PGE_2 (0.2%) and (B) an exaggerated pattern of breathing following PGE_2 (1.0%).

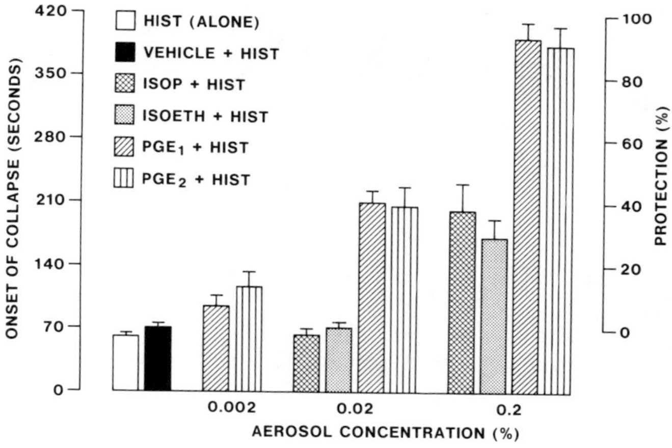

Figure 8* - Comparison of the protection afforded by aerosols of PGE_1, PGE_2, isoproterenol (ISOP) and isoetharine (ISOETH) against histamine (HIST) aerosol-induced asphyxial collapse in conscious, normal guinea pigs. Each bar represents the mean ± SE from 10 animals.

*(Reprinted with permission of The Williams and Wilkins Co.; Wasserman et al., J. Pharmacol. Exp. Ther. 214: 68-73, 1980).

When OA-sensitized animals encountered the aerosolized antigen, signs and symptoms of anaphylaxis ensued usually within 150-200 sec. Aerosol bronchodilators (same as above) provided antianaphylactic actions of approximately 60-100% (Figure 9). Thus, aerosol bronchodilators of the PGE and sympathomimetic classes are effective vs. immunologic challenges in sensitized animals (Wasserman et al., 1980a).

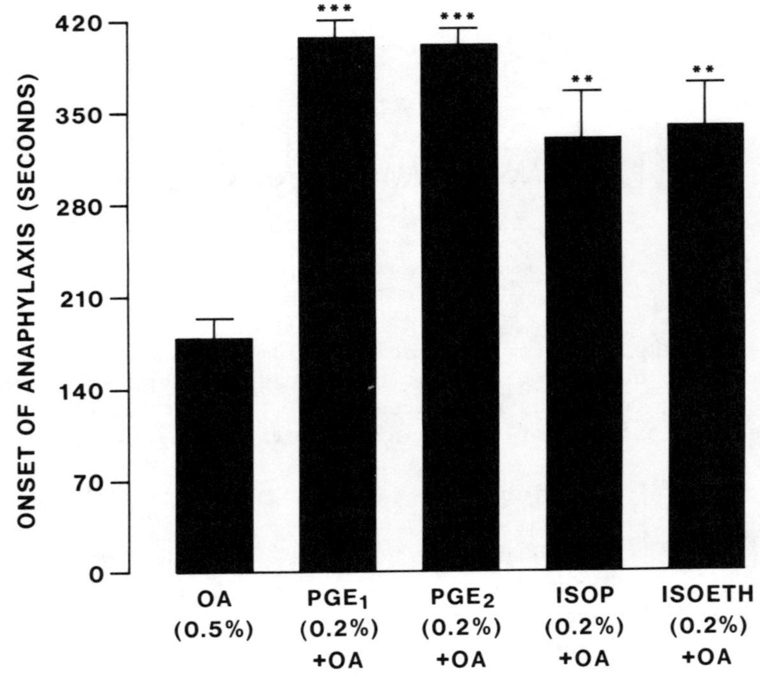

Figure 9 - Comparison of the anti-anaphylactic effects of aerosolized agents (see Figure 8) in ovalbumin (OA)-sensitized, conscious guinea pigs. Each bar represents the mean ± SE response of eight animals. $^{**}P<0.01$; $^{***}P<0.001$ when compared to OA alone.

Lastly, aerosolized bronchoconstrictors can also be analyzed and compared quantitatively. In the concentration range 0.001-1.0%, various known bronchospastic agents: acetylcholine, histamine, serotonin, and methacholine produced concentration-dependent effects on the onset of collapse in normal guinea pigs (Figure 10). Most curiously, $PGF_{2\alpha}$, a potent canine, monkey, and human bronchoconstrictor, was without effect in the guinea pig in concentrations up to 10.0% (Figure 10).

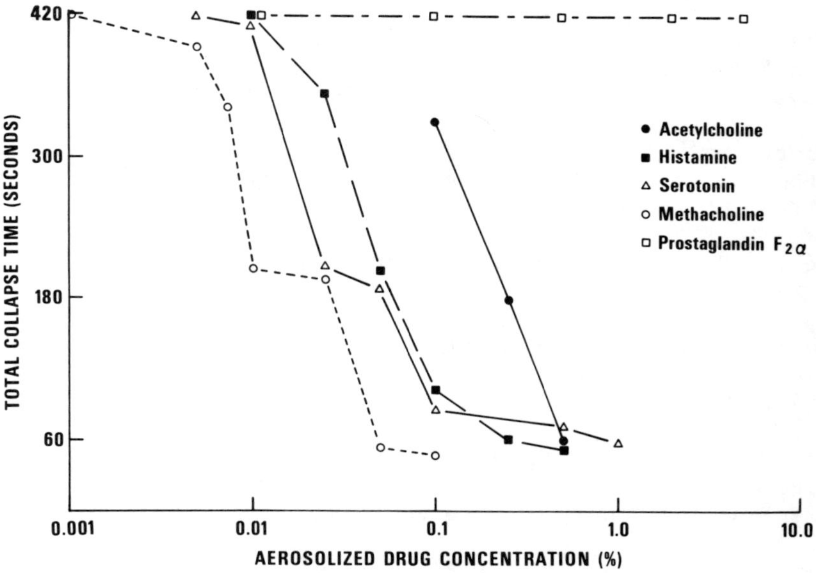

Figure 10 - Comparison of the bronchoconstrictor effects of several known aerosolized spasmogens in the guinea pig system. The time to asphyxial collapse is indicative of the ability of these agents to produce bronchoconstriction.

CONCLUSION

Aerosolization of test agents for local effects in the lung experimentally or clinically would be the most direct, accurate, and prudent method to avoid the harmful systemic actions of oral or parenteral routes.

REFERENCES

Amdur, M.O. and Mead, J. (1958). Mechanics of respiration in unanesthetized guinea pigs. Amer. J. Physiol. 192:364-368.

Brain, J.D. and Valberg, P.A. (1979). Deposition of aerosol in the respiratory tract. Amer. Rev. Resp. Dis. 120:1325-1373.

Colebatch, H.J.H., Olsen, C.R., and Nadal, J.A. (1966). Effect of histamine, serotonin, and acetylcholine on the peripheral airways. J. Appl. Physiol. 21:217-226.

Cuthbert, M.F. (1971). Bronchodilator activity of aerosols of prostaglandins E_1 and E_2 in asthmatic subjects. Proc. Roy. Soc. Med. 64:15-18.

Davies, D.S. (1975). Pharmacokinetics of inhaled substances. Postgraduate Med. J. 51 (Suppl.7):69-75.

Diamond, L. (1972). Potentiation of bronchomotor responses by beta-adrenergic antagonists. J. Pharmacol. Exp. Ther. 181: 434-445.

Eppinger, H. and Hess, L. (1915). Vagotonia: A clinical study. In Vegetative Neurology, trans. by W.M. Karus and S.E. Jelliffe, The Nervous and Mental Disease Publishing Co., New York.

Gardiner, P.J., Copas, J.L., Elliott, R.D., and Collier, H.O.J. (1978). Tracheobronchial irritancy of inhaled prostaglandins in the conscious cat. Prostaglandins 15:305-315.

Giles, R.E., Finkel, M.P., and Mazurowski, J. (1971). Use of an analog on-line computer for the evaluation of pulmonary resistance and dynamic compliance in the anesthetized dog. Arch. Int. Pharmacodyn. Ther. 194:213-222.

Gold, W.M.: Cholinergic pharmacology in asthma. In Asthma-Physiology, Immunopharmacology and Treatment, ed. by K.F. Austen and L.M. Lichtenstein, Academic Press, N.Y., p. 168-184.

Herxheimer, H. (1952). Repeatable microshock of constant strength in guinea pig anaphylaxis. J. Physiol. 117:151-155.

Herxheimer, H. and Roetscher, I. (1971). Effects of prostaglandin E_1 on lung function in bronchial asthma. Europ. J. Clin. Pharmacol. 3:123-125.

Kawakami, Y., Uchiyana, K., Irie, T., and Murao, M. (1973). Evaluation of aerosols of prostaglandins E_1 and E_2 as bronchodilators. Europ. J. Clin. Pharmacol. 6:127-132.

Solomon, A., Hershfus, J.A., and Segal, M.S. (1955). Aerosols of epoxytropine tropate methylbromide for the relief of bronchospasm. Ann. Allergy 13:90-95.

Wasserman, M.A. and Griffin, R.L. (1979). Bronchospasmolytic effects of methscopolamine bromide. J. Pharmacol. Exp. Ther. 211:159-166.

Wasserman, M.A., Griffin, R.L., and Marsalisi, F.B. (1980a). Inhibition of bronchoconstriction by aerosols of prostaglandins E_1 and E_2. J. Pharmacol. Exp. Ther. 214:68-73.

Wasserman, M.A., DuCharme, D.W., Wendling, M.G., Griffin, R.L., and DeGraaf, G.L. (1980b). Bronchodilator effects of prostacyclin (PGI_2) in dogs and guinea pigs. Eur. J. Pharmacol. 66: 53-63.

Yu, D.W.C., Galant, S.P., and Gold, W.M. (1972). Inhibition of antigen-induced bronchoconstriction by atropine in asthmatic patients. J. Appl. Physiol. 32:823-828.

Intranasal Toxicity Testing in the Rabbit Via Nasal Spray

GEORGE A. ELLIOTT, EDWARD N. DEYOUNG, ANDREJS PURMALIS, PAUL A. TRIEMSTRA, and BARBARA A. WHITED
Pathology and Toxicology Research
The Upjohn Company
Kalamazoo, Michigan

ABSTRACT

A system for evaluating the safety of intranasal sprays using the rabbit as the test animal is described. In this system the spray is delivered by a modified commercial atomizer powered by a portable compressor. Tissue blocks are obtained systematically so that all structures of the nasal cavity can be examined histologically. Results of the study of several compounds in this system are presented and suggest that some of the changes, particularly those frequently seen in the maxilloturbinals, may be non-specific responses. Alterations occurring in the olfactory epithelium of the ethmoturbinals may be more specific and of greater overall importance. Results also suggest that it is possible to distinguish compounds that will produce changes in one type of epithelium but not in another.

INTRODUCTION

For several years we have used a spray system to deliver drugs in intranasal toxicity testing (Elliott and DeYoung, 1970). We first decided to investigate the use of a spray technique because the compounds to be tested were to be administered as sprays in the clinic. We have been able to achieve a more uniform distribution throughout the nasal cavity with sprays than we could with drops.

This paper describes that system and some of the findings in the evaluation of several compounds.

MATERIALS AND METHODS

The spray system we have used was developed from a standard, commercial atomizer, a DeVilbiss 151 (figure 1).

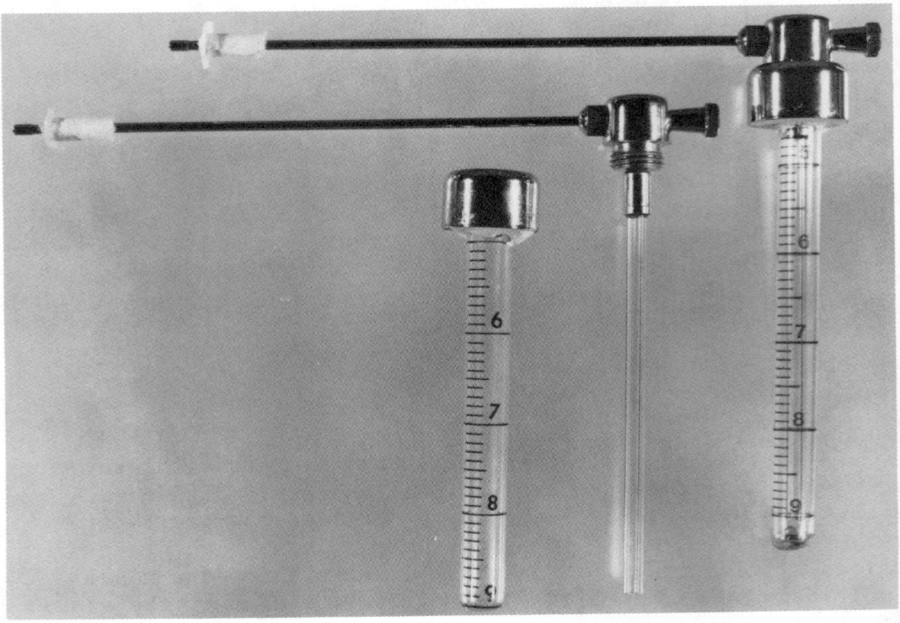

Figure 1. Commercial atomizer modified as used.

The fluid reservoir supplied by the manufacturer is replaced by one made from a 10.0 ml pipette (glass or plastic) calibrated in 0.1 ml. The pipette is cut so that the reservoir will hold about 4.0 ml and will accomodate the supply tube furnished by the manufacturer. The upper end of the cut pipette is cemented into the original collar with plaster of Paris. A plastic baffle, placed 1.0 cm from the tip of the delivery tube is used as a stop when the tube is inserted into the nasal cavity. The atomizer is powered by a portable air compressor set at 6-7 psi.

For the test species we have used New Zealand White rabbits, preferably weighing a little more than 3 kg. The rabbit was chosen because: (1) with a few exceptions the lining of the nasal cavity is similar in type and distribution to that of the human (Negus, 1958); (2) the same per nostril volume (0.1-0.2 ml) was used in clinical studies; (3) it can be handled with relative ease - we place the rabbit in a standard canvas cat bag obtained from a veterinary supply house; and (4) the cost per animal is low when compared with other non-rodent species.

Usually we have avoided problems with the sinusitis and rhinitis frequently found in the rabbit by having a knowledgeable and cooperative supplier and by careful screening during the pretest observation period.

At necropsy the nose and head are bisected anteriorly-posteriorly by a sagittal cut made slightly off the midline with a heavy knife and hammer (figure 2).

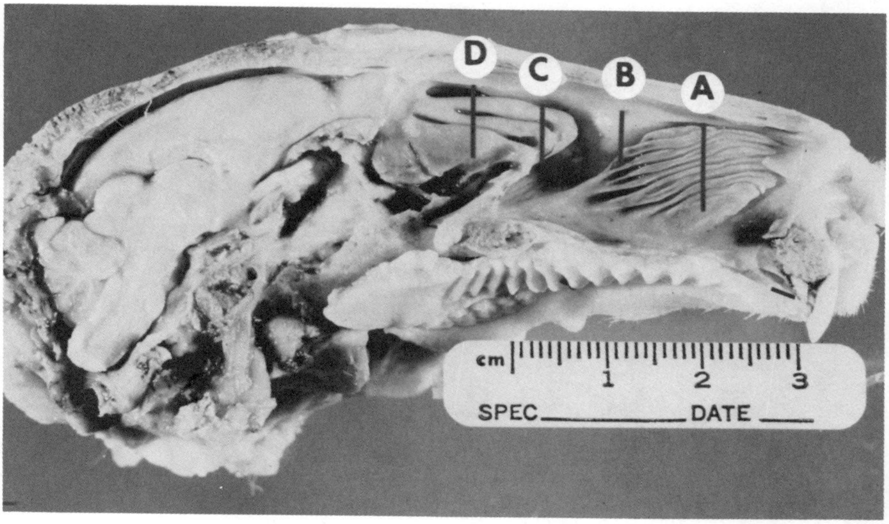

Figure 2. Interior of nasal cavity showing sites from which tissue blocks are obtained: maxilloturbinal (A); nasoturbinal (B); and ethmoturbinal (C & D).

This approach leaves the nasal septum intact on one side and exposes the entire nasal cavity on the other. The mandible is removed; the brain also may be removed or it may be left *in situ*. Following fixation and decalcification, transversely cut tissue blocks are removed from each turbinate. This technique affords examination of the various turbinates and their epithelial coverings, the septum and the paranasal sinuses.

The first block is obtained from the maxilloturbinal, the large structure on the lateral wall in the anterior part of the nasal cavity (figure 2). Block 2 permits examination of the nasoturbinal and paranasal sinuses. Sections from blocks 3 and 4 allow one to examine the ethmoturbinals at two points, and also, posterior segments of the paranasal sinuses. These two blocks are cut in such a way that the molar teeth are excluded from the section, thus shortening the time needed for decalcification. The septum may be examined simultaneously with the sections obtained from the other structures.

The maxilloturbinal of the rabbit is seen in cross section (figure 3) as a branched structure covered with two layers of low epithelium (Negus, 1958).

This is in contrast to the primate in which the structure is a single scroll covered with ciliated columnar epithelium. Functionally, the maxilloturbinal takes care of air humidification needs and temperature control in most mammals. This is made possible, at least in part, by its heavy vascular bed.

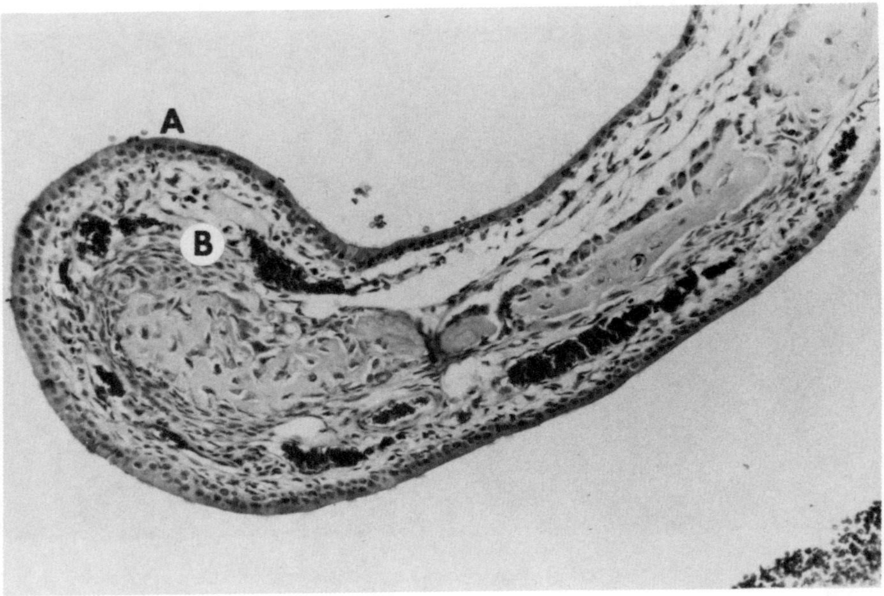

Figure 3. Normal maxilloturbinal showing low epithelium (A); lamina propria (B). Hematoxylin and eosin stain; X500.

The nasoturbinal and the medial septal aspect of the ethmoturbinal are covered primarily by olfactory epithelium (figure 4). In contrast, in the human the ethmoturbinals are lined primarily by ciliated columnar epithelium. Olfactory epithelium in man is found in small areas anterior to the middle turbinal, on the superior turbinal, the nasal septum, and the roof. However, the total area of olfactory epithelium is reasonably similar. In man it is reported as 10.0-12.5 cm^2 and in the rabbit as approximately 7.5 cm^2 (Negus, 1958).

The septum of the rabbit, and to a great extent that of man, is lined largely by ciliated columnar epithelium, as are the paranasal sinuses. The other principal locations of ciliated columnar epithelium in the rabbit are the anterior lateral aspects of the ethmoturbinal scrolls.

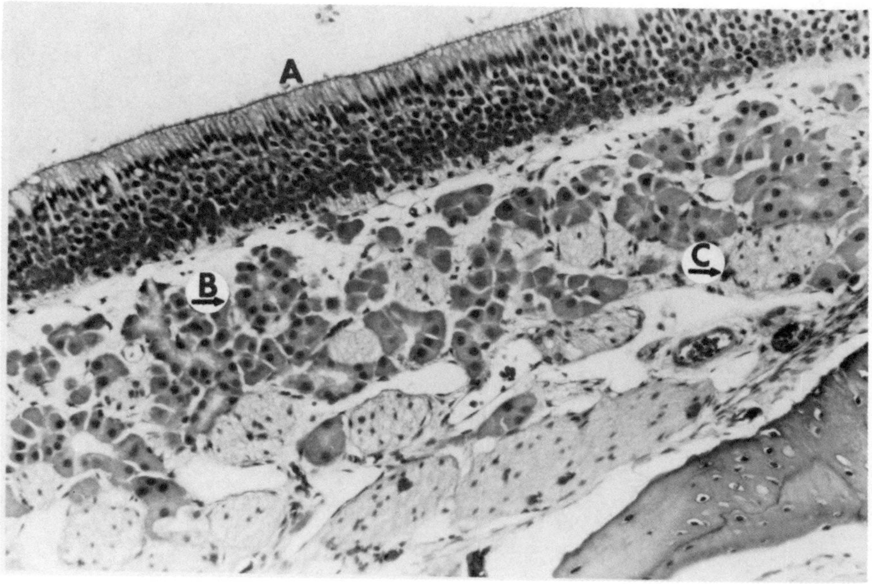

Figure 4. Normal ethmoturbinal showing olfactory epithelium (A); Bowman's glands (B); nerves (C). Hematoxylin and eosin stain; X500.

RESULTS AND DISCUSSION

In the evaluation of compounds of developmental interest we have studied several reference compounds. Some of these agents have appeared to be rather selective as to the types of tissues which they attack. Several workers have reported that a 1% solution of $ZnSO_4$ will severely damage the olfactory mucosa in various species (Matulonis, 1975; Mulvaney and Heist, 1971; Schultz, 1960; and Smith, 1938). This damage often is seen as a coagulation necrosis in which segments of the entire epithelial layer loosen and pull away from the underlying lamina propria (figure 5). The lamina propria with its prominent nerves and Bowman's glands usually remains intact. In some instances a mild-to-moderate hyperplasia of the maxilloturbinal epithelium occurs, but the maxilloturbinals are never damaged to the extent that the ethmoturbinals are.

In contrast, during a 7-day study with one of the more commonly used over-the-counter (OTC) nasal sprays, a rather pronounced hyperplasia of the epithelium of the maxilloturbinals developed (figure 6), while only minimal changes were seen in the ethmoturbinals.

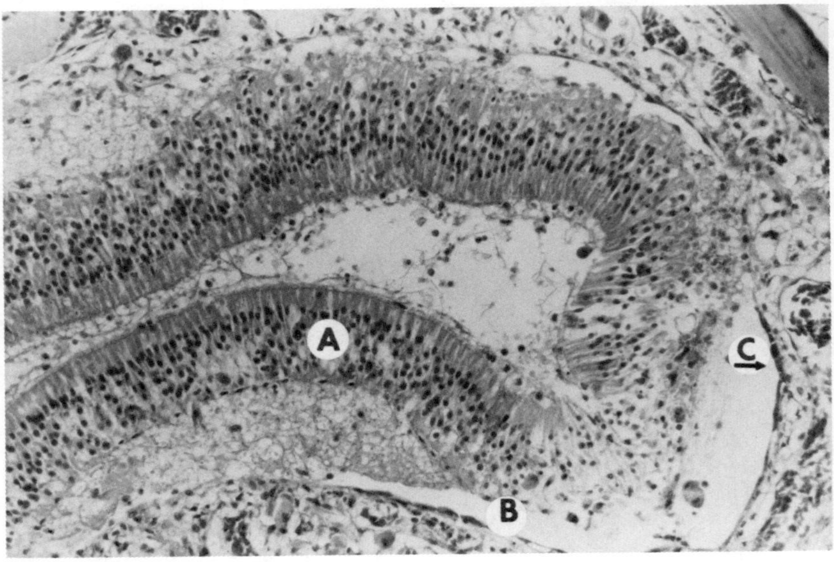

Figure 5. Ethmoturbinal at 21 days after two days of spraying with 0.5% $ZnSO_4$. Olfactory epithelium (A) has pulled away from lamina propria at (B); early regrowth of epithelium at (C). Hematoxylin and eosin stain; X500.

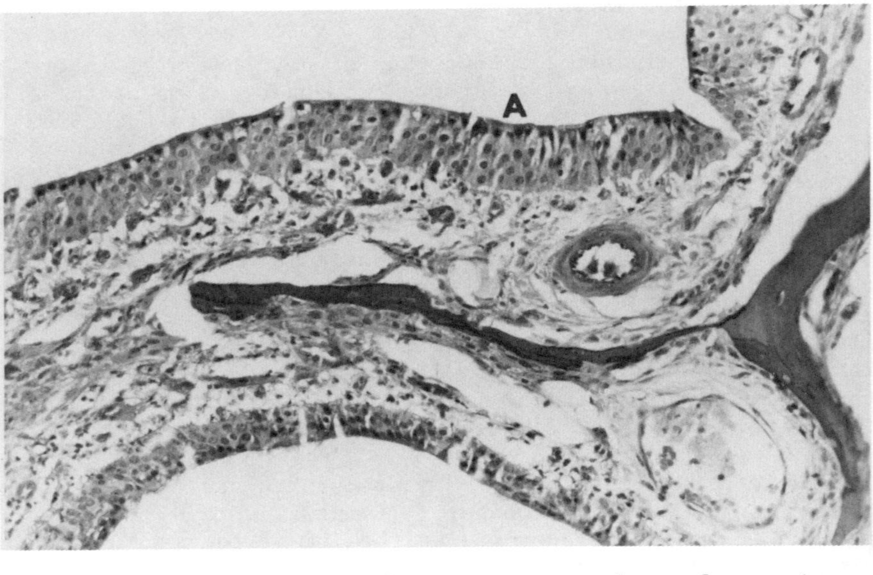

Figure 6. Maxilloturbinal following seven days of spraying with a common over-the-counter spray showing hyperplastic changes in the epithelium as at (A); epithelium is taller and cells are more numerous than in Figure 1. Hematoxylin and eosin stain; X500.

When sprayed twice daily for five days, a 0.1% solution of histamine diphosphate produced changes in both the maxilloturbinals and the ethmoturbinals. In some areas the maxilloturbinal epithelium underwent a patchy squamous metaplasia. In other areas there was marked hemorrhage and congestion of the lamina propria with vascular necrosis and necrosis of the overlying epithelium (figure 7). There were frequent, heavy, purulent, lumenal exudates, and the ethmoturbinals also were severely damaged. The olfactory epithelium was markedly distorted; in some areas it was necrotic and appeared to be sloughing in intact sheets, similar to that seen in $ZnSO_4$ treated rabbits. In other areas the epithelium was flattened.

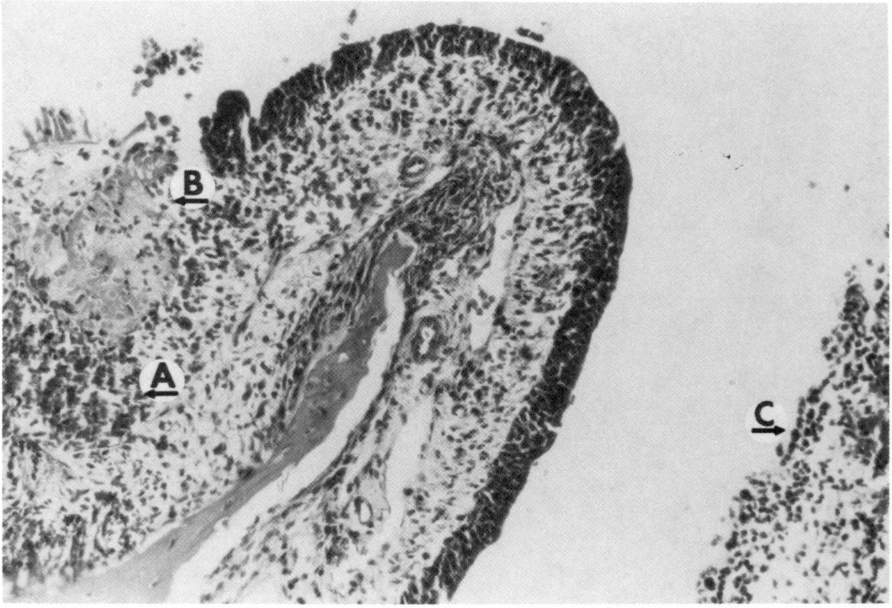

Figure 7. Maxilloturbinal after five days of treatment with 0.5% histamine diphosphate showing hemorrhage and congestion of the lamina propria (A) with necrosis of the overlying epithelium (B) and a heavy purulent lumenal exudate (C). Hematoxylin and eosin stain; X500.

A 1% spray of a methyl quinazoline administered for four days also was accompanied by changes in both the maxilloturbinals and the ethmoturbinals. The maxilloturbinal epithelium (figure 8) was both hyperplastic and metaplastic, and resembled that seen following use of the OTC preparation in the 7-day study described previously. Again, the alterations seen in the olfactory epithelium were severe, consisting of epithelial distortion with squamous metaplasia, fusion or adhesion of adjacent scrolls, patchy epithelial erosion, and fibrosis in the lamina propria.

A 0.6% concentration of calcium elenolate, sprayed for 14 days, also produced changes in both the maxilloturbinals and the ethmoturbinals. However, these changes were not nearly so severe as those accompanying the use of histamine or the methyl quinazoline. The maxilloturbinal epithelium was more columnar than usual and goblet cells were more numerous. The olfactory epithelium frequently was flattened and appeared thinned and irregular.

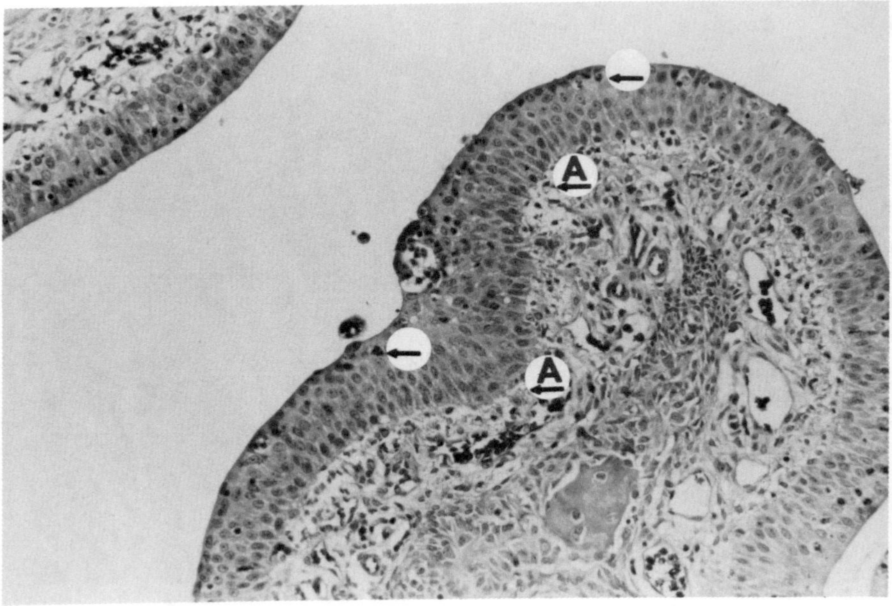

Figure 8. Maxilloturbinal after four days of treatment with a 1% methyl quinazoline showing hyperplasia and squamous metaplasia of the epithelium (A) and a few inflammatory cells (arrows). Hematoxylin and eosin stain; X500.

The use of normal saline sprays also may not be entirely innocuous. On several occasions we have seen a moderate hyperplasia of the maxilloturbinal epithelium after repeated spraying in saline control animals (figure 9). This observation suggests that to some degree this type of response in the maxilloturbinals may be nonspecific; therefore, it should be taken into consideration in the evaluation of test compounds.

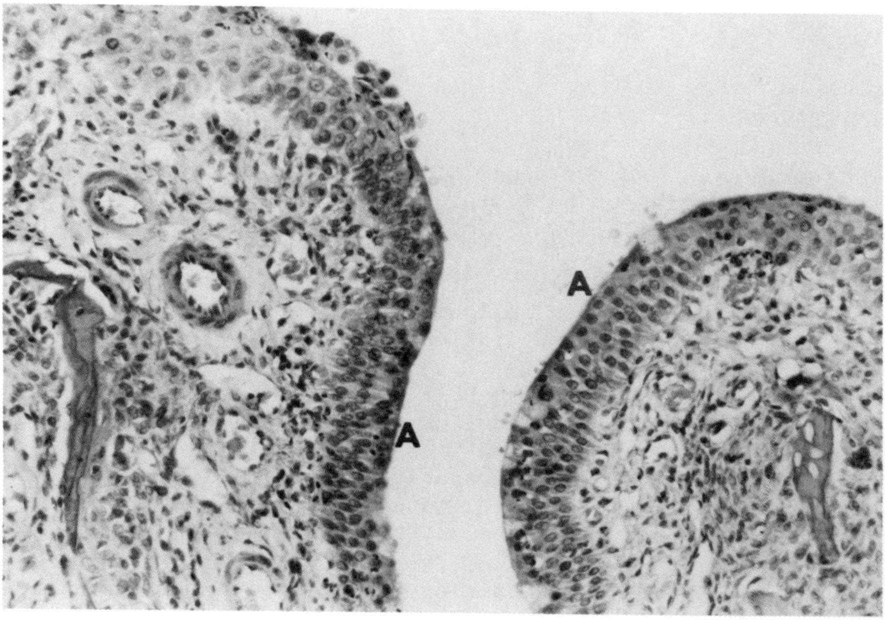

Figure 9. Maxilloturbinal of saline control showing moderate, diffuse epithelial hyperplasia (A). Hematoxylin and eosin stain; X500.

CONCLUSIONS

In summary, there are three primary points:

A. A simple and relatively inexpensive technique for the testing of intranasal sprays has been described. This technique lends itself to multiple dose as well as to single dose studies.

B. A procedure for obtaining specimens from the various structures of the nasal cavity for histologic examination also has been described.

C. Some of the histologic changes seen following the administration of several compounds have been presented. Some compounds have appeared to be selectively toxic for different types of nasal epithelium.

Furthermore, based on several clinical studies, we believe that the system described may, to a considerable degree, be predictive for man.

REFERENCES

Elliott, G. A., and DeYoung, E. N. (1970). Intranasal toxicity testing of antiviral agents. Annals New York Acad. Sciences. 173:169-175.

Matulonis, D. H. (1975). Ultrastructural study of mouse olfactory epithelium following destruction by $ZnSO_4$ and its subsequent regeneration. Am. J. Anat. 142:67-89.

Mulvaney, B. D., and Heist, H. E. (1971). Regeneration of rabbit olfactory epithelium. Am. J. Anat. 131:241-251.

Negus, V. (1958). The Comparative Anatomy and Physiology of the Nose and Paranasal Sinuses. E. and S. Livingstone, Ltd., Edinburgh and London.

Shultz, E. W. (1960). Repair of the olfactory mucosa. Am. J. Pathol. 37:1-19.

Smith, C. G. (1938). Changes in the olfactory mucosa and the olfactory nerves following intranasal treatment with one per cent zinc sulfate. Canad. Med. Assn. J. 39:138-140.

Lung Clearance of Particles and Its Use As A Test in Inhalation Toxicology

J. FERIN
Department of Radiation Biology and Biophysics
University of Rochester
Rochester, New York 14642

ABSTRACT

Pulmonary clearance of particles is one of the defensive functions of the lung essential for the maintenance of respiration. Particle clearance is closely related to environmental health effect considerations because toxic inhalants are obviously prime suspects regarding interference with clearance. It is generally accepted that alveolar macrophages have a key role in clearance of particles from the alveoli. Additional clearance pathways and mechanisms have also been recognized. Some substances are preferentially handled by some mechanism of clearance at least during some part of the post-exposure period. If such substance has a low toxicity and its clearance pattern has a high reproducibility, than a deviation from the established pattern may serve as an indicator of a functional change in clearance. In our experience, TiO_2 particles have these characteristics and can be used in an experimental clearance test.

INTRODUCTION

With the inhaled air various substances of the environment reach the lung where they may affect vulnerable structures, interfere with lung functions, provoke pathological processes or penetrate into other tissues and organs. It is now generally accepted that pulmonary clearance of particles is an important defensive response of the lung, essential for the maintenance of respiratory functions. Various structures (e.g., mucociliary system, alveolar macrophages) and factors (e.g., absorption, solubility, particle size) have been identified as participants in this complex nonrespiratory function. It has been realized that pulmonary clearance of various materials differ substantially. The Task Group on Lung Dynamics (1966) attempted to organize in its deposition and clearance model the available information and divided the various compounds into three classes with clearance half-times around one day, a few days to a few months and around 6 months to several years. It can be assumed that the different clearance half-times of various particles are the result of the combinations of clearance pathways and mechanisms involved. An explanation can be envisioned in some instances (e.g., extremely soluble or insoluble particles) in others the reasons are obscure.

METHODS

Testing of particle clearance, which may involve measurement and characterization of kinetics, pathways or mechanisms, require particle deposition in the lung. Usually at different time intervals after aerosol inhalation the particle content of the lung or of its subdivisions (e.g., lobes, lymph nodes, trachea) is determined by measuring the radioactive label, using chemical, microbiological or other techniques depending on the particles used. Some methods can be used <u>in vivo</u> (radioactive labeling, magnetometry) others require analysis of lung tissue. A test particle should have a low toxicity, its clearance pattern must be reproducible, the clearance pathways and mechanisms should be known and the analytical technique involved should be sensitive and simple. Some substances are preferentially cleared by some mechanism at least during some part of the postexposure period. Experiments which such particles may yield information on specific clearance pathways or mechanisms (e.g., bronchiolar or alveolar clearance, clearance by alveolar macrophage involvement).

We used extensively TiO_2 particles for testing clearance (Ferin, Leach, 1976,1977). TiO_2 particles have a very low toxicity and solubility. In these experiments the rats were killed in groups of ten at various days postexposure, usually at day 1, 8, 25 and 130. The TiO_2 of the lungs was determined photometrically using 4,4-diantipyryl methane monohydrate. The method is sensitive to 0.5 μg/sample and the reproducibility, especially for amounts greater than 5 μg, is excellent. The average median aerodynamic diameter of the TiO_2 particles of the exposure aerosol in the various experiments was ~1.0 μm with an average geometric standard deviation of ~2.3. After a

6-hour inhalation exposure in a 2 m^3 Rochester type chamber, using an aerosol concentration of about 15 mg/m^3, the alveolar deposition in a male Long-Evans rat (360 g) is about 155 µg TiO_2/lung. This clearance assay tests alveolar clearance of particles via the airways and with the involvement of alveolar macrophages. Solubility or lymphatic clearance play a minor role at least in the first 25 days postexposure. The lung TiO_2 content of an unexposed rat is negligible. For more details see Ferin, Feldstein (1978) and Ferin, Morehouse (1980).

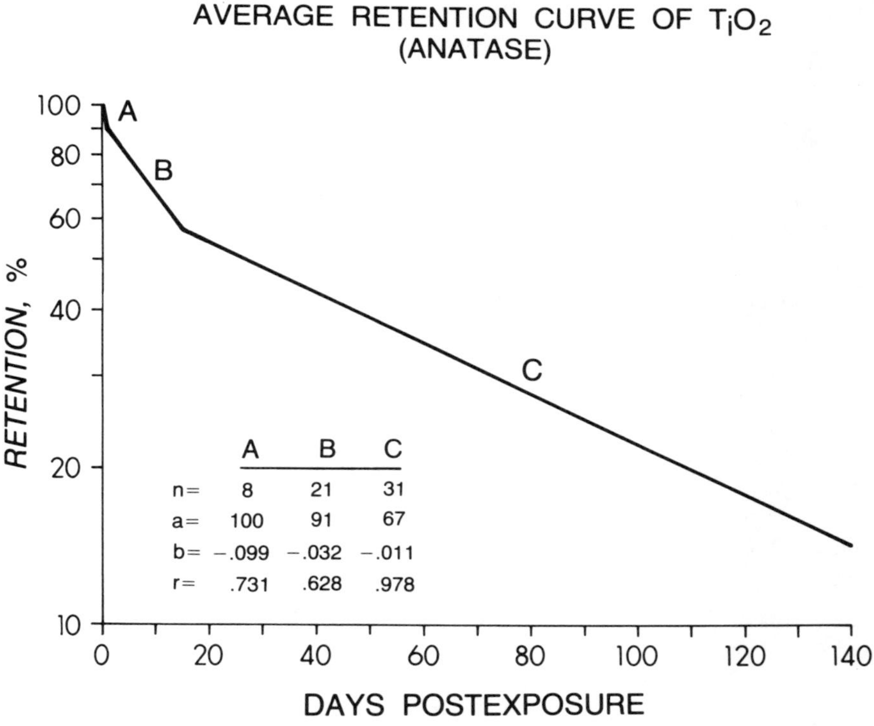

FIG. 1 Retention curve after a 6 hour aerosol exposure. The curve indicates TiO_2 particle removal from the lung. It can be subdivided into three exponential components. n = number of experiments, each experiment involving about 10 rats, a = intercept, b = slope, r = correlation coefficient.

An average retention curve (Fig. 1), generated from control groups of various experiments, shows that in 31.2 days postexposure 50 percent of the originally deposited amount is still retained in the lung and 50 percent has been cleared. The retention curve can be subdivided into three exponential components: Component A represents bronchial, B and C alveolar clearance. A clearance half-time can be computed for each component which participated in the overall $t_{1/2}$ of 31.2 days (Fig. 2).

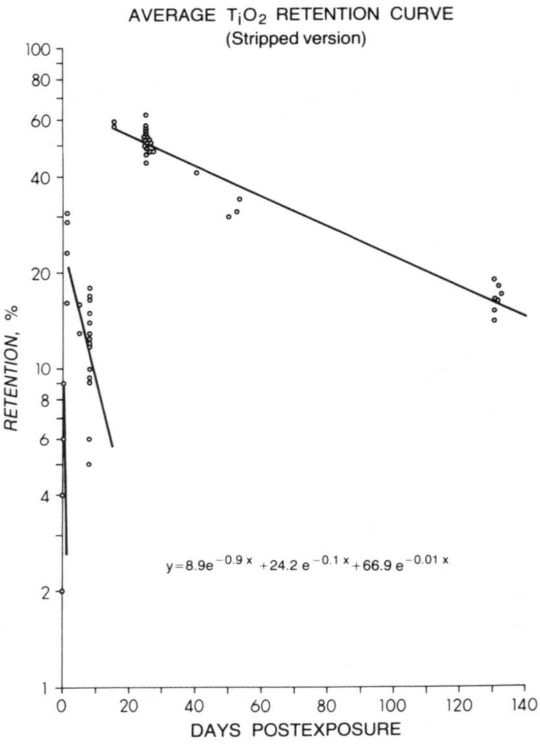

FIG. 2 Stripped version of the retention curve with individual components. The clearance half-times are 0.77, 6.9 and 69.3 days, respectively. The circles indicate individual experiments, average of about 10 rats.

Particles deposited during exposure in the bronchial tree are cleared very fast (component A, $t_{1/2}$ = 0.77 days). The short-term alveolar clearance (component B) has a $t_{1/2}$ of 6.9 days and the long-term alveolar clearance (component

C) a $t_{1/2}$ of 69.3 days. If one is concerned with alveolar clearance only, than for practical purposes the starting point of the retention curve can be set at day 1 post-exposure (Fig. 3). It can be assumed that the amount of particles determined at day 1 represents the particles deposited during exposure in the alveoli. The particles deposited during exposure in the bronchial tree have been cleared in the first day ($t_{1/2}$ = 0.77 days). The overall alveolar clearance half-time is 60 days.

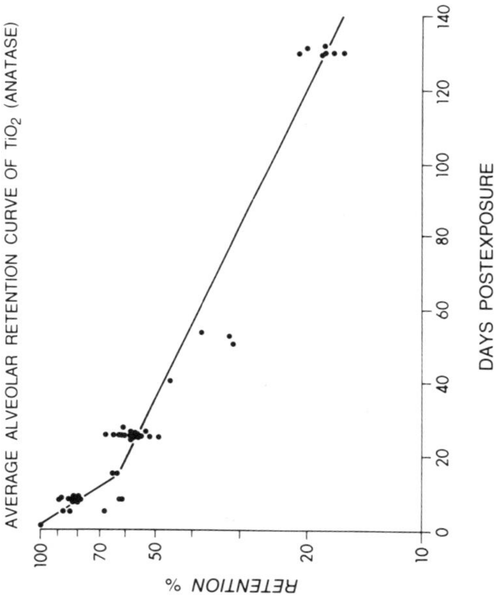

FIG. 3 Alveolar retention curve after 6 hour aerosol exposure. The circles indicate individual experiments, average of about 10 rats. First component: N = 35, a = 103, b = -0.035, r = 0.81, $t_{1/2}$ = 20 days; Second component: N = 31, a = 74, b = -0.011, r = 0.98, $t_{1/2}$ = 64 days. (For code see Fig. 1).

CONCLUSIONS

We studied the effects of SO_2, NO_x (Ferin, Leach, 1977) and of asbestos (Ferin, Leach, 1976) on TiO_2 particle clearance by comparing clearance in control and treated animals. In all three instances the effect was dose dependent and we could find a response ranging from negligible effect to substantial depression of clearance.

Recently we have reported that particle clearance capacity in two strains of rats may differ (Ferin, Morehouse, 1980). Two strains of commonly used experimental rats were compared. The Fisher 344 inbred rats, because of the smaller size, retained predictable fewer particles after a 7-hour exposure than the larger outbred Long-Evans rats. This can be expected in view of the different lung size of the two strains. In addition, clearance of the retained particles was significantly slower in Fisher 344 rats. Therefore, not only differences in animal species but also in strains should be considered when lung clearance experiments are performed.

ACKNOWLEDGEMENT

This paper is based on work performed partially under support from US-EPA and partially under Contract No. DE-AC02-76EV03490 with The U.S. Department of Energy at the University of Rochester Department of Radiation Biology and Biophysics and has been assigned Report No. UR-3490-1974.

REFERENCES

1. Ferin, J. and Leach, L.J. (1976). The effect of amosite and chrysotile asbestose on the clearance of TiO_2 particles from the lung. Env. Research 12: 250-254.

2. Ferin, J. and Leach, L.J. (1977). The effect of selected air pollutants on clearance of titanic oxide particles from the lungs of rats. Inhaled Particles IV. Ed. by W.H. Walton, Pergamon Press, Oxford and New York, pp. 333-340.

3. Ferin, J. and Feldstein, M.L. (1978). Pulmonary clearance and hilar lymph node content in rats after particle exposure. Env. Research 16: 342-352.

4. Ferin, J. and Morehouse, B. (1980). Lung clearance of particles in two strains of rats. Exp. Lung Research 1: 251-257.

5. Task Group on Lung Dynamics. (1966). Deposition and retention models for internal dosimetry of the human respiratory tract. Health Physics 12: 173-207.

REGULATORY GUIDELINES

Regulatory Guidelines for Inhalation Toxicity Testing*

S.B. GROSS
U.S. Environmental Protection Agency (EPA)
Washington, DC 20460

ABSTRACT

A wide variety of laws in the U.S. and in other countries have been passed requiring evaluation and control of potentially toxic chemicals. Four sets of national and international guidelines for toxicological testing in animals have been in development over the past several years. These include the EPA's pesticide testing guidelines as required by the Federal Insecticide, Fungicide, and Rodenticide Act (FIFRA); EPA's chemical testing guidelines required by the Toxic Substances Control Act (TSCA); the interagency testing guidelines being developed by the Interagency Regulatory Liaison Group (IRLG); and the international testing guidelines being developed by the Organization of Economic Cooperation and Development (OECD). This paper briefly considers the development of toxicological testing guidelines and focuses on some of the requirements for acute, subchronic and chronic inhalation testing.

*Since none of the guidelines have been officially approved as final, this summary is based on the author's personal view of the anticipated final guidelines. He has participated with others in the overall development of the Guidelines within EPA, has represented the Agency as a member of the IRLG, and has contributed to the OECD guidelines through the Agency's representatives to the OECD. He has also served as the leader for the inhalation guidelines testing team within the Agency and as a consultant to the IRLG.

INTRODUCTION

Over the past several years the Environmental Protection Agency (EPA), a number of federal agencies (cooperating through the Interagency Regulatory Liaison Group [IRLG]), and a number of countries worldwide (cooperating through the Organization for Cooperation and Development [OECD]) have been involved in developing guidelines for toxicological testing in animals. Such testing is carried out as part of the process of evaluating the possible toxic effects chemicals may have on people, wildlife and domestic animals. The inhalation toxicity testing guidelines are part of the battery of toxicity tests shown in Table I.

Table I. TOXICITY TEST PROTOCOL BATTERY*

Acute Tests	Chronic Tests
Oral LD_{50}	12 months to lifetime
Dermal LD_{50}	Oral, dermal, inhalation
Inhalation LC_{50}	Lifetime oncogenicity
Skin irritation	
Eye irritation	**Miscellaneous**
Delayed Neurotoxicity	Toxicokinetics/Metabolism
Dermal sensitization	Immunotoxicity
	Behavioral
Subchronic Tests	Short-term
90-day oral	Step sequence
14, 28 and 90-dermal	
28 and 90-day inhalation	
90-day neurotoxicity	
Teratology	
Reproductive effects (2 and 3 generations)	
Perinatal	

*Proposed or under development as EPA's FIFRA/TSCA, IRLG and/or OECD guidelines.

This discussion will first briefly review the development of the guidelines in EPA, IRLG and the OECD and will outline some of the general and then deal with the specific requirements for toxicological testing by the inhalation route.

I. Need for Toxicological Testing Guidelines

More than 50,000 chemicals are now on the world market and it is estimated that 1,000 new chemicals are commercially introduced each year (O.E.C.D., 1980). These chemicals permeate all aspects of life on this planet. As a result, numerous laws have been passed at the national (Table II) and international (Table III) levels in an effort to evaluate the toxicity and to control potentially hazardous materials.

The current guidelines effort (Preston, 1980) grew out

Table II. FEDERAL LAWS DEALING WITH TOXIC SUBSTANCES
Taken from Temple (1979)

Statute	Responsible agency	Sources covered
Toxic Substances Control Act (TSCA)	EPA	Requires premarket notification evaluation of all new chemicals (other than food, food additives, drugs, pesticides, alcohol, tobacco)
Clean Air Act	EPA	Hazardous air pollutants
Federal Water Pollution Control Act	EPA	Toxic water pollutants
Safe Drinking Water Act	EPA	Drinking water contaminants
Federal Insecticide, Fungicide, and Rodenticide Act (FIFRA)	EPA	Pesticides
"Miller Act" of July 22, 1954 (codified as §346(a) of the Food, Drug and Cosmetic Act)	EPA	Tolerance for pesticide residues in human food and animal feeds
Resource Conservation and Recovery Act	EPA	Hazardous wastes
Marine Protection, Research and Sanctuaries Act	EPA	Ocean dumping
Food, Drug and Cosmetic Act	FDA	Basic coverage of food, drugs and cosmetics
Food Additives Amendment	FDA	Food additives
Color Additive Amendment	FDA	Color additives
New Drug Amendments	FDA	Drugs
New Animal Drug Amendments	FDA	Animal drugs and feed additives
Medical Device Amendments	FDA	Medical devices
Wholesome Meat Act	USDA	Food, feed and color additives and pesticide residues in meat and poultry
Wholesome Poultry Products Act	USDA	
Occupational Safety and Health Act	OSHA	Workplace toxic chemicals
Federal Hazardous Substances Act	CPSC	"Toxic" household products (equivalent to consumer products)

Table II. FEDERAL LAWS DEALING WITH TOXIC SUBSTANCES Taken from Temple (1979) (Continued)

Statute	Responsible agency	Sources covered
Consumer Product Safety Act	CPSC	Dangerous consumer products
Poison Prevention Packaging Act	CPSC	Packaging of dangerous children's products
Lead Based Paint Poison Prevention Act	CPSC	Use of lead paint in federally assisted housing
Hazardous Materials Transportation Act	DOT (Materials Transportation Bureau)	Transportation of toxic substances generally
Federal Railroad Safety Act	DOT (Federal Railroad Administration)	Railroad safety
Ports and Waterways Safety Act	DOT (Coast Guard)	Shipment of toxic materials by water
Dangerous Cargo Act		

of a request by industrial representatives in the late 1960's and early 1970's that the Agency provide additional guidance to applicants for the testing requirements for pesticide registrations. This was followed in 1972 by a mandate from Congress when FIFRA was modified to respond to environmental needs. The guidelines became an attempt to identify the state-of-the-art methods for testing which are used in qualified industrial and commercial laboratories. Many laboratories, most notably within the pharmaceutical industry, have a considerable degree of sophistication in toxicology testing; however, many other laboratories do not and have not provided toxicological data which would meet even minimum standards. With the increased concern for evaluating the large number of chemicals of commercial and

Table III. INTERNATIONAL TOXIC CHEMICAL CONTROL LAWS Obtained from Page (1980)

Country	Law
United States	Toxic Substances Control Act
Canada	Environmental Contaminants Act
European Economic Community	Sixth Amendment to EEC Hazardous Substances Directive
Japan	Chemical Substances Control Act
Sweden	Action Products Hazardous to Man or the Environment
Switzerland	Law on Trade in Toxic Substances
United Kingdom	Health and Safety at Work Act Control of Pollution Act
France	Chemicals Control Act
Norway	Product Control Act
Denmark	Law on the Work Environment

environmental concern, there has been an exponential growth of laboratories involved with toxicological testing and an increase in the numbers of studies which now have to be evaluated. The guidelines provide needed guidance to reviewers as well as registration applicants.

II. Development of the Toxicology Testing Guidelines

One of the early and more comprehensible guides for toxicology testing has been the booklet "Appraisal of Safety for Food, Drugs and Cosmetics" published by the Association of Food and Drug Officials of the U.S. in 1959. This booklet (which did not include inhalation toxicity testing) has formed the basis for testing standards used under the Food and Drug and Cosmetic Act over the years but it did not represent legal requirements as such.

EPA Guidelines. In response to industry's request and in response to government's need to set consistent standards, Dr. Edward Carter, a plant pathologist in the pesticide program (then part of USDA), began an effort in 1969 which resulted in the publication of EPA's first set of proposed guidelines (EPA, 1975). Congress wrote into Section 3 of the 1972 Amendments of FIFRA, and later into Section 4 of TSCA (1976), the requirement that the Administrator further develop and promulgate guidelines or test standards. As a result of an extensive effort, proposed pesticide guidelines were published in 1975, and the toxicology guidelines were reproposed on August 22, 1978 (EPA, 1978). The first sets of proposed TSCA guidelines were published on May 9 and July 26, 1979 (EPA, 1979 a and b). The FIFRA requirements are referred to as "guidelines" and the TSCA requirements as "standards"; however, the testing requirements for both FIFRA and TSCA are to be identical.

Public Participation. Hundreds of scientists within and outside of the Agency have helped with the development of the EPA guidelines. Initially, scientists within the Agency identified the regulatory needs for toxicity testing, studied the literature, and consulted with experts within government, industry and academia. Public meetings were held to discuss drafts of the guidelines with the latter experts in attendance. Final drafts of the proposed guidelines were published and the public was invited to comment. At least 323 submissions (Page, 1980) were received from the public in response to both the FIFRA proposal of August 22, 1978 (EPA, 1978), and the two TSCA proposals of May 9 and July 26, 1979 (EPA, 1979 a and b). The comments came from industry (116), trade associations (27), universities (10), professional societies (16), U.S. government agencies and scientists (34), foreign government bodies (10), private testing or consulting laboratories (44), individual scientists and concerned citizens (53), public interest organizations (10), and legal firms (2). Each of the comments has been carefully analyzed and the guidelines revised as appropriate.

IRLG Guidelines. The many different federal laws concerned with the control of chemical substances are administered by different departments and agencies as illustrated in Table II. Four regulatory agencies - the Consumer Product Safety Commission, the Food and Drug Administration, the Occupational Safety and Health Administration, and the EPA - agreed to work together to reform the regulatory process and to improve protection of workers, public health and the environment (IRLG, 1977). They formed the IRLG to implement their agreement. In January 1979, the Food Safety and Quality Service of the Department of Agriculture also joined the IRLG. The Testing Standards and Guidelines Work Group of the IRLG (which also had representatives from the Department of Energy, the National Cancer Institute, and the Department of Commerce) had the responsibility to develop the guidelines for toxicological testing. It also cooperated with the EPA and the OECD in the development of their respective guidelines. As part of its external review, the IRLG published drafts of its guidelines, held public meetings and also invited comments from the participating federal agencies.

OECD Guidelines. Since potentially toxic substances may cross national boundaries via export or pollution, there was an obvious need for approprite controls on an international basis. Different regulatory approaches would place a strain on critical testing resources and might lead

Table IV. OECD EXPERT GROUPS OF THE ENVIRONMENT COMMITTEE/CHEMICALS GROUP
Obtained from Page (1980)

Expert Group	Lead Country	Expected Completion Date
Eco-Toxicology	Netherlands	Early 1980
Degradation/Accumulation	Japan/Germany	Early 1980
Good Laboratory Practices	United States	1981
Physical-Chemical Properties	Germany	Early 1980
Long-term Effects on Human Health	United States	Late 1980
Short-term Effects on Human Health	United Kingdom	Early 1980
Step-Sequence Testing	Sweden	Late 1980
Glossary of Key Terms	Germany	1981
Confidentiality	France	1981

to non-tariff barriers to trade. The OECD Chemicals Testing Programme was established by the Chemicals Group of the OECD to deal with the issues of international cooperation in these matters. The OECD consisted of 18 European countries, Canada and the United States when it was formed in 1961 from the Organization for European Economic Cooperation. Japan, Finland, Australia and New Zealand joined OECD in later years. Two expert groups from the Chemicals Programme - the Long-term Effects and Short-term Effects on Human Health Expert groups (Table IV) - were given responsibilities for developing the toxicity testing guidelines. Representatives from Belgium, Canada, Denmark, France, Germany, Italy, Japan, Netherlands, Norway, Switzerland, United Kingdom, United States, as well as the European Economic Community, and the World Health Organization met on numerous occasions in various parts of the world to develop a set of testing guidelines which were, as of December 1980, being reviewed by the various OECD member countries in near final form.

OVERVIEW OF THE GUIDELINES

Although the format for the different guidelines will vary, there are three areas of requirements which are common to all of the different guidelines shown at the left side of Table V: 1) the Good Laboratory Practice (GLPs), 2) the general testing considerations and 3) the requirements which are specific to individual studies. The other types of requirements shown on the right side of Table V can vary from law to law and country to country.

An overview of the GLPs is presented in Table VI. The GLPs apply to the quality of the studies by requiring that they be carried out by appropriately trained individuals

Table V. OVERVIEW OF TOXICITY TESTING GUIDELINES

Common to All Guidelines	Regulation/Country Specific Requirements
1. Good Laboratory Practice	1. When Required
2. General Considerations	2. Application of the Results
3. Test Specific Requirements	3. Reference to Other Guidelines
Purpose(s)	Chemical and physical property characterization
Definition(s)	
Test Substance	
Test Animals	Risk Assessment
Test Procedures	Environmental fate studies
Test Results	
Test Reports	Other

who have clearly defined responsibilities; the work is carried out in suitable facilities using appropriate equipment and methods; data and specimens are retained for possible future inspection, and the planned procedures, results and records are maintained under acceptable control by a Quality Assurance Unit.

The general section requirements provide general guidance on the specific requirements for individual tests. These are addressed below in the discussion of the inhalation testing requirements.

An overview of the test report is provided in Table VII. Specific requirements for the test report are provided in all three sections (the GLPs, the general section

Table VI. OVERVIEW OF GOOD LABORATORY PRACTICE REQUIREMENTS

a) General provisions: Scope and purpose; applicability; definitions

b) Organization and Personnel. Personnel qualifications; facility organization and responsibility assignments; study director responsibilities; quality assurance unit responsibilities and personnel.

c) Facility Requirements: Overall; animal care and supply facilities; facilities for safe handling and storage of test agents and hazardous materials; adequate laboratory operation areas; provisions for specimen and data storage; administrative and personnel facilities.

d) Equipment: Appropriate for the study: Maintenance and calibration of equipment.

e) Testing Facilities Operation: Experimental design; standard operatng procedures; reagent and solutions; animal care.

f) Test and Control Articles: Test and control article characterization; test and control article handling; mixture of article with carriers.

g) Procedural Requirements: Clearly documented procedures for conduct of the studies; identification of responsible staff.

h) Records and Reports: Reporting of nonclinical laboratory study results; storage and retrieval of records and data; retention of records.

i) Disqualification of Studies and/or of Testing Facilities: Purpose; grounds for disqualification; notice of and opportunity for hearing on proposed disqualification; public disclosure of information regarding disqualificaton; alternative or additional actions to disqualification; suspension or termination of a testing facility by a sponsor; reinstatement of a disqualified testing facility.

and in the specific test protocols). Overall, the test report is required to identify responsible staff and an adequate description of the experimental conditions and test results.

"Harmonization" of the Various Guidelines. Although, as already indicated, the various laws administered by different governmental bodies from different countries may require testing of the same chemicals for different purposes and/or to differing degrees, the procedures and quality control requirements necessary to carry out a particular test are to be the same. Thus, the procedures for an oral acute study on a chemical or chemical mixture required for a specific law in one country may be used to meet the needs of any other law of cooperating countries which requires an oral acute test on the same substance. The quality standards for the testing laboratory themselves (the GLPs) carrying out the acute oral study is also being "harmonized."

Table VII. OVERVIEW OF TEST REPORT REQUIREMENTS

a) Cover: Title - type of study, name of compound; laboratory; sponsor; date.

b) Laboratory Data: Responsible personnel, titles, signature dates.

c) Study Summary: Type of study, guidelines used; summary of results; "important disclaimers"; study dates - beginning, end.

d) Study Design
   1) Test substance: Chemical name, synonyms and trade names; molecular structure; composition: purity, methods of analyses; source.
   2) Vehicles or diluents: Identification of agents used, purity, source, methods of incorporation.
   3) Test animals: Species and strain, source, age, sex, body weights; rationale for use; preconditioning; method of assignment to experiment; animal care - special to study; satellite or interim groups.
   4) Test Procedures
      i) Limit test methods (if applicable).
      ii) Control groups - type, animals (sex, numbers, selection process).
      iii) Preparation of the test animals.
      iv) Administration of the test materials: route, duration and frequency of exposure; fasting.
      v) Observations of Animals: post exposure period; frequency and types of observations (signs of toxic responses - nature, onset, severity, duration); body weights; food and water consumption as indicated.

Table VII. OVERVIEW OF TEST REPORT REQUIREMENTS (Continued)

vi) Clinical Laboratory Testing: hematology; blood chemistry; urinalyses; special testing.

vii) Pathology:

A) Necropsy: body weights; organ weights; organ, cavity, orifice, surface pathology and conditions; fixation of tissues.

B) Histopathology: preparation of sections - routine and special.

5) Test Results: Summary data primarily - individual data only when necessary to illustrate or support summary information.

i) Animal data: body weights; mortality; toxicity.

ii) Study objectives - as appropriate:

A) Limit test results if applicable.

B) Median lethality - limits, slope, methods; observed toxicity.

C) No-Observable-Effect-Level (NOEL); dose response observations - observed toxicity clinical laboratory results, pathology.

6) Quality Control Data: Methods, results.

7) Discussion and Evaluation: Deviations from guidelines; problems which arose, solutions used, effects of solutions.

8) References: Guidelines used, methods, etc.

e) Laboratory Facilities Summary: Rooms, facilities, animal care; waste disposal.

f) Archival Information: Storage of data, specimens, reports.

National (interagency) and international agreements to these conventions are nearly completed for many of the testing protocols. However, the Good Laboratory Practice agreements are not as far along. Thus, the GLPs, and the general and specific testing requirements are to be essentially the same from agency to agency and country to country, but written in the context of the requirements of different laws. The harmonization process has been made easier since many of the scientists from EPA and IRLG participated in the development of the OECD Guidelines and have had to deal with the same comments and concerns of scientists from regulatory agencies and industries through the world.

Waivers and the Revision of the Guidelines. The guidelines are not intended to be the "final word" in toxicological testing. All of the guidelines have mechanisms whereby improved and innovative methods may be substituted for those prescribed in the formalized guidelines. Generally, it is assumed the guidelines apply only to new chemicals; however, they are expected to be applied to the evaluation of old chemicals when the current use of such chemicals raises questions of safety and when the older studies are not adequate compared to today's requirements. On the other hand, old studies will not have to be repeated if they do not quite meet the current requirements, providing the results from such studies are consistant with the results of related studies, and the use patterns of the chemicals do not suggest any obvious hazards.

INHALATION TESTING STANDARDS

Tables VIII through XII (as well as some of the other tables presented in this paper) provide the testing requirements in the form of overviews. The text below provides some discussion of the tabular materials.

Inhalation toxicity testing is normally required when

Table VIII. COMPARISONS OF INHALATION TESTS

Acute	Purpose: LC_{50}, statistical limits, slope. Exposure: Single 4 hour generally, longer if indicated by exposure conditions, 14 days post-exposure observation. Animals: Rat preferred; 5 animal/sex/level. No controls. Limit test: 5 mg/l if achievable, 5 animals/sex. Necropsy desirable.
Subchronic	Purpose: Toxicity due to repeat exposures, NOEL. Exposure: 14, 28 or 90 day exposures, 6 hours/day, 5 days/week. Animals: Rat preferred; 10 to 20 animals/sex/level at termination; recovery groups, 14 to 28 days, suggested. Controls: At least one control-sham or vehicle. Clinical laboratory testing: Hematology, blood chemistry, urinalyses and possible special tests. Necropsy and histopathology required.
Chronic	Purpose: Toxicity due to extended repeat exposures, NOEL. Exposure: 12 or more months, lifetime for rodents; 6 hours/day, 5 days/week, up to 23 hours/day and 7 days/week. Animals: Usually rat; 20 to 50 animals/sex/level at start. Clinical laboratory testing required. Necropsy and histopathology required.

there is a possibility of exposure by the inhalation route. Thus, testing is required when a chemical or its conversion products are: 1) a gas, 2) a vapor of a volatile liquid or solid, 3) an aerosol of a liquid (spray), or a solid (dust) or, 4) a combination of aerosol and vapor. The test substance should not be substantially different from the use chemical in its physical or chemical form but may, in the case of aerosols, need to be reduced to particles which are inhalable for the test animals. Exposures are provided using whole-body dynamic flow inhalation chambers; however, newer methods may be used (such as face or head only) which preclude the added dermal and oral exposures due to the test materials depositing on the animal's fur.

There are three types of inhalation studies which may be required and they are briefly compared in Table VIII and discussed in Tables IX and X. The purpose of the acute inhalation study is to determine the median lethal concentration (LC_{50}), its statistical limits, and its slope, using a single short exposure of 4 hours and a post-exposure period of 14 days. This test is usually used as a measure of relative toxicity for the purposes of classification and labeling and may provide information on the mechanisms of action and susceptible target organs. Usually five animals/sex/test level are used. No controls are required for the acute studies; however, if a vehicle is required to aid in generating the atmosphere, it ideally should not substantially alter the chemical or toxicological properties of the test substance.

Table IX. OVERVIEW OF ACUTE INHALATION TOXICITY TESTING

1) When Required: Potentially significant exposures to gases, vapors of liquids or solids, aerosols of liquids (sprays) or solids (dusts), combination of these.
2) Purpose: Determine LC_{50}, confidence limits, slope; relative toxicity for labeling; define target organs and mechanism of action if possible.
3) Definitions: LC_{50}, mass median aerodynamic diameters, optical diameters, inhalable and respirable diameters.
4) Standards
   - Test Substance: Technical, manufacturing, formulation products, and/or use dilutions; test same physical and chemical form as expected exposure; must be respirable for test animal.
   - Vehicle: If required, should be characterized; ideally should not significantly alter chemical or toxicological properties.
   - Test Animals: Young adult laboratory rats preferred (125 to 250 gm), other species with justification;

Table IX. OVERVIEW OF ACUTE INHALATION TOXICITY TESTING (Continued)

males and females (nulliparous, non-pregnant), 5 animals/sex/test level.

Limit Test: If 5 males and 5 females, exposed for 4 hours to 5 mg/L actual concentration of inhalable test substance unless not achievable because of the characteristics of the test agent, causes no deaths, no further acute inhalation testing will be necessary.

Controls: None required.

Exposure Levels: Usually 4 or more levels, a minimum of three concentrations possible, should bracket the LC_{50} (between 10% and 90% mortality), only one 0% and one 100% adjacent mortality levels should be used to calculate the LC_{50} and slope.

Duration of Exposure: Minimum of single 4 hour, longer if indicated by human exposure; allow added time for equilibration of chamber.

Exposure Conditions: Whole body exposures in dynamic flow chambers preferred, uniform atmosphere distribution, single caging preferred, animal volume equal to or less than 5% of chamber; alternative methods with approval.

Chamber Measurements

- *Air Flow: At least 12 volume changes/hour, monitor frequently, record every 30 minutes.
- *Temperature: 22° +/- 2°C, monitor frequently, record every 30 minutes.
- Humidity: 40% to 60% unless altered by generation of chamber atmosphere, monitor frequently.
- Concentrations: Nominal; analytical (gaseous and/or particulate) from the breathing zone; *two times during run (after equilibrium and during last hour of exposure), minimum suggested.
- Particle Size for Aerosols: Should characterize during development of the generation system and confirm at least one time during run depending on the expected variation within chamber; sampled from breathing zone of animal; must be respirable for test animal.

Observations: Close observations during and just after exposures; daily (early AM and late afternoon) for 14 days; record abnormalities (nature, onset, duration); body weights before exposure, weekly and at sacrifice.

Necropsy: All animals whether dying or sacrificed, desirable.

Histopathology at option of study director.

5) Test Reports

*Constant electronic monitoring desirable.

Table IX. OVERVIEW OF ACUTE INHALATION TOXICITY TESTING (Continued)

Summary of Findings

GLP: Facility and personnel information, quality assurance, storage of samples, records.

General Section Requirements: Tests substance identification, characteristics; animal data; animal care, deviations from guideline procedures; statistical methods used: quality assurance.

Test Specific Information

Test Substance: Vapor pressure, boiling point, flammability, explosivity and stability.

Exposure Chambers: Design, operation, make-up air, waste disposal, equipment for controlling temperature, humidity, the generating system, methods for analytical concentrations, particle sizing.

Operation Data: Individual and summarized (means, SD's) - air flow, chamber temperature and humidity, nominal concentrations (without SD's), analytical concentations, and for aerosols, median particle sizes and geometric SD's specifying the % of respirable and non-respirable based on weight.

Limit Test Results: When applicable.

Response Data

Toxicity observed, onset, duration, animals involved, time to death, body weights, necropsy findings, LC_{50}, 95% confidence limits and slope of the dose mortality curve for each sex, method of calculation.

References for methods and equipment used.

Discussion and Evaluation

Table X. OVERVIEW OF 90-DAY INHALATION TOXICITY TESTING

1) When Required: Repeat exposures to products containing inhalable chemicals (as gases, vapors, aerosols or combinations).
2) Purpose: Provides information on the types chemically induced toxicity and establishes a no-observed-effect level (NOEL) under the test conditions; used in determining allowable exposure, mechanisms of toxicity.
3) Definitions: Same as acute inhalation toxicity testing.
4) Standards

Test Substance: Technical grade of active ingredient(s).

Vehicle: If required, should be characterized; ideally should not significantly alter chemical or toxicological properties of test substance.

Test Animals: Young adult laboratory rats preferred (125 to 250 gm); other test species with justifica-

Table X. OVERVIEW OF 90-DAY INHALATION TOXICITY TESTING (Continued)

tion, start with enough animals (15 to 20 sex/level) so as to have at least 10 animals/sex/level at end of experiment for clinical testing, necropsy and histology; add additional animals if interim sacrifices or recovery groups are planned.

Exposure Concentrations

At least 3 levels plus controls, concurrently.

High level - definite signs of toxicity.

Low level - no toxicity (responses similar to controls).

Intermediate level(s).

Control: One vehicle or chamber (air) control; air and vehicle controls with use of uncharacterized vehicles.

Duration of Exposure: 6 hours/day, 5 days/week; extend exposure if indicated by exposure conditions.

Exposure Conditions: Whole body in dynamic flow chambers preferred, uniform air distribution, animal volume equal to or less than 5%, single caging preferred; alternative methods with approval.

Chamber Measurements

*Air Flow: At least 12 changes per hour, adequate oxygen (19% or more), etc.; record every hour.

*Temperature: 22°+/-2°C; record every hour.

Humidity: 40% to 60% unless altered by generation of atmosphere.

Concentrations: Nominal for each run.

*Analytical (gaseous and/or particulate), sampled at breathing zone; two times - once after equilibration, once during last hour, desirable.

Particle Sizes for Aerosols: Sampled at breathing zone; at least one sample per run desirable; must be inhalable for test animal.

Observations: Daily (early AM and late afternoon); body weights weekly; food consumption if indicated.

Clinical Laboratory Testing

Ophthalmological examination at end of study on at least high level and control groups, other groups with positive findings.

Hematology routine on all animals at end of study; specific tests as indicated by observed or expected toxicity.

Blood Chemistry routine on all animals at end of study, appropriate to evaluate electrolyte balance, carbohydrate metabolism, liver and kidney function; pulmonary function and other tests as indicated by observed or expected toxicity.

*Constant electronic monitoring desirable.

Table X. OVERVIEW OF 90-DAY INHALATION TOXICITY TESTING (Continued)

Urinalysis routine based on non-rodent species; on rodents, only as indicated based on observed or expected toxicity.

Gross Necropsy: Complete necropsy on all animals; organ weights on liver, kidney, adrenals, and testes in all animals; preserve organs and all lesions for possible future histopathological examination; perfusion of lungs with fixative considered desirable.

Histopathology: Examine microscopically all gross lesions; complete histopathology for high level and control animals; for the intermediate and low level groups, examine screen organs (liver, kidney and heart), target organs and organs with positive findings from the high group and the controls.

5) Test Report

Summary

GLP and General Section Requirements

Test Specific Information

Test substance Vapor pressure, boiling point, flammability, explosivity and stability.

Exposure Chambers Description, operation.

Chamber Operation Data Tabulation and summary by test groups: - air flow, temperature, humidity, nominal concentrations, analytical concentrations, particle size measurements - percent respirable and non-respirable based on weight.

Response Data Tabulations and summaries by test groups: Toxicity observed, onset, duration, animals involved, body weights, food consumption if obtained, clinical laboratory findings, gross and microscopic findings, NOEL.

References

Discussion and Evaluation

The purposes of the repeat exposure tests are to establish a no-observable-effect-level (NOEL), to determine the types of toxicity and the target organs which might result from repeated exposure. Usually three exposure levels in addition to controls are used: 1) a high exposure level in which there are demonstrated definite toxic effects; 2) a low dose level equivalent to the NOEL which produces either no toxic effects or effects which are not significantly different from any effects which are seen in the control groups; and 3) an intermediate exposure level which should help demonstrate the dose-response nature of toxic effects due to the test agent. The subchronic tests usually involve exposures of 3, 4 to 13 weeks, while the chronic tests are carried out over one year periods and may last for periods up to the average life-times expected for the test animals. Exposures are frequently at least 6 hours per day, 5 days a week but may involve almost continuous exposures (approximately 23 hours per day) and 7 days per week depending on the amount of exposure expected with the use of the test chemicals. Studies of 3 or 4 weeks usually require that 10 animals per sex per level survive to be included in the clinical laboratory testing and pathological evaluation, while the 13-week studies require 20 animals per group. The chronic study requires additional animals (usually 50 per group) in order to have enough animals survive the exposure period and to improve the ability to separate statistically spontaneous disease from disease caused by the test agents. By applying a "safety factor" (better described as an "uncertainty factor" [NAS, 1977]) to the NOEL, one attempts to determine acceptable levels of exposure for humans and "non-target" organisms. In the case of carcinogenicity and other non-threshold effects, quantitative risk analyses are used to determine what levels may be allowed which should reduce the risk of cancer to some acceptable level.

Toxicity vs. Hazard. The inhalation tests attempt to determine the toxic effects of an agent on biological systems which are inherent property of the chemical rather than a measure of toxic hazards. Hazard is a combination of exposure and toxicity. A significant toxic hazard occurs when an individual's exposure is such as to produce a toxic effect. If there is no exposure (regardless of how toxic the agent is), there is no hazard. Any product - a technical or manufacturing use product, a final use product or an intermediate use product - which requires a label for shipping purposes generally requires acute toxicity testing. In some cases in which there is expected exposure to metabolic products or degradation products, the conversion product may need to be tested when such products are expected to produce a significant hazard. Subchronic and chronic studies are carried out generally using the technical grade of the product only. Therefore, synergistic or antagonistic effects due to materials which are added to the chemical to aid in its application are generally not assessed, as this would make testing requirements prohibitive.

Test Animals. Young adult rats of both sexes are generally preferred for testing. This is primarily due to the availability, cost and convenience of using these animals. Other species which handle the test substance in a manner more nearly similar to man based on metabolism and kinetics of absorption, distribution, and excretion may be preferred to the rat and can usually be substituted for the rat with approval by the government agency.

Exposure Conditions. The concentration levels and durations of exposure were discussed above. The chamber conditions, except for the concentrations of the test material, should be essentially the same among the different test chambers during the different runs on each study. The exposure chambers should provide for an evenly distributed atmosphere throughout the chamber. Crowding should be minimized, preferably one animal to the cage, and the total volume of the test animals should not exceed 5% of the volume of the chamber. Air flow should be allowed for at least 12 chamber volumes per hour in order to assure at least 19% oxygen, avoid excessive animal heat and humidity build-up and avoid the excessive accumulation of waste gases. The atmospheres to which the animals are to be exposed should be adequately characterized as to the concentrations, the temperature, humidity, and in the case of aerosols, the particle sizes. Aerosols should be generated such that the particles can be inhaled and have the opportunity to be deposited along the complete pulmonary system, that is, from the trachea to the alveoli of the deep lung.

Observations and Measurements of the Test Animals. The animals should be viewed periodically throughout the day during normal maintenance and should be examined carefully at least once each day, including week-ends and holidays. Except for the acute studies, moribund animals should be sacrificed when found in order not to have excessive animal losses due to cannabalism and autolysis. Animals should be weighed initially, at the termination of the experiment, and weekly or monthly depending on the duration of the experiment. Clinical laboratory testing (Table XI),

Table XI. POSSIBLE ROUTINE CLINICAL LABORATORY TESTS

Hematology: Hematocrit, hemoglobin, erythrocyte count, total and differential leukocyte counts, clotting potential such as clotting time, prothrombin time, thromboplastin time or platelet count.

Blood Chemistry: Measure of electrolyte balance, carbohydrate metabolism liver and kidney function such as calcium, phosphorus, chloride, sodium, potassium, fasting glucose, lactic dehydrogenase, serum glutamic pyruvic transaminase, serum glutamic oxaloacetic transaminase, serum alkaline phosphatase, urea nitrogen, albumin, blood creatinine, total bilirubin, and total protein. Might consider analyses of lipid, hormones, acid/base balance and carboxyhemoglobin.

Urinalysis: Volume, color, specifc gravity or osmolarity, pH, protein, glucose, ketones, formed elements (RBC's, WBC's epithelial cells), casts, crystalline and amorphous materials, and blood pigments.

Table XII. COMPLETE GROSS NECROPSY AND HISTOPATHOLOGY EXAMINATIONS

Grossly examine external surface of the body, all orifices and the cranial, thoracic and abdominal cavities and their contents.
Grossly and histologically examine following organs: Brain (at least 3 levels), spinal cord (at least 2 levels), pituitary, salivary glands, thymus, thyroid/parathyroid, heart, aorta, esophagus, lung (with mainstem bronchi), trachea, liver, stomach, small and large intestines, spleen, kidneys, adrenals, pacreas, urinary bladder, gonads, accessory genital organs, mammary gland, skeletal muscle, lymph node, sternum with bone marrow, and peripheral nerve, skin for dermal tests.

including hematology and blood chemistries are to be carried out on the repeated exposure studies but are not required for the acute studies. Urinalyses should be done routinely on non-rodents and only on rodents when the urinary tract is adversely affected based either on observed or expected toxicity. Every animal in repeat exposure experiments should receive a complete gross necropsy (Table XII), and histological examinations are expected on the high exposure and control groups, and on the key organs of the intermediate test groups. Any organs found to have pathological changes in any one group, should be examined in the animals of the other test groups in order to determine possible dose-related changes.

Test Report. The general requirements for the tests report are presented in Table VII. The requirements specific to inhalation studies are presented in Tables IX and X.

IMPACT OF THE GUIDELINES DEVELOPMENT

Almost every single requirement as proposed was subject to much discussion and question. The inhalation team dealt with over 600 individual comments or questions on inhalation testing alone. A detailed discussion of the issues is beyond the scope of this paper; however, a few points might be made here.

Clearly, it was apparent that different scientists favored many different approaches. Too often, scientists did not understand what was being required and why. Many critics questioned the need for any guidelines, protesting that they would stifle originality and detract from the quality available in many laboratories. Many complained that such requirements cost too much and contributed substantially to the country's inflationary problems. Some scientists wanted fewer animals to be used and others wanted considerably larger numbers to improve statistical estimates. Some wanted no preferred species in order to use only those species which best approximated man. Some scientists wanted to use only one sex if the limit test was negative for one sex. And so forth.

The guidelines efforts thus have caused many scientists to examine the scientific basis for the testing methodologies that are currently in place and have provided for a public airing of important issues. If the guidelines induce scientists to examine more closely the validity of toxicological testing methods as they are used to predict hazards for mankind, they will have provided an additional significant benefit to the field of regulatory toxicology. In the author's view, they should be further examined from the standpoint of false-negatives - that is, a finding of no toxicity when there will be a hazard to humans with the use of the chemical - and also the possibility of false-positives - that is, a finding of toxicity due to unrealistic exposure conditions or using excessively sensitive test systems - which may exclude the use by humans of important, and in some cases, life-saving chemicals.

REFERENCES

EPA (1975), Guidelines for Registering Pesticides in the United States. 40 FR 26802, June 25, 1975.

EPA (1978), Proposed Guidelines for Registering Pesticides in the United States; Hazard Evaluation: Humans and Domestic Animals. 43 FR 37336, August 22, 1978.

EPA (1979 a), Proposed Health Effects Test Standards for Toxic Substances Control Act Test Rules. 44 FR 27334, May 9, 1979.

EPA (1979 b), Proposed Health Effects Test Standards for Toxic Substances Control Act Test Rules and Proposed Good Laboratory Practice Standards for Health Effects. 44 FR 44054, July 26, 1979.

IRLG (1978), Interagency Regulatory Liaison Group Notice of IRLG Work Plans and Public Meetings. 43 FR 7174, February 17, 1978.

NAS (1977), "Drinking Water and Health," National Academy of Sciences, Washington, D.C., pg. 803.

OECD (1980), OECD High Level Meeting on Chemicals 19th/21st May, 1980, Press Release, Paris, 21 May. Organization for Economic Co-operation and Development, Chateau de la Muette -2, rue Andre-Pascal, 75775 Paris Cedex 16 - 524 82-00.

Page, Norbert N. (1980), Personal communications.

Preston, William (1980), Personal communications.

Temple, T. (1979), Controlling Toxics, EPA Journal, pp 10-19, July-August, 1979.

POST-SYMPOSIUM CORRESPONDENCE

Post Symposium Correspondence

Editor's note

The Symposium provided an opportunity for inhalation toxicologists to report their latest achievements and to identify and discuss existing problems. Indeed, the discussions continued in the post symposium correspondence which was stimulating and useful. To share the benefit and intensity of the discussions, several excerpts have been prepared for the Symposium participants and the readers of this book. What follows came from letters Dr. Moss wrote in response to Dr. MacFarland's presentation: "Overview: A problem and a nonproblem in chamber inhalation studies" and Drs. Alarie and Drew's comments following that response.

On Uniformity of Chamber Atmosphere

(If) all that Drs. MacFarland and Alarie said about fluid dynamics of concentration build-up in a box and our ability to monitor aerosol, vapor or gas levels is correct. There (should be) no hot spots regardless of the streams of exposure atmosphere through the chamber and the resulting stagnant zones. The measured concentration within the chamber must ultimately reach a steady state and must be uniform throughout so long as the exposure atmosphere generation continues to deliver a uniform mixture to the chamber air inlet.

But why am I and why are others so concerned about uniform mixing throughout an exposure chamber? My concerns can be boiled down to just two statements:

1. As an inhalation toxicologist, I am faced with one minimum requirement: to give each animal in an exposure group as accurately as possible the same inhalation dose.

2. Animals clean the air they breathe.

The recent Lovelace work (Beethe et al. Evaluation of a recently designed multi-tiered exposure chamber, LE-67, available from NTIS, Springfield, VA 22161) demonstrates that regardless of variation in biological response, giving an exposure group of animals doses that vary less than 8% is possible.

Chamber fluid dynamics as Dr. MacFarland presented them require that the concentration of the inhalation dose be even more uniform than the 8% variation.

Then how could animals possibly get less than an equal dose of aerosol? The answer: they exhale clean air, and an animal in a stagnant region of the chamber will partially inhale the bubble of clean air he has just exhaled. The animal in the stagnant zone fools us. He reduces his dose simply by not moving. This phenomenon will probably be noted frequently as more and more toxicology laboratories expose animals to the recommended $5 g/m^3$ dust loads. From the few animals not obscured by such dense aerosols, the movement of clean exhaled air is visible.

This seems like a small point, but that's it. I believe that much of the variability in the biological response within any one animal exposure group will be isolated and explained once the variability in inhaled dose is reduced.

Owen R. Moss
November 3, 1980

On Chamber Atmosphere and Aerosol Concentration

In my opinion, conducting an experiment at $5 g/m^3$ is not appropriate simply because solid aerosol systems are not stable or even quasi-stable at this concentration. Sadly, such experiments conducted in exposure chambers are being called *INHALATION TOXICOLOGY*. Using a particle size of about 1 to 2 μ and other principles Dr. MacFarland outlined, I have operated chambers with nonvolatile liquid droplet aerosol concentrations of up to 100 mg/m^3 without difficulty. At concentrations above this and especially when particles are bigger, problems arise. I offer the following considerations about the problems Dr. Moss listed in his letter above:

1. With a dust concentration of $5 g/m^3$, particle size of 3μ or 1μ and unit density sphere, we will have about 3.5×10^8 and 9.6×10^9 particles/cm^3 respectively. This is a lot of particles, and coagulation will be

a major problem, I simply cannot see how a stable or quasi-stable aerosol could exist in all parts of the chamber under such circumstances. The concentration would be $5g/m^3$ as specified, but the number of particles and their sizes in different areas of the chamber would vary greatly. Since

$$\frac{-dn}{dt} = Kn^2$$

where n is the number of particles and K is the coagulation constant (0.5×10^{-9} cm^3/sec), I can't see how coagulation can be avoided, regardless of chamber configuration, airflow, etc. To think that all animals no matter where they are in the chamber will receive identical doses of aerosol when the chamber concentration is $5g/m^3$ is absurd. At that concentration, nothing can be done to ensure that all animals in a group receive the same inhalation dose. Coagulation will change particle size which will then influence deposition which in turn will influence the dose received.

In fact the solution Dr. Moss proposes will make things even worse. In coagulation of aerosols, not only n^2 is important but air turbulence, eddies, swirls, etc., increase coagulation. The turbulence also increases deposition on surfaces, and mass concentration and particle number and size will change.

Quite frankly, I have no solution for the problems that arise when rats are exposed at $5g/m^3$. That seems like throwing rocks at rats. The coagulation changes for that load could be calculated for the residence times for Moss' chamber. To see how the aerosol changes from the top of the chamber to the bottom would be interesting.

2. A chamber should be operated at 12 air changes per hour, i.e., the airflow should be equivalent to the volume of the chamber. Thus, for a 100-liter chamber, the airflow should be 100 liters/minute. If this is provided, t_{99} would occur in about 5 minutes. The airflow can be reduced by about one-quarter without much trouble, but reducing it by one-tenth is asking for problems unless the animal loading is very low.

3. Assuming that a rat weighs 200 grams, in the chamber described above, the maximal number of rats would be 25, and for each rat the volume of space occupied will equal 0.2 liter.

4. With 5% loading, the rats will breathe 5 liters/minute (25 rats x 2 ml (VT) x 100 (f) = 5 liters/minute). A 5% loading is of no consequence. Remember that 5% loading is not used frequently; usually 1% loading is used. Therefore, I don't see your suggestion that the animals clean the air they breathe, a problem if the chamber is operated as outlined above.

I suggest that a group of experts in the field should get together for one day to examine in detail the problems of exposing animals at $5g/m^3$ and to see if this can be called inhalation toxicology. Some superficial thinking about the coagulation problem indicates that the particle size will become so large that, in fact, rats cannot inhale such particles. This reminds me of Amdur's demonstration that sulfuric acid mist at 7μ did not affect guinea pigs while the 0.2 and 2μ were very potent. To conclude that sulfuric acid mist is nontoxic on the basis of the 7μ experiment would be a bad mistake. I am afraid that similar mistakes will occur if the particle size is not specified for experiments run at a concentration of $5g/m^3$.

Yves Alarie
November 24, 1980

On Chamber Atmosphere Equilibration

It is an important contribution to the science of inhalation toxicology by showing us that with certain designs, catch pans can be used in inhalation chambers while maintaining a uniform concentration throughout the exposure area. This had not been adequately documented, and I am glad that someone has made this important contribution.

I need to better understand Dr. Alarie's point about 12 air changes per hour in a 100-liter inhalation chamber with an airflow of 100 liters per minute. With the conditions specified, I consider the rate to be 60 not 12 air changes per hour. I might add that I find these air flow rates abnormally high for long term inhalation studies when I consider atmospheric clean-up and contaminant use.

In Silver's original article (Constant flow gassing chambers: Principles influencing design and operation. J. Lab. Clin. Med. 31, 1153-1161, 1946), he derived the general form of the build-up and decay equation:

$$t_x = K \frac{a}{b}$$

where x is the percentage nominal concentration attained in time, t; K is a constant; a is the chamber volume; and b is the airflow, for t_{99}, K=4.6; for T_{95}, K=3.

Silver made the case that misinterpretation of the term *AIR CHANGE* contributes most to large errors. An air change occurs when a volume of air equal to the volume of the chamber has passed through the chamber. However, one air change does not completely renew the chamber air since dilution occurs. Silver predicted that one air change would change the concentration by only 63%. He suggested that the term *AIR CHANGE* be eliminated from gassing terminology. However, in the ensuing 35 years, the term continues to cloud the issue.

I agree with Dr. Alarie that inhalation studies at $5 g/m^3$ are absurd. If a group of experts can meet for a day and convince the regulatory agency of the absurdity of this concentration, I will be happy to participate and to help.

Robert T. Drew
December 9, 1980

On Terminology

I agree with Dr. Drew that the ventilation engineers would say 60 air changes per hour. This is their standard terminology, and I don't think we will be able to change it. However, the air has not been changed 60 times; from Silver's equation, the air has been changed 12 times. We can avoid this terminology if we state the chamber volume and airflow.

I also agree that changing the air 12 times per hour may create problems with the atmospheric clean-up equipment and the amount of contaminant, but it is not abnormally high flow. Dr. MacFarland has suggested a flow rate of 0.1 times the chamber volume which is one-tenth the rate I suggested of 1.0 times the chamber volume. I always tell students to try for 1.0 but if technical problems such as clean-up or amount of contaminant interfere, reduce the air flow to 0.25 or possibly 0.1 depending on the animal load. I don't like 0.1 or any less air flow because of the time requred for t_{99}. At 0.1 this will be about 50 minutes.

Maybe together we can establish some minimum value to serve as a guideline. Can we establish an acceptable amount of time to reach t_{99} for chronic exposure lasting 6 hours/day? Is 1/6 of 6 hours OK? Long ago I gave up trying to convince regulatory agencies, but if we can agree on some guidelines, the inhalation toxicology community may welcome them. Perhaps we should promulgate guidelines before the agencies do.

Yves Alarie
December 18, 1980

On Appropriate Flowrate

On the question of the appropriate flowrate to utilize with a chamber of given volume, it is pointed out that investigators generally work in the range: F(l/min) = 0.1 to 1.0 V(liter) and that the duration of exposure, t, should be at least 13 x t_{99} for a satisfactory study. It is true, of course, that the suggestion that t should be at least 13 x t_{99} is a matter of opinion and further discussion of this point might prove of value. It is difficult to understand why the phrase "air changes" persists. It conveys no immediate meaning that is not deceptive. To illustrate this, imagine being informed that there are 100 ppm of a contaminant in the air in a chamber and that the chamber is now flushed with clean air for 30 minutes at a rate of 10 air changes per hour. What is the concentration of the contaminant when this operation is performed? It is immediately evident that one has no conception of the answer to this question. To find the answer, it is necessary to return to the general equation: $t_x = K\frac{a}{b}$.

In the example, 10 air changes per hour means that if the volume of the chamber is a liter, the flowrate, b, is 10a per hour, or $\frac{10a}{60}$ per minute. Thus,

$$t_{99} = 4.6 \times \frac{a}{\frac{10a}{60}}$$

$$= 27.6 \text{ minutes.}$$

It is now immediately evident that, after 30 minutes of flushing with clean air, the concentration of the contaminant will be slightly below 1% of its initial value of 100 ppm, i. e., the concentration will be slightly below 1 ppm. The point to note in this example is that the statement in terms of "air changes" per unit time conveyed no direct meaning, but the description of the relationship between volume of chamber and total flow through it, given in terms of t_{99}, gave an immediate estimate of the concentration after performing the specified operation of flushing for 30 minutes. Despite all this, Alarie is undoubtedly correct in saying that ventilation engineers will not change their ways. But inhalation toxicologists should use a form of expression that conveys an immediate conception.

H. N. MacFarland
May 13, 1981

Editorial Remarks

Silver described the build-up and decay of a gaseous contaminant in a chamber containing no animals. However, to the best of my knowledge, no similar study has been conducted with aerosol or dust atmospheres. As Dr. MacFarland suggested at the symposium recorded here, theoretically Silver's equation should apply to respirable particles so the distribution of an airborne contaminant should be uniform once equilibration occurs. Indeed, Schreck et al. (this volume) observed nearly uniform distribution of a diesel aerosol of submicron particle size at mass concentration of approximately 40 mg/m^3.

On the other hand, when dealing with a deisel aerosol of submicron particle size but at mass concentration of up to 20 g/m^3, Holmberg et al. (this volume) showed that the aerosol stream entered from the top of a Rochester chamber as a discrete plume and impinged preferentially on the animals in the top center tier of cages. The possibility of nonuniform exposure of animals was great and a uniform concentration built up slowly. Similarly, Leong et al. (this volume) showed that the distribution of diatomaceous earth particles, of about 3 μm size and at concentrations up to 5 g/m^3, were more concentrated in the center than in the periphery of the exposure chamber. The higher the chamber airflow, the higher the concentration of the dust deposited in the center than in the periphery.

To avoid the creation of hot spots in the chambers, Holmberg used perforated plates while Leong used wide-angle air nozzles to disperse the airborne contaminants at the air inlet side of the chamber into a "uniform" front before the particles reached the animals. Doe and Tinston (this volume) rotated the animal exposure cages to attain a uniform exposure pattern.

The main factors contributing to the nonuniformity of aerosol distribution are aerosol concentration followed by aerosol particle sizes. As Alarie pointed out in his letter, coagulation and change of particle size cannot be avoided at high chamber aerosol concentrations.

Unfortunately, inhalation toxicologists dealing with product safety evaluations have to comply with the 5 g/m^3 analytical concentration set by regulatory agencies. In addition, many products have a wide range of particle size from submicron to much bigger than 10 μm. In a typical aerosol inhalation experiment, only 4 to 13% of the aerosol with a mass median diameter of 2 to 7 μm could be found in the chamber atmosphere. Most aerosol particles were lost on the animal fur or chamber walls (Sachesse et al. Measurement of inhalation toxicity of aerosols in small laboratory animals in experimental model systems in toxicology and their significance in man. Proceedings of the European Society for the Study of Drug Toxicity, Vol. XV, Zurich, Lane 1973 ISBN 90-219-0248-6). Similarly, Leong et al. (this volume) recovered 25 to 73% of diatomaceous earth particles in a nominal chamber concentration of 0.49 to 2.9 g/m^3. The percent of particles remained airborne is low. In order to attain a 5 g/m^3 analytical concentration will require the generation of the aerosol at a much higher nominal concentration. Thus, the demand for a 5 g/m^3 analytical concentration by the regulatory agencies is unrealistic.

Concerning suitable chamber airflow, Dr. MacFarland talked about the flow being 0.1 to 1.0 times the volume of the chamber, and Alarie prefers 1.0 times the volume. The t_{99} for a flow ratio of 0.1 would be 46 minutes and that for the ratio of 1 would be 4.6 minutes. A t_{99} of 46 minutes would be reasonable for a 6-hour exposure study but too long for a 1-hour exposure study. On the other hand, a t_{99} of 4.6 minutes would be suitable for an acute 1-hour study using a small chamber but would cause a high consumption of test material in a chronic study using a large chamber. Therefore, the use of a fraction of exposure duration instead of a fraction of chamber volume as a criterion for setting chamber airflow seems reasonable, e.g., by adjusting the chamber airflow to provide a t_{99} of not more than 10% of the total exposure time. Thus, the chamber airflow would be such that the t_{99} for a 1-hour exposure should be no longer than 6 minutes and that for a 6-hour exposure should be no longer than 36 minutes. Then the ratio of chamber concentration build-up time and the exposure duration is always 1:10, regardless of the size of the chamber used.

The chamber concentration build-up and decay can be regulated to a nearly square wave pattern by using the differential metering method. For example, 300 ml/min of a gaseous agent can be added to an airflow of 600 l/min to provide a concentration of 500 ppm in a 6000 liter chamber in 46 minutes (t_{99} for 300 ppm). The t_{99} can be reduced to about 6.9 minutes by initially metering the agent at 600 ml/min for 6.9 minutes (t_{50} for 1000 ppm) and then decreasing the agent flow to 300 ml/min thereafter. This way, the concentration of the agent in the chamber can build up quickly without excessive waste. Other methods for effecting rapid equilibration in dynamic chambers are possible (MacFarland, Respiratory Toxicology. IN: "Essays in Toxicology" _7_, 121-154, 1976).

Regarding the proposed regulatory guideline that the chamber airflow should be "at least 12 chamber volumes per hour in order to assure at least 19% oxygen, avoid excessive animal heat and humidity build-up" (Gross, p. 296, this volume). Such regulatory requirement appears to be excessive. Actually, the chamber airflow can be as low as 6 chamber volumes per hour without causing the aforementioned problems. For example, in a typical chronic inhalation study, usually 100 rats are exposed in a chamber of approximately 6000 liter volume (6 foot cube). The minute volume of a rat weighing 250 grams is about 0.25 l/min. The total air consumption for 100 rats would be 25 l/min. If the chamber airflow is 6 chamber volumes per hour, the airflow would be 600 l/min which far exceeds the 25 l/min to be consumed by 100 rats in the chamber. Therefore, the probability of oxygen deficiency is negligible.

If the 12 volume changes are required to dissipate the heat the animals produce, the requirement is still excessive. Bernstein and Drew (The major parameters affecting temperature inside inhalation chambers, Am. Ind. Hyg. Assoc. 41, 420-426, 1980) show that "with the chamber air supply at room temperature, heat transfer through noninsulated stainless steel walls was effective in removing approximately 90% of the heat generated by the animals as compared to only 10% removed by the air stream." Therefore, the use of high airflow for heat dissipation is unnecessary.

The only problem generated by a 6 chamber volumes per hour airflow is a slow t_{99} which would be 46 minutes. However, the t_{99} can be expedited by using the differential metering method previously described.

Basil K. J. Leong

INDEX

Index